CHILDREN'S HOSPITAL

CHILDREN'S HOSPITAL

Peggy Anderson

1817

HARPER & ROW, PUBLISHERS, New York

Cambridge, Philadelphia, San Francisco, London

Mexico City, São Paulo, Singapore, Sydney

This book is for the children in it,
or to their memories,
and for all who love those children or remember them with love.

FIRST EDITION

Designer: Sidney Feinberg

Library of Congress Cataloging in Publication Data

Anderson, Peggy.
   Children's hospital.

   1. Children—Hospitals—Psychological aspects—Case
studies.   2. Terminally ill children—Psychology—Case
studies.   3. Terminally ill children—Family relation-
ships—Case studies.   4. Chronically ill children—
Psychology—Case studies. 5. Chronically ill children—
Family relationships—Case studies.   I. Title.
RJ27.A57   1985   362.1'9892   81-47650
ISBN 0-06-015089-0

85 86 87 88 89 RRD 10 9 8 7 6 5 4 3 2 1

Preface

This book is first and foremost about six children. Over a certain period not long past, these youngsters were patients at one of America's finest hospitals for children. Three of the six continue to return to the hospital for treatment or occasional monitoring.

When I began my research on these patients, they ranged in age from fifteen years to nine days. Their stories as set down here are as true to fact as I have been able to make them given that I could not be at every child's side at every moment and given, too, that though the six were not all patients at the same time, a unified narrative demanded that they appear to have been hospitalized simultaneously. The real first names of five of the children have been retained in accordance with their wishes or their parents'.

My intention from the start was to explore the responses of those involved when a child is struck down by serious illness or injury: to discover how—or whether—the child, the family, and the hospital staff members attempting to save or cure the child are able to tolerate the intolerable. I took those soundings in a single hospital. I did not set out to write a portrait of that institution per se but rather to describe situations that, while they might differ in detail, could have taken place at almost any hospital specializing in pediatrics. For this reason I have deliberately blurred the specific identity of the children's hospital referred to in the text and have used pseudonyms for all the characters but one, French physician Paul Tessier, who pioneered the techniques now used throughout the world in craniofacial reconstructive surgery.

But I did my research at Children's Hospital of Philadelphia, and I owe a huge debt of gratitude to the staff there. Researching, organizing, and writing this book took five years. Throughout that period, the staff members I interviewed at Children's spent countless hours on the job and off helping me to understand not only their own roles, feelings, and motivations but also physiology, medicine, the sociology of the hospital, and the principles involved in caring for very sick children, and helping me further to track down or verify innumerable small details critical to an accurate representation of the cases I was following. In short, I was accorded the staff's fullest cooperation and unfailing courtesy.

This says much about Children's of Philadelphia, for in exchange I promised administrators nothing more than an advance look at the finished manuscript solely as a means for them to decide whether they wished their institution identified in the preface. The administrators accepted these terms out of faith that the hospital they run could withstand the close scrutiny of an outsider. Without question the quality of care given at this institution, the research conducted there, and of course the encouragement given these enterprises by both the administration and the board have made CHOP one of the most highly regarded hospitals of its kind in the world. It is not flawless and does not purport to have all the answers. The imperfections I saw and the reservations I have about Children's will be plain to any reader, as they were to those at Children's who reviewed the finished manuscript. It is to the credit of CHOP decisionmakers, I believe, that they have seen fit nonetheless to stand behind their institution: to claim their flaws as well as their triumphs.

I owe very special thanks to a number of people now or once at Children's who were exceptionally generous with their time or insights or both: chaplain Jack Rodgers; nurses Pat Bush, Mary Donar, Linda Gerstenhaber, Pixie Groh, Helen Lewis, Jody McGhee, and Mary Lou Mesmer; physicians Derek Bruce, Marty Eichelberger, Audrey Evans, William Fox, Steve Halpern, Robert Kettrick, C. Everett Koop, George Peckham, Russell Raphaely, Harley Rotbart, Luis Schut, Edward Sewell, William Sharrar, Ann Showan, Larry Stephenson, John Templeton, Edward Walsh, Linton Whitaker, and Elaine Zackai; public relations director Pat Usner; respiratory therapist Ethel McIntyre; social worker Nancy Stefacek; and vice-president Shirley Bonnem, who was instrumental in securing the hospital's support for this project, who saw to it that I got both the assistance and the freedom I needed to pursue my investigations, and who blessed my efforts with her enthusiasm.

Others once or now on staff who helped me in a great variety of ways number in the dozens and include doctors, nurses, and nurses' aides; administrators and supervisors; play, physical, occupational, and speech therapists; secretaries; housekeeping personnel; public relations specialists; researchers; social workers; nutritionists and dietitians; unit clerks; a medical technologist; a psychologist. I would like to thank Paul Addonizio, Diane Amato, Lester Baker, Jane Barnstiner, Steve Barrer, David Beele, Janie Bellamy, Peter Berman, Judy Bernbaum, Winnie Betsch, Betty Betteridge, Harry Bishop, Marianne Boegli, Maryann Bolton, Spencer Borden IV, John Bowman, Dolores Braxton, Ann Cavaliere, Henry Cecil, Edward Charney, Sue Cheetham, Helenterese Coffee, Mary Collins, Donna Console, Robin Cooke, David Cornfeld, Jean Cortner, Drew Costarino, Marie Crimmins, Giulio D'Angio, Ruth Davenport, Laura Dawson, Cindy DeFeo, Susan DeJong, Betty Devlin, Tina DiMarcantonio, Jerry Dinger, Elizabeth Doolan, Joann Dorsey, John Downes, Shahnaz Duara, John Duckett, Henry Edmunds, Ron Ellis, Miriam Farber, John Fisher, Don Fitzpatrick, Nancy Ford, Joel Frader, Ellie Furlan, Marie Gallagher, Vic Garcia, Frances Gill, Jean Gingrich, Erna Goulding, Jeff Gross, Marge Gualtiere, Susannah Harris, Wendy Hart, Karen Hartpence, Marybeth Helfrick, Richard Herron, Brenda Hicks, Charles Howell, Klaus Hummeler, Charles Ingersoll, Diane Jacobowski, Marguerite Johnson, Naomi Katsch, Lorraine Kitchen, Herb Klar, Colleen Kraus, Donna Krell, Brenda Krill, Peggy Kroger, Kay Kurbjun, Mary Kurzeknabe, Lida Kwart, Beverly Lang, Pam Larson, Kathy Lewis, Michelle Lloyd, Ted Lockwood, Lorrie Lombardo, Stephen Ludwig, John Macoviak, Peggy Majernick, Tony Mauro, Carol Lynn Maxwell, Harold McCoy, Sharon McCoy, Barb Morray, Sharon Moscowitz, Deidre Mullin, Donald Norris, Beatrice Parker, Pat Pasqueriello, Bev Paul, Jennifer Pearce, William Potsic, Dale Price, Nancy Quigley, Graham Quinn, Peggy Rafferty, Debbie Raiken, William Rashkind, Margaret Reford, Sheryl Resha, Darnell Reynolds, Vivian Rhoads, Carol Ritter, Fran Ritter, Sheryl Rosen, Judy Ross, Chuck Rubin, Rich Ruddy, Jane Runkel, Marianne Ruskavich, Tom Scanlin, Susan Scarvalone, Elias Schwartz, Stanton Segal, Cinda Seigworth, Conchita Sheldon, Bonnie Simon, Barry Slavan, Betsy Smith, Betty Smith, Pauline Smith, Janet Spiker, Allen Spitzer, Linda Spungen, William Squires, Elaine Stevens, John Stevenson, Kathy Swan, David Swedlow, Rosalind Ting, Stuart Toledano, Marion Viglione, Jan Walker, Jo Walker, Hugh Watts, Jeff Weiss, Steve Weissman, Charlotte Welch, Linda Wilson, Camillus Witzleben, Jeannie Woodward, Barbara Wriston, Linda Wright, Moritz Ziegler, and Tim Zietz.

Valuable information was also given to me by two staff members now deceased, Mary Ames and Mary Taylor; by psychiatrists Lee Graham, Gordon Hodas, and John Sargent from the Philadelphia Child Guidance Clinic and Michael Pertshuk from the Hospital of the University of Pennsylvania; and by nurses Kay Fury and Linda Vansickle from Children's Seashore House in Philadelphia.

The main story in this book is about a boy I have called Mark Price. Important contributions were made to Mark's story by his friend Rosalie McDevitt, now deceased; by Pastor Ralph Eberle of the Jordan Lutheran Church of Orefield, Pennsylvania; and by certain people affiliated with the Allentown and Sacred Heart Hospital Center in Allentown, Pennsylvania, now called the Lehigh Valley Hospital Center: Bengy Guerriere and the nurses on her staff who cared for Mark; physicians John Farrell, Jack Lenhart, and John Shane; and chaplain Edward B. Connolly. For useful conversations I also wish to thank Mark's friend Chris Gearhart.

My understanding of pediatrics in general and of present-day issues in that field was greatly enriched by Thomas Cone's definitive and beautifully written *History of American Pediatrics* and by the following people: Frank Bowen, M.D., Head, Newborn Pediatrics, Pennsylvania Hospital; Gary Brickner, M.D., an obstetrician-gynecologist in private practice in Lawrenceville, New Jersey; Alfred De-Lorimier, M.D., pediatric surgeon, University of California San Francisco Medical Center; Donald C. Drake, medical writer, *Philadelphia Inquirer;* Carol Levine, editor, *The Hastings Center Report;* Vanessa Merton, associate professor, New York University Law School; Thomas H. Murray, Ph.D., associate for social and behavioral studies, The Hastings Center; and Victor C. Vaughan, M.D., former medical director, St. Christopher's Hospital for Children, Philadelphia.

I am particularly indebted to Barbara Schraeder, R.N., Ph.D., associate professor of nursing, Thomas Jefferson University, Philadelphia, for thoughts on pediatrics which invariably broadened my own perspective and never once let me forget that at the center of every issue and every theory is a child in crisis.

I am also grateful to Michael Denworth for telling me how it felt to recover from a severe injury; to Joann and Charles Patton for telling me how it felt to watch a daughter recover from a severe illness; to Cynthia Williams for consistently producing virtually flawless interview transcripts and for being interested in what I was doing at a stage when few others knew; and most certainly to Renée C. Fox, professor of sociology, psychiatry, and medicine at the University of Pennsylvania, who took time from her own work to review part of my manuscript when I sorely needed an expert opinion and who honored me with her confidence.

I've gotten through this long project with a lot of help from my friends. Sue Nicholson, my first friend in kindergarten, transformed my drafts into clean text with dispatch, absolute dependability, and always a warm word for the author. Joyce Corlett did careful research on contemporary pediatrics when I despaired of ever getting at it myself; she and Mary Fish spent long hours making sure that the interview tapes and transcripts were in perfect accord; David Fish helped me understand critical medical details when I couldn't bring myself to call Children's one more time; Don Drake, Bernie Fleury, Barbara Leff, Barbara Schraeder, and Elaine Tait read and commented on pieces of the manuscript when I needed certain kinds of feedback; Connie Rosenblum offered sensitive editorial suggestions that helped me solve problems and stave off fears; editor Fredrica S. Friedman, an old friend, gave me invaluable technical assistance and ways to believe in myself when my courage faltered.

Moral support came to me in abundance from those friends and others: Lois and Joel Belsky, Judith Braun, Diana Burgwyn, Jean Byrne, Maureen Carroll, David Craig, Shyrlee Dallard, Doris and Howard Darnell, David Fineman and Linda Loyd, Alice Gilliam, Alvia Golden, Bob Hamburger, Gloria Hochman, Ralph Keyes, Pat and Joe Kelly, Keith Knost, Martha Weinman Lear, Lynn Luria-Sukenick, Tom Maeder, Bob Maris, Clifton Ogburn, Mike Pakenham, Margaret Robinson, Joyce Russe, Olaf Saugen, Nora Sayre, Loretta Schwartz-Nobel, Bob Shogan, Dorothy Storck, Mary Walton, Bill Wartman, Barbara Wilson, and "Mr. 80%." No support has meant more to me these past five years than that provided me by the close friends I saw regularly who never failed to show real interest in how this project was progressing no matter how many reports they'd already heard: Anne Boysen, Joyce Corlett, Carol Horner, and Barbara Leff.

When I signed the contract for this book, I promised Harper & Row a manuscript within a year. Another house might have run out of patience. If H&R came close, I was protected from that knowledge by Larry Ashmead, an attentive, wise, enthusiastic editor and all-round lovely man who stuck by me in the face of pressures I know he must at times have felt quite keenly. The shaping of *Children's Hospital* would have been a far tougher task had I not been able to lean heavily on Larry's considerable talents.

Jay Acton, my agent, who has guarded my best interests with diligence, acuity, and foresight, has been simply wonderful.

My mother, Kay McMillan, who has never to my knowledge doubted me, has also been simply wonderful.

Among all the people who helped make this book a reality, none deserves more credit or more thanks from me than the children and parents who were willing for their stories to be told. Some of the children were too young or too sick to be interviewed. Of the others, and of all the mothers and fathers, I asked a huge commitment of time and energy and candor during the worst or some of the worst days of their lives. All of the parents and the oldest of the children made this commitment saying they hoped their doing so would help others going through similar tribulations. They talked with me for hours and hours and hours, in some cases over many months. What they gave me was the most moving and most humbling material it has ever been my privilege to work with.

I did research on eight children. As the manuscript grew thicker and thicker, it became obvious to me that I could not do justice to eight stories in a volume of publishable length. I am very grateful to Beau's parents, Joan and Jim Baldwin, and to David's parents, Shelly and Joel Schneeweis, for all that they shared with me and for their gracious understanding of a decision I made with the utmost reluctance.

Finally, I want to say a special word of thanks to Mark's mother, who was in a position to appreciate better than anyone else could what I faced here at the typewriter day after day. Her encouragement was a great gift.

The real first names of five of the children in this book have been retained. All other names in the text are pseudonyms, except that of French physician Paul Tessier.

DECEMBER

Saturday, December 1

With considerable difficulty, because he was breathing with considerable difficulty, Mark Price eased himself off his bed in the Adolescent Unit, slipped into his Children's Hospital bathrobe, grasped his IV pole, and, wheeling the pole in front of him, leaning on it for support—because he was so short of breath now that he could hardly stand—he left his room and started down the hall for the nurses' station.

He was fifteen and looked twelve: a small, pale stick figure whose clothing hung from his bones. Sixty-four pounds, as of his admission on Thursday, and barely five feet tall. His body bore other marks of his disease. His teeth were discolored from years of antibiotics. His fingernails were enlarged from chronic oxygen deprivation. His chest was deformed. Most of Mark's energy in recent years had been spent on drawing breath and trying to cough up mucus. The effort had been strenuous enough to reshape his rib cage, giving him pigeon breast. Only his hair and his eyes looked healthy. His hair was his vanity. It was straight, blond as oak, and cut in a Dutch-boy bob. He kept it shining. His eyes were blue and clear and alive. They would have seemed large in his thin face even without the glasses that magnified them.

His chest felt as if a belt were tightening around it. He could not understand why he was having so much trouble breathing. After two days on antibiotics, he had felt well enough earlier this evening to go downstairs to the Children's cafeteria for Supper Club. Back on the floor, he had started feeling pain.

Kate had called the resident, Dr. Barth, Darryl, and they had taken him into the treatment room for a rhythm strip. It was like an electrocardiogram, they had explained, only shorter and faster than a regular EKG. That had scared him. He had problems enough with his lungs. He didn't need problems with his heart too. Fortunately the rhythm strip had been normal.

But his breathing had continued to get worse, and so had the pain. His 8:00 breathing treatment hadn't helped. Percussion hadn't helped. Yet his nail beds were pink, and Kate had said his lips were pink, so he knew he was getting enough oxygen, and when she'd listened to his chest just a few minutes ago, she had told him she'd heard nothing unusual.

He wondered if he were going crazy. When he'd asked his mother to bring him in on Thursday, he'd been having unusual trouble breathing then too, though not as much as he was having now, but Dr. Griffin had said he thought the reason for the trouble was not medical but psychological. Anxiety. A blood test done on Adolescent an hour later had shown nothing unusual in Mark's oxygen levels. So were his problems tonight also psychosomatic?

He'd been telling himself for two hours that maybe they would go away if he stopped thinking about them. Instead he'd had to breathe faster and faster to get the air he needed, and now it almost seemed to Mark that the faster he breathed, the less air he got.

Finally, at 8:40 he had been able to stand it no longer.

Kate stood in the nurses' station trying to convince Darryl Barth to order a chest x-ray for Mark. She was twenty-three, a tall, blue-eyed, black-haired, freckle-faced Irish Catholic dressed this evening in a corduroy jumper and a plaid blouse. She was not as concerned about her patient as he was about himself. She only knew that when she had listened to his lungs at 8:30, his left had sounded very slightly different than it had at 8:00—a difference so slight that Kate had been unwilling to describe it even to herself as a decrease in breath sounds. But she had gone immediately to page the resident.

"I can't put my finger on it," she had told Barth on the phone, "but something on that side doesn't sound right to me. It sounds . . . far away."

He had returned to the floor reluctantly. Four weeks into a six-week rotation on Adolescent, Darryl Barth knew Kate McDevitt well enough to recognize worry in her voice but not yet well enough to read that worry. She had been worried earlier too; yet neither she nor he had heard anything unusual in Mark's lungs, and the rhythm strip had been fine. Besides, the boy had been basically okay for two days. Out of his first-year-resident's insecurity, however, Barth had made it a rule to always pay attention when a nurse expressed concern to him about a patient.

Tonight as usual he wore a rumpled green scrub suit. He was twenty-six, not very tall, a little too heavy, with fine, dark hair falling over his forehead to the rims of his tortoiseshell glasses. He faced Kate now, listening attentively to her urgings without feeling persuaded. Dr. Griffin had felt so strongly on Thursday that Mark's breathing problems derived from anxiety. The normal blood study that afternoon had seemed to back him up. Why subject the child to unnecessary x-ray?

Kate persisted. "I know what Dr. Griffin said. But I know Mark. I just can't believe anxiety is his problem right now." She coaxed. "Come on, Darryl, you don't have to pay for it!"

"Kate . . ." Mark stood in the hallway next to the nurses' station, breathing very fast and pulling for air. "It's really getting worse."

Kate heard fear in his voice. Until this admission, she had never known him to be fearful.

"Darryl, why don't you take a listen to Mark's lungs," she said lightly, "since he obviously doesn't trust my judgment?"

The boy did not smile. She rolled a chair from the nurses' station into the hallway and helped him onto it. The resident put his stethoscope to Mark's chest.

The difference between what he had heard earlier and what he was hearing now was stark.

It was a difference in volume. Barth could hear sounds on the right, but the boy was not aerating well on the left side. Could the child's lung be slowly collapsing? The resident had never heard a pneumothorax occurring. Somehow this didn't sound as acute as Barth thought a lung collapse would sound. But something was definitely wrong. He was seized with admiration for the nurse.

He did not see the situation as a dire emergency. The boy was not cyanotic; his lips and nail beds were pink. Not wanting to upset the patient, the young doctor said calmly, "Well, Mark, you're obviously having trouble, so I think we'll get a chest x-ray and see what we can find out."

Barth stepped to the desk, dialed a phone, and quietly told a senior resident that he was taking a patient to Radiology with a possible pneumothorax. Moments later he and Kate had Mark on the elevator in a wheelchair hooked up with oxygen. The Radiology Department was three floors down. A technologist was waiting at the reception desk.

"Give me a lead apron," Kate said to her. "I'm going in there with him. I don't care if my babies do have three heads." The patient's faint smile encouraged her.

But in the long minutes it took for the x-rays to be shot and processed, his respirations grew increasingly labored. His whole body went up and down with his effort to take in air. Kate found out why when the technologist called her into the file room where Darryl Barth and the senior resident were laying out the films.

"Kate, look at this, look at this!" Darryl grabbed her. "His lung is more than twenty-five percent collapsed! You made the save of the decade! If you hadn't picked it up . . ."

The congratulations got lost in hurried decisionmaking. Pneumothorax is the accumulation of air in the chest cavity. It may occur traumatically when the chest wall is punctured from without, as in a bullet or knife wound, or it may occur spontaneously, as Mark's apparently had, when a bleb, or bubble, in the lung wall breaks. Either way, as air leaks into the chest, taking up more and more space, the sides of the lung flatten against each other, and the organ becomes useless. The speed at which this occurs depends on the size of the hole. It may take minutes or hours. Spontaneous pneumothorax is not unusual in persons who are young and healthy. Joggers, for example, may collapse an entire lung. People in good physical condition can usually maintain bodily function on the strength of the other lung long enough to pick themselves up, hail help, and get to a hospital.

In a healthy person, a twenty-five percent pneumothorax would not automatically be treated. Some physicians prefer to see if the problem will take care of itself. Often it does. The hole in the lung seals off, the air in the chest cavity is absorbed into the tissue, and the person returns to normal function. With Mark, who needed maximum support from both lungs just to get through a day, the question was not whether to treat but where.

Emergency treatment for a collapsed lung is to insert a needle into the chest and draw out the air with a syringe. Once the immediate danger is past, a tube must be inserted into the pleural cavity to keep it free of air and give the lung a chance to reexpand. If necessary, these procedures could have been done on Mark right there in Radiology. But the preferable course was to get the patient back to the Adolescent treatment room where backup equipment and supplies were within instant reach of nurses who knew the room cold. Assessing Mark quickly, the doctors decided to make the trip.

They took him on a rolling stretcher, Darryl on one side, Kate on the other, the senior resident pushing from the rear, walking fast. Mark sat heaving for breath and begging for help. Darryl tried his best to reassure him.

"We'll have you feeling better in five minutes, Mark. We know what's wrong, and we know what to do about it." In two sentences the resident explained lung collapse. Thanks to the x-ray technologist, a security guard was holding an elevator for them.

Between the third floor and the sixth, Mark got suddenly worse. He became sweaty and began to turn blue. He felt as if he were suffocating. While relieved to learn that his problem was something real, not just his imagination, he wondered if he could possibly last five more minutes. Sweat poured down his face. He was scared as he had never been scared in his life.

Darryl Barth had begun to sweat himself. Except in medical school, where he had had a few opportunities to pump adults under supervision during cardiac arrest, he had never played a big role in an emergency before. From his first day at Children's he had known that pneumothorax is treated initially by a needle through the chest wall. Barth had never done the procedure or seen it done.

Hoping the patient would not notice that her hands were shaking, Kate pulled his robe to his waist and unbuttoned his pajama top. "Okay, Mark, hang in," Kate said as the elevator doors parted on Six. "We're almost there."

They ran him to the treatment room. There, as the senior resident indicated a spot on Mark's left side under his arm and Kate scrubbed the skin with iodine soap, Barth took out of its sterile paper wrap a large-bore needle sheathed in a thin plastic catheter and, with step-by-step instructions from the senior resident and explanations to Mark at every step, shoved the needle into the boy's chest, then withdrew the needle back through the catheter, leaving one end of the flexible narrow tube in the pleural cavity. In his struggle to get air, Mark barely reacted. Barth attached a 50 cc. syringe to the other end of the catheter and pulled back on the stopper. Mark sagged and let out a grunt.

"What's the matter?" Barth spoke in fear that he'd done something wrong. He was sweating profusely. His legs felt dizzy.

"Nothing," Mark gasped. "It feels better already."

All told, Darryl Barth extracted 600 cc. of air from the inside of Mark's chest. With every moment that passed, the boy grew more comfortable, more animated, more talkative. Barth had never seen a change as dramatic.

"I feel *so* much better!" Mark kept saying. He wiped his face with tissues held out to him by Kate. "I can't believe how much better I feel! I was so scared! It's such a scary feeling not to be able to breathe!" Though still inhaling with effort, he was ebullient with relief. He looked at Barth. "You saved my life!"

"Kate saved your life. She's the one who picked up that your lungs didn't sound right."

The boy turned to the nurse. "*You* saved my life!"

"Luck of the Irish!" Kate was able to reply. Her heart had only just left her throat.

A cardiothoracic surgery resident arrived in the treatment room and inserted a tube in Mark's chest. This procedure, similar to needling, is far more painful. For one thing, a chest tube is bigger than the narrow catheter Barth had used: the sharp-edged metal tip that pierces the flesh is almost as big around as a pencil. For another thing, the tube must go in at least six inches under ribs and into space surrounded by tissue that is exquisitely sensitive. It must be put in carefully, meaning slowly.

To minimize Mark's pain, the surgeon injected a local anesthetic into the boy's skin below his left shoulder blade and asked Kate to give him morphine through his IV line. Even so, the tube going in felt to Mark as if a burning rod were being shoved into his body.

He was unable to keep from shedding tears. Holding him, Kate felt his tears on her neck and thought her heart was going to break. An x-ray showed that the chest tube was in too far. When the surgeon pulled it back, the patient cried out. In the year and a half she had known Mark, Kate had never seen him so vulnerable.

He was moved back into his own bed at 11:00 P.M. The tube exiting his side had been hooked to a suction-drainage device called a Pleur-evac, which was pinned to hang down from the edge of his mattress and would keep his chest cavity free of air. The Pleur-evac in turn was plugged into wall suction. Until the chest tube was removed, the patient would be confined to the immediate vicinity of his bed.

Darryl Barth explained to Mark that a healthy person with a collapsed lung usually needs a chest tube for only a few days. How long it would take for a diseased lung to reexpand the resident could not say. He explained that while the tube was in place, Mark would probably experience discomfort, for which he could have pain medications.

When Barth had gone out to the nurses' station to call Mark's parents and his primary physician, Dr. Daniel Earnshaw, Kate pulled the yellow curtain around her patient's bed and began carefully to swab the dried blood and iodine soap from his chest, wanting to settle him for sleep if possible. But Mark had his own plans. He knew his parents would come in as soon as they'd heard the news, and he wanted to wait up for them. So far as he knew, his mother had never heard of a pneumothorax either. It would scare her, he told Kate. He wanted to reassure his mother that he was all right.

Kate protested. "It'll take them two hours to get here." But the patient was adamant.

It was obvious to her that physically the boy was miserable. A chest tube is painful in the healthiest patient, and in Mark the pain was exacerbated by every breath and every cough. The tube made it almost impossible for him to find a comfortable position. The codeine and Tylenol he'd been given were proving only somewhat helpful. Barth had been reluctant to prescribe stronger drugs because analgesics depress respiratory function and are risky for persons with bad lungs.

Kate felt sure that Mark was also very frightened. He was unusually bright, fifteen going on thirty, the nurses would tell each other, and he lived with his disease by knowing a great deal about it—so much that newer nurses on Adolescent actually felt intimidated by him, though not after they'd gotten to know Mark and found out how much fun he was. He knew so much that he could almost have written his own orders at Children's. Kate teased him about it: "Yes, sir, Dr. Price!" His knowledge gave him a sense of control. It allowed him to monitor his own condition and to understand what was happening from one month to the next. Now something had happened that he'd never heard of. Who wouldn't be scared?

He hadn't acknowledged fear, but Kate would not have expected him to do so. Insofar as she was aware, he never divulged his deepest feelings about his illness, not even to his parents. It was for precisely this reason that Dr. Griffin had offered Mark the opportunity to talk to a psychiatrist on this admission. The boy had not liked the psychiatrist, and his parents and the doctors had agreed that he would not have to see him again. Staff members who knew Mark thought this too bad. So did the patient's mother.

Yet Kate had come to read Mark's silence about the hard truths of his life as a reluctance to burden anyone with his problems. In fact, he had always given her the impression that he didn't feel he had many problems—a sign of denial, perhaps, which given the circumstances was understandable and even healthy.

He seemed determined to live in the fullest sense of the term. Illness had diminished his enthusiasms little if at all: for reading, for coins, for music, for televised sportscasts, for clowning and high jinks. Once he and his roommates on Adolescent had fixed up their room to look like a massage parlor! Sick as he was, Mark was always a lift for the staff, especially after the first few days of each admission when he'd begin to feel better. He loved to sit out at the nurses' station and joke with the nurses. They'd respond by pretending to fight over him.

"See this black eye, Mark?" one nurse would say. "Well, we had a little fistfight, and this is what I got. Trish got you, but that means I'll get you tomorrow!"

"I don't care if you do get to take care of him. You're only his nurse. I'm his girlfriend."

"I'm his nurse *and* his girlfriend!"

"That's okay," Kate would say, "because he and I are getting married!"

The first time she had said this, Mark had suggested that they marry on her birthday. This past June he had been readmitted just two days before her birthday. "Mark, if this is your way of getting out of the wedding, you can forget it," she had told him, "because I have the hospital chapel reserved, and we're getting married as planned!"

Though plainly in respiratory distress, he had picked up on this immediately. "Oh, God, I thought I could get out of it! I'm getting cold feet!" On the day itself the other nurses had given Kate a party and a cake, and somebody had had a camera, and Mark had said, "Let's get a wedding picture!"

The resulting snapshot had shown no cake. But the photographer had captured the nurse and the patient poised with a knife, and the patient was smiling. No matter how awful he looked or felt, Mark always managed a smile.

At the sink in his bathroom, the nurse filled a small plastic basin with warm water. She set the basin on the bedside table and began to sponge Mark's face with a clean washcloth. Wanting to give the boy whatever peace she could, she addressed his new problem out of her limited knowledge of it.

"Mark, we've had kids on the floor who've had pneumothorax from stab wounds. They've always cleared up in a few days."

"Yeah?" He seemed interested. His voice was raspy but earnest and perky—like the chirp of a bird, Dr. Earnshaw had remarked once. "Well, I know that's what Darryl said about healthy lungs." He added, "At least I didn't get stabbed!"

She put her arms around his shoulders and hugged very lightly. His right arm hugged her back. "I love you," he said with feeling. "Thanks for sticking by me tonight."

"Oh, Mark. I love you too. If it had to happen, I'm glad I was there."

"Me too."

"If you just weren't such a rotten kid."

"Yeah." He smiled briefly but grew suddenly grave. "Kate, I do appreciate what you did. Geez, you saved my life! But I can't believe you lied to me."

The accusation took her breath away. "What do you mean?"

"After you heard the decreased breath sounds, you told me everything was fine with my lungs."

"Mark . . ." She took his hand. "Mark, you know how much I care about you. To be very honest, I couldn't cope right then with the fact that something seemed to be wrong with your lung, and I didn't want to alarm you unnecessarily. At that point I hadn't even given a name to what I'd heard. We gave you answers as soon as we had them."

"I was really scared." It was not a reproach but something he wanted her to understand. "I didn't know what was going on. I thought I was going to die."

"Oh, Mark, I was scared too. You know I'd never hold the truth from you. . . ."

"That's why I couldn't understand why you did this time. But I can see why you didn't want to tell me anything you weren't sure about."

"I didn't *want* anything to be wrong."

He nodded. They looked at each other until at last Kate said lightly, "Mark, I'm not a pro on lungs, you know. If this was the first time in twenty-three years I was wrong about anything, I didn't want it to be about your lungs!"

"Well, now you still haven't been wrong! I'm just glad you found it. I'm not anywhere near ready to die."

That she knew. He had always said he was going to fight.

She emptied the basin in the bathroom and returned to Mark's bedside to fluff the pillows behind him. As he moved, he winced. He looked drained and exhausted.

"I'm going to stay on the floor until your parents get here," she said gently, "but I'll leave you alone now and let you get some rest."

"I'm going to wait up!"

"Okay, I'll leave you alone and let you wait up! Do you need anything?"

"I don't think so."

"Darryl's going to be here checking on you pretty frequently through the night, and I'll make sure the night nurse knows about your pain meds."

"Thank you."

She left the room dark except for the small reading light just above Mark's head. When she had gone, he opened his Bible.

He was fighting cystic fibrosis. It was a battle he knew he would lose. His fate had been sealed at the moment of his conception. CF is incurable and fatal. The most common hereditary disease among Caucasians, it kills more young Americans than does any other genetic disorder. At least half of those affected now live to celebrate their twentieth birthdays. When Mark was diagnosed at the age of nine months, his prognosis was thought to be five years.

For all the scientific breakthroughs that have revolutionized medicine in recent decades, cystic fibrosis remains, from a researcher's standpoint, one of the most recalcitrant, most frustrating diseases of modern times. It is known to be a dysfunction of the exocrine system in which the sweat, salivary, and mucus glands produce abnormal secretions. It is thought to result from an inborn error of metabolism, the error being the absence of whatever element would trigger the glands to produce normal secretions. No one knows what that element is. The cause of CF remains a mystery.

An infant born with this disorder has received a CF gene from each parent. But carriers can be identified only after they have given birth to an affected child. As the disease can elude diagnosis for years, parents may not discover that they are carriers until they have two or three affected children. Cystic fibrosis cannot be detected in utero.

Severity of symptoms varies from child to child. The cruelest manifestations result from the mucus, which is exceedingly thick. The mucus inhibits digestion by blocking the flow of enzymes from pancreas to intestine. Children with CF often have huge appetites but are nevertheless malnourished because their bodies digest only small amounts of what is eaten.

Worse, the mucus clogs the lungs. This not only makes breathing difficult but fosters infection. Normal mucus is a thin, slippery substance that washes the lungs and helps to keep them free of dust and germs. The heavy, sticky mucus of a CF child does just the opposite. It builds up in the lungs and retains dust and germs. Bacteria colonize in the mucus. The longer they flourish, the worse the infection. The bugs become resistant to one antibiotic after another. Repeated infections damage the lung tissue and afflict the child with chronic progressive pulmonary disease.

Symptoms can be treated. Until the infection becomes acute or the patient is otherwise in crisis, they are treated at home. In fact the goal of CF specialists is to keep the children out of the hospital and in school as much as possible for as long as possible. But even home care is expensive and disruptive of family routine.

The most time-consuming of the treatments is percussion and postural drainage. While the child lies or sits in positions designed to encourage the flow of mucus out of the lungs, the parent claps and vibrates the child's chest and back to shake the mucus free of the lung walls so it can be coughed up and spit out. Some children like to thin the mucus with an aerosol mist during this treatment. Some like to do part of the percussion themselves. Each treatment lasts at least ten or fifteen minutes. As many as four a day may be necessary.

Further, these youngsters must take large doses of certain vitamins and must adhere as strictly as possible to a diet low in fats and high in calories, protein, and salt. Finally, to compensate for the pancreatic enzymes that never get where they are supposed to go, CF children take pills containing extract of animal pancreas at every meal.

What usually brings them into the hospital is pneumonia. The lung infection develops until breathing becomes too difficult to manage at home. In the hospital the kids get aggressive chest toilet and intravenous antibiotics to reduce the pneumonia. The frequency of admissions increases as the child gets older and his or her condition worsens. The typical admission lasts ten to fourteen days. At Children's, by patients and staff alike, it is called a tune-up.

Mark's birth had been the easiest of his mother's three deliveries. In the hospital he had appeared to be fine. At home Ellen had been unable to satisfy his hunger. Very soon he was guzzling down the full contents of eight-ounce bottles. Often he would bring a lot of it back up, loaded with mucus. He'd fill his diaper with a loose, greasy mass that smelled positively foul. As much as he ate, he had remained scrawny. After a few months his appetite had fallen off. He'd grown congested. He'd begun to wheeze. The family doctor had thought allergies. He had put Mark on antibiotics and promised to do tests when the baby got older.

Late in Mark's seventh month, he'd developed a cold which had eventually turned into pneumonia. He had been hospitalized and put on oxygen. When he recovered, the pediatrician caring for him had done tests and given the baby's mother and father the grim news.

Ellen had discovered the CF Clinic at Children's by asking around. Dr. Earnshaw had admitted Mark, confirmed the diagnosis, and answered every question the baby's parents had had. In subsequent months he had educated and guided Ellen until caring for Mark had become routine for her.

For years Mark had done well. Once in treatment, he had gained weight and thrived. His two-year-old baby picture was beautiful. He'd had no trouble keeping up with a brother thirteen months

older. Ellen and her husband had more or less raised the boys together as healthy children.

Eventually Mark had realized that other children did not take
pills or get percussion four times a day. Perhaps because his parents
never dwelled on these differences, the boy had simply accepted
them. He had come to CF Clinic at Children's every three months
and needed to be hospitalized no more than once a year. Meanwhile
researchers had made improvements in the treatment of cystic fibrosis which improved the outlook for patients, though not their
ultimate destiny. It became common for children with CF to live
into their teens.

The disease had begun to restrict Mark's life when he was ten.
He had had to stop pitching for Little League. He had found it
increasingly difficult to ride his bike. Playing had left him tired,
without strength. He had begun to read more, and to spend more
time with his turtle. His height had leveled off. Inch by inch, his
classmates had grown taller around him.

Yet his symptoms had remained less severe than those of other
CF children his age. Ronnie, Mark's best friend in Clinic, had died
when both boys were twelve. Crushed, frightened, angry, Mark had
confronted a doctor about his own prognosis. The doctor had assured him that his case was not nearly as severe. Mark had let it be
known at the time that he did not intend to die of cystic fibrosis.
The following year he had missed several weeks of school and been
hospitalized twice. Even so, until after his fourteenth birthday, he
was still considered a mild case.

Then he had begun having trouble breathing. He had missed a
lot of school. He had begun attending Clinic monthly. Sometimes
he would be admitted to the hospital directly from Clinic, often
needing oxygen.

In the last few months, his condition had become a source of
great sorrow to his parents. Mark could not lie down anymore. He
couldn't breathe lying down. He slept with his body slumped against
pillows at his back, or he'd sit cross-legged and bowed over pillows
in front of him. Unless someone helped him, he was restricted to
one floor of the house. He could not ride his bike anymore. As of
early November, he had stopped going to school full-time.

He had put that decision off until his disease had forced his
hand. Through all of August he hadn't felt well. By the third week,

his mother had thought without saying so that he ought to be in the hospital. One afternoon he had said to her, "You know, Mom, the first week of school is very important, because that's when you get to know what's expected of you and what kind of teachers you're dealing with."

Ellen had understood perfectly why her son was hanging on at home. Mark loved school. In the classroom he could compete. He couldn't play baseball or basketball, but he always made the honor roll. School this year had promised an end to isolation. Bob, Mark's second father, had taken a new job in June. The family had moved about a hundred miles northwest to a town where they knew no one. Randy and Denise had ridden their bikes to the swimming pool every day and made friends that way. Unable to join in on such play, Mark had spent a lonely summer teaching tricks to Taffy, his dog.

So when school opened in September, Mark had begun his sophomore year. He had gone every day that first week. To cushion his thin buttocks against the hard wood seats, he had worn an extra set of underpants. His mother's suggestion that he take a pillow had exasperated him. "Mom! You can't carry a pillow around!" Because his bowel movements were so foul-smelling, he had used the toilet in the school nurse's office. His brother had helped him from class to class.

Mark had used as little help as possible. The new housing development in which the Prices lived topped a low hill surrounded by fields. A single road led out to the main highway. Every morning, the school bus picked children up where the road met the highway, and every afternoon it dropped them off there. Labored though his breathing had become by September, Mark had insisted on walking home. Or, more precisely, on dragging himself up the hill.

On the Saturday following the first week of school, he had asked his mother to call Dr. Earnshaw and get him a bed—the first time he had ever offered the information that he felt bad enough to be hospitalized.

After fourteen days in the hospital, he had returned to school full-time. Within three weeks, he had been in trouble again. He had come back to Children's in October and stayed ten days. He had grown very depressed during that admission. For a week he had barely talked—not to Ellen, not to Bob, not to the nurses.

What had finally brought him around was his mother's inspiration to get a two-hour pass and take him to a nearby Italian restaurant for a change of scene. When he checked out of Children's on Halloween Day, he had been himself again.

But that first evening home, when his parents had finally dared suggest to him that he consider going to school part-time, he had seemed almost grateful.

Earlier that day, while the nurses prepped the boy for discharge, Dr. Earnshaw had called Ellen to his office.

"I think you realize that Mark is in the final stages of his illness."

"Yes."

"I can't give you any amount of time, really. It could be a year. It could be two. Things don't look good now, but these children are unpredictable. I've been fooled more than once."

On Thanksgiving Ellen had fixed all the things Mark had always loved for Thanksgiving dinner. He had picked at his meal. On Friday he had been scheduled to visit his natural father's new family. Mark had missed his father's wedding in September because he'd been in the hospital. On Thanksgiving night Ellen had asked him whether he thought he was up to going.

"I want to go," he had told her, "but I'm not going to push myself."

The weekend had turned out wonderfully for him. His father's house was surrounded by woods. Mark had spent hours playing in the woods with the children of his father's new wife. He had visited with his oldest and dearest friend, Carl, the son of his mother's best friend, Sandy. He had felt as strong as he'd ever felt and been able to do as much as he had ever felt capable of doing. He had returned home in a happy frame of mind.

On Monday he had been too uncomfortable to go to school. On Thursday he had been readmitted to Children's. He'd told Dr. Griffin that he knew he needed a tune-up and wanted to get it over with before Christmas.

On Thursday evening Darryl Barth had gone into Mark's room to become acquainted with his new patient. The boy's breathing had eased. Both he and his mother had seemed less anxious than when they had appeared on Adolescent a few hours earlier. Mark had wanted updates on other cystics the doctor might know about.

When Barth had asked the Prices about their Thanksgiving, Mark had talked with obvious pleasure about his visit to his father's.

The scenes he described had stuck in the resident's mind. Restoring Mark to that level of activity had seemed a reasonable goal for this admission: more weekends in the woods, more fun times with the people who loved him. The challenge as Barth had seen it Thursday evening was to assuage anxiety in both the child and his family: to convince the Prices that Mark would return to school, to support them, and to give them the appropriate amount of hope.

Now Mark's lung had collapsed. That event had changed the whole character of his hospitalization. He was to remain in the Adolescent Unit for seven weeks and one day.

More than a thousand youngsters would be treated as inpatients at Children's during that period. Some twenty thousand more would be treated as outpatients, either in the Emergency Room or in one of the hospital's many specialty clinics. Most of those children would reside in the neighborhood or the region. But the youngsters admitted as inpatients would be flown in from as far away as Europe, Latin America, and Asia, referred to Children's because of its reputation as one of the best institutions of its kind in the world and because of the youngsters' own desperate circumstances.

The patients at Children's Hospital are very sick indeed. They are sick not with the common, transient illnesses of normal childhood but with illnesses or injuries that may deprive them of normal childhood, or of life itself. They are far too sick to be cared for in pediatricians' offices, too sick even to be cared for on pediatric wards of general hospitals, too sick to be cared for by anyone except consummate experts in the care of sick children. This expertise is precisely what Children's offers them. To most youngsters born or stricken with serious medical problems, this hospital and others of its caliber offer hope that is simply unavailable anywhere else. Children's can feel like the saddest place on earth. It can also feel like the happiest.

One of the youngsters treated at Children's Hospital while Mark Price was there this time was Candy Rudolph, a lively, loving six-year-old as yet apparently unaware of the malformed face that had prompted her parents voluntarily to submit her to life-threatening reconstructive surgery. Another was Brandon Gregory, admitted to

Children's a few hours after his premature birth weighing just a pound and a half. Another was Freddy Eberly, a sweet-natured fourth grader who would never again be the same after a car had sent him skyward but who nonetheless would recover from his multiple injuries when he might easily have died.

Jody Robinson was a patient at Children's while Mark was there. In fact, Jody had been a patient at Children's for his entire eighteen months of life—an amazing little boy with major birth defects, no family, and the personality of a star. Gina DeRose was a star too, in her own way—an effervescent eight-year-old in remission with leukemia who tended to land on Oncology Clinic like a meteor shower.

Mark never met those children. Nor did they ever meet each other. But over a season or two one year, their lives and fortunes were all in the hands of the experts at Children's Hospital.

The Prices' home stood a mile outside a small town whose rural environs were interrupted by factories. From town to Children's Hospital was eighty miles. Bob Price took advantage of the empty roads and zipped along somewhat faster than he usually drove. He was a big man, blond and balding, an easy, kind-faced person who could have hired out as Santa Claus. His wife sat beside him smoking, silent in the darkness as he himself was silent. Dr. Barth's call had awakened them at 11:30. A few minutes later, Dr. Earnshaw had called to reassure them and to urge them not to go into the hospital till morning. But Ellen had been too upset to wait. They had been dressed and rolling within fifteen minutes.

Bob was not nearly as worried as his wife was. Dr. Earnshaw had said that the pneumothorax was not a catastrophe. Bob could trust this statement not only because he trusted Earnshaw but also because by great coincidence a young man he knew from the church softball team had suffered a lung collapse recently, and within three weeks the man had been out playing ball again. Furthermore, Bob was by nature more relaxed and optimistic a personality than Ellen was.

He had owned the building into which she had moved with her three children after her divorce. Like her he had been newly divorced and the parent of three children, though they lived with his ex-wife; like her he had known the grief of having an unwell child.

Bob's youngest was autistic. After a two-year courtship, Bob and Ellen had married the day after Mark's twelfth birthday.

Two years later Bob Price had adopted Mark. The impetus had been the child's medical expenses. The assistance available from insurance policies held by Mark's natural father had been minimal. Bob was an industrial chemist for a company with an exceptionally good insurance plan. Mark and his stepfather had developed an extremely close relationship. Bob had become Mark's friend when the boy's activities with other youngsters had begun to be restricted by his physical condition. So when Bob had suggested that he adopt Mark to make him eligible for superior medical coverage, the boy had been very much in favor of the idea.

Their relationship consisted of good times. Mark took his troubles to his mother. He came to Bob entirely for fun, and fun they had, the boy's deterioration notwithstanding. For some reason Bob drove now thinking back on a coin auction he and Mark had attended this past summer. Silver prices had gone up, but on one of the auction tables Mark had come across an Eisenhower coin priced at $4.50 that he knew to be almost pure silver and worth twice or three times that amount.

"Hey, Bobby," he'd said in a conspiratorial whisper, "look at the bargain I got!" With a straight face he had gone to the proprietor to purchase the coin. The man, realizing instantly that he'd been caught by his own inattention, had burst out laughing.

"You little thief!" he'd said to Mark, putting an arm around his shoulders. He had even called his wife over. Mark had bought the coin for $4.50, and he and Bob had laughed all the way home.

They had arrived at the entrance to the state turnpike. As Bob opened his window to pull a toll ticket from the machine, cold air irritated his nostrils and turned his breath to fog. Closing the window, heading south, he took his wife's hand. "How are you, honey?"

"Okay." Her smile was an effort. "I just want to get there."

She was thirty-eight, five years younger than he and average in build, but there was a weariness in her face and a vulnerability in her bearing that made her appear older and smaller than she was. Life had hurt Ellen Price. Though she tried to be happy and did feel blessed in some very important ways, pain stuck with her like a shadow. Others saw her as emotional, warm, empathic. She thought of herself as nervous. She was darker blond than her kids and had a small raised mole on her forehead.

Bob asked gently, "Are you worrying about the lung collapse?"

She was wondering what further complications they had to look forward to. Just six months ago they had found out totally by accident about hemoptysis. On a list of meetings posted on the Adolescent bulletin board one morning while he was in the hospital, Mark had read of a talk on CF to be given that afternoon by a doctor visiting from another state. Attending with Dr. Earnshaw's permission, Ellen and her son had discovered that CF patients may hemorrhage from the lungs.

"Actually I'm worrying more about his emotional state. He must be terribly frightened."

"I know. I'm so glad Kate was working tonight. At least he was with somebody he cares about."

Ellen looked over at Bob wondering if he would ever know how grateful she was that he had entered their lives. After the children, he was the best thing that had ever happened to her. Her childhood had been miserable for reasons she discussed rarely. Two years out of high school, she had married for security and found just the opposite. Ending the marriage had made life easier in some respects but had left her on her own with no career, no college degree, and three children to raise, one having a fatal disease.

She had gone to live near the one person in her life Ellen had known she could count on: her high school friend Sandy. With a husband, four kids, and a house, Sandy had had stability to spare. Ellen had been able to relax and recover in the priceless atmosphere of a friendship she trusted. In Sandy's children her own had had good companions. Ellen had found a job she loved as a full-time teacher's aide and then had found a soulmate in her landlord.

He swung off the turnpike shortly before 1:00 A.M. After paying the toll, he picked up the expressway that would take them to within a few blocks of Children's.

"Thank God it happened at the hospital," she said.

"I was about to say that myself."

She lit another cigarette. Thank God for the hospital, period. It was a sanctuary for all youngsters who were different from what most people would consider normal. This thought had come to Ellen during Mark's last admission when he had become so depressed. Walking the halls one day, passing the medical library, she had gone in on impulse and looked up the word in a dictionary. Sanctuary: a place of refuge. A place to run for help, and did they ever! Sanctuary: asylum. No questions asked. Sanctuary: immunity. Oh, yes. A place for Mark and all the other children to be immune from the cruelties of ignorance, of complacency. A place where they had to make no explanations. Ellen had observed that her son sometimes seemed relieved to go into the hospital. There he had friends. There he felt completely comfortable—so comfortable that after the first few days, when he'd begin to feel better, he'd say to her, "You don't have to hang around, Mom. Don't you have other things to do? Go on home; I'm okay."

There were times at Children's when she had to turn her eyes from painful sights. But she had observed that Mark and the other youngsters didn't seem to see each other's scars or bandages or abnormal shapes. They saw only the person. The staff likewise. At Children's Hospital deformities and diseases were an accepted part of life. The place wasn't perfect, Ellen knew. But what or who was perfect? Without this sanctuary, where would the children be?

Mark was loved at Children's. They would take care of him at Children's until his mother got there.

Hard as he fought it, he succumbed to sleep before his parents arrived. When he finally dropped off, both Kate and Darryl felt huge relief. The boy's discomfort had made him nearly distraught.

His parents met briefly with his nurse and his resident in the Adolescent head nurse's office. Ellen Price greeted Kate with a kiss and thanked her for saving Mark's life. Barth reviewed the events of the evening. Bob Price was struck by the young doctor's humility. Instead of saying, "I did this, and then I did that," Barth gave a lot of credit to Kate. Bob was also struck by the regard Barth showed for Mark as a person.

The Prices had come prepared to stay. Before Kate left for home, she helped them set up a small rollaway cot next to Mark's bed for Ellen and another in the patient lounge for Bob. Soon thereafter Mark woke up. He was very glad to see his parents and gave them every detail of his lung collapse as if doing instant replay of an exciting moment on the field. To his mother he seemed less upset than she was.

But he was awake and in pain off and on throughout the night. All night long Darryl Barth and a nurse went in and out of Mark's room to medicate and comfort the boy.

Kate got home about 2:00 A.M. feeling that everything she had gone to school for had paid off. She had wanted to be a nurse since the age of five. Never before had she personally rescued a patient from death. And Mark, of all people. He had always been one of her favorites.

She didn't know yet that as of tonight he would become for her like a book she had started and couldn't put down.

Settling into bed, Kate said a novena prayer and cried her eyes out.

Sunday, December 2

The Admissions Office at Children's is located in a quiet corner of the ground floor, away from the noise and bustle of the lobby. Glassed in, carpeted, comfortably furnished, and soothingly lit, it resembles a travel agency except in decor. A giraffe painted on one wall nibbles happily at a border of flowers painted just beneath the ceiling. On the wall of one admitting cubicle, a red cartoon car heads toward a brown building that is obviously Children's. On the wall of the second cubicle, a smiling family of three adult mice presents a smiling child mouse to the admitting clerk. The youngster holds a mouse doll. One end of Admissions is a play area containing a child-sized table and chairs and littered with books and games and toys.

The Rudolphs arrived about 11:30 A.M. with their coats over their arms. Yvonne's mother was with them. Handing her coat to her grandmother, Candy scampered immediately over to the play area, sat down at the little table, and began to dress the paper dolls that were lying there. She was six years old and small for her age. Her cute, slender body was clad today in Sunday best: a flowered dress of peach and pink and white, a peach pinafore, white tights, new black patent-leather shoes. From neck to toes, the child looked perfectly normal.

But her face looked odd. Though the planes were smooth and the skin was unblemished beneath the bowl-cut brown bangs, the middle of Candy's face receded as if the whole structure from eyebrows to upper lip had been pushed in, leaving her with bulging eyes, no bridge above the button of her nose, and the appearance of a jutting lower jaw. Actually the upper jaw simply fell short of the lower. For Candy to keep her mouth closed required effort which the child often did not bother to make.

Her parents and her grandmother took seats near the admitting cubicles. Yvonne Rudolph was a short, small-boned woman in her late twenties with a tight mass of brown curls drawn back behind her ears. She wore a pink blouse, new gray slacks from Sears, and very little makeup. On her lap lay Candy's "security blanket," grubby, well-worn Baby Diaper Rash. Thanks to time and twisting, the doll's ropy yellow hair stood straight up on her head in spikes, as if from a bad scare. Bill Rudolph was lanky and bespectacled, a few years older than his wife and nearly a foot taller. He had on green corduroy trousers and a matching sport shirt. His mother-in-law was a tall, attractive, coiffed woman in a suit whose nails were long and polished.

The three adults attempted conversation. The one admitting clerk on duty was busy with another parent.

Candy's mother pulled at the doll's tresses and prayed for no delays. Because of the plastic surgeon's schedule, the operation had been arranged a year in advance. For one whole year she and Bill had been preparing themselves emotionally for an event that could be, as they saw it, a critical factor in Candy's future happiness and in their own peace of mind. Yvonne knew that the surgery would be a success. Because Candy was a special child, she knew that God would not let anything happen to her unless it was His will. She also had the utmost confidence in Dr. Rolfe Lorimer. Despite all his re-assurances, however, Yvonne still feared that the operation would somehow impair the child's mental function. She couldn't wait to put this fear behind her, couldn't wait for her firstborn to be done with the traumas that were about to beset her.

Dr. Lorimer was going to make Candy's face look more normal. He would do this by shaving her head, opening her scalp from ear to ear, peeling down the flesh of her face, retracting her brain through a window cut into her skull by a neurosurgeon, breaking and rearranging bones, and then sewing up her scalp again. The operation would involve rib grafts taken from Candy herself.

She would have bandages over her eyes for several days. Because of swelling, she would probably not be able to see for at least several days after the bandages came off. Barring complications, she would be in the hospital about a week. The swelling would not disappear for six months or more. The new face would take a full year to settle. Each person heals differently, Dr. Lorimer had emphasized. He could not guarantee that the change would be permanent. Repairs sometimes had to be done over. Though he himself had not lost a patient from surgery of this kind, there was a worldwide two percent death rate from infection. Of course, he had warned them, anesthesia always carries a risk.

The decision to go ahead with such an operation for their daughter had not actually been difficult for the Rudolphs. Strangers stared at Candy on the street. Salespeople assumed she was Mongoloid or otherwise retarded and sometimes made comments to this effect, which triggered in the child's mother an urge to kill. Other children teased Candy, especially another kindergartner she called Mean Brian who made her cry by coming at her eyes with fingers crawling like snakes. If this was how the world received Candy Rudolph at age six, how would it treat her when she was sixteen? Yvonne had wanted her daughter's face reconstructed within an hour of discovering that such a thing was possible.

"Candace Rudolph?" The admissions clerk motioned the family to his desk. A moment later Bill Rudolph and his daughter were on their way to a laboratory on the other side of the building where a technician would type her blood.

The child skipped ahead apparently oblivious of the notice she aroused in one or two visitors who passed her. Sometimes now she seemed self-conscious when she saw strangers looking at her. Her father was never unaware of the looks Candy got from strangers. An engineer by trade, a man who virtually never permitted his emotions to drive him off a steady course, Bill Rudolph could nonetheless be upset by the way people reacted to his older daughter. At home he usually forgot that there was anything different about her. In the streets, at the playground, at the store, he could never forget. When people stared at Candy, they disturbed her father's tranquility.

On a recent visit to Children's for a preoperative checkup, Candy had been given a tour. An older nurse had shown her the operating room holding area where she would wait for surgery, the lounge where her parents could sit while she was having surgery, the intensive care unit where she would go when the operation was over, and the sixth-floor surgical unit where she would be transferred after a few days when she no longer needed intensive care. She had even met the nurse who would take care of her there. Candy had liked Tammy Torrence. Because of Tammy, and because the older nurse had told her she could bring Baby Diaper Rash with her, and because she was only six, and an immature six at that, Candy had come to the hospital this morning in a relatively happy frame of mind.

The sight of the laboratory made her stop skipping.

The lab was full of strange equipment. There was no play area. When a young male technician greeted the Rudolphs jovially and invited Bill to sit down in the chair beside his desk, Candy clung to her father and hid her face against his shoulder. Ordinarily she was afraid of nothing.

The young man began to explain to her that he was going to take a little bit of her blood by sticking her finger quickly with a tiny blade.

The child began to squirm and to whimper. The technician suggested sympathetically that she sit on her daddy's lap. Though she did so, her fear grew.

But the technician had been trained in the techniques of taking blood from fearful children. Firmly yet without force, he took Candy's hand and touched her finger to a disposable syringe to show her that when he collected the blood, it wouldn't hurt. Next he touched her finger to a glass slide to show her that that wouldn't hurt either. She showed interest in what he was doing and seemed somewhat palliated. But the instant he said, "There'll just be a little prick, and that's the only thing that will hurt," she tried hard to pull her finger out of his hand. Failing, wailing in protest, she buried her head in her father's neck.

The technician gave her finger a quick jab. "That's all, Candy," he announced.

She sat up astonished.

"It's all over. You were such a good girl!"

As the technician drew blood into his syringe from the drop at the tip of her finger, Candy watched in fascination.

He might have let it go at that. Instead, finishing up, the young man told her tales about drawing blood from kids who hadn't been nearly as good as she had. A sixteen-year-old had spit at him! A female technician weighing two hundred pounds had grabbed the kid and made him wipe off his spit! Another kid had put up a fuss in the lab, and her mother, who weighed *three* hundred pounds, had sat on her! When the technician opened up a Snoopy Band-Aid, Candy actually offered her finger. She skipped all the way back to Admissions. Asked by her grandmother if the finger hurt, the child assured her that it did hurt and boasted that the man had said she was a good girl.

The admissions clerk directed the family to the surgical unit on the sixth floor. There Candy was disappointed to learn that Tammy had the day off. The nurse taking care of her instead led the Rudolphs to a four-bed room in which one of the beds was empty and freshly made. By 1:30 Candy Rudolph was sitting cross-legged on that bed wearing a new pink nightgown with a big lace collar and taking full advantage of her special status.

"I need a pillow," she told the nurse, who went to find one.

"Where's Teddy?" Candy demanded of her mother.

"We didn't bring him," Yvonne replied, "but here's Baby Diaper Rash, and we also have Fuzzy." She took a fat blue dog from a canvas sack of Candy's things and laid the dog down next to Candy.

"Mommy, get that dog off and put that blanket on me! I'm hungry!" Asked by the nurse if she would go to the bathroom for her, the child rejected the suggestion with one word. *"No!"* This embarrassed her mother and also surprised her. Candy was usually very cooperative.

But when she had gone with the nurse to get weighed, and when she had drunk some Coke from a paper cup, and when her parents had promised to bring her a sandwich from the cafeteria, and when the nurse had shown her a two-way stethoscope, letting her hear the sounds in her own chest, Candy began to calm down. When the nurse proceeded to ask her questions and to write down her answers, the child responded politely.

She liked hot dogs, hamburgers, and soup, she told the nurse. She did not like spinach or Brussels sprouts. She took a bath three times a week. She brushed her own teeth. At home she had her own room. She did not need to sleep with a light on. Her favorite toy was Baby Diaper Rash. She liked to swim. For going to the toilet she said pee-pee and poo-poo. Usually she wore glasses, but she needed a new prescription, and she wasn't going to get it till after the operation. She had one sister, Amy, who was three years old. When the nurse had finished her questions to the patient, Candy snuggled down under the covers with Baby Diaper Rash and put her thumb in her mouth.

The nurse turned to the child's parents and took a medical history.

Yvonne had given it so many times that she thought she could do it in her sleep. It was always painful.

She and Bill had moved west to California just a few months before the baby was due. The pregnancy had continued without incident. Labor had begun on schedule. But ten hours later when the doctors directed Yvonne to push, she had felt no urge. The infant had been delivered by emergency Caesarean. In the recovery room somebody had told Yvonne that she had a little girl.

The Rudolphs had been warned in prenatal classes that newborns are not pretty. When they'd first seen Candy, neither had noticed anything wrong. The next day their pediatrician had told them that there was "a slight problem." A day later, after doing x-rays, he had informed them that there were more serious problems than he'd thought. The baby's head had developed abnormally. Ordinarily, the doctor had explained, the bones of an infant's skull meet along lines called sutures, which remain open to allow for the growth of the brain. Ordinarily the sutures do not close completely until the child is a year old. Candy's had closed in utero, a malformation called craniosynostosis. While he himself had never seen a case like it, the pediatrician knew that the baby needed one or more operations if her brain were to grow.

Of course it was dangerous to give anesthesia to an infant. Candy could die from the surgery. But without it, the doctor had warned her parents, she might be brain-damaged or blind or both.

She had had her first craniectomy at the age of ten days. The surgeon had removed a strip of bone along the coronal suture, which runs across the top of the skull from ear to ear. Five months later, discovering that the suture had closed again, he had reopened it with a second craniectomy. This time the surgeon had painted the edges of the bone with a chemical fixative intended to prevent them

from growing back together immediately. Since then Candy had undergone no further surgery on her cranium.

But she had had other problems. At the age of two months she
had begun having seizures. Tests and electroencephalograms had
failed to yield an explanation. Eventually the child had been put on
phenobarbital. She was still taking it. Astigmatic, she had begun
wearing glasses at the age of three—thick lenses shaped specially to
accommodate the protrusion of her eyeballs. She had subsequently
needed muscle surgery on both eyes to correct a squint. Thanks to
the malformation of her facial structure, her breathing was slightly
labored, and her speech was nasal and difficult to understand. She
continued to need speech therapy.

Just before Candy's fifth birthday, the Rudolphs had taken her
back to the original surgeon for a routine checkup. The doctor had
expressed concern about the coronal suture. He had expected the
treated edges of bone to grow together eventually. Instead, the gap
between the front and back of the child's cranium had filled in with
soft tissue. If Candy were to fall off her bike or be struck in the
head in an auto accident, she'd be unprotected, the surgeon had
felt. He'd suggested the insertion of a metal plate.

The Rudolphs had resisted. While understanding the doctor's
reasoning, they'd had questions he had not been able to answer to
their full satisfaction. Would the presence of a metal plate in
Candy's head harm her in some unpredictable way? Would they
have to keep replacing the plate as she grew? She'd been doing just
fine. Why put her through any more surgery? At the very least the
child's parents had wanted a second opinion.

Yvonne had grown up across the city from Children's Hospital.
Her parents still lived in the old neighborhood. Her father, a
Lutheran minister, still had a church there. As the Rudolphs had
planned to fly east for Christmas in any event, they had asked
Yvonne's father to make an appointment for Candy with a neu-
rosurgeon at Children's.

They had been extremely impressed with Guillermo Perez.
Yvonne had once taken Candy to a neurosurgeon who had studied
her as if she were a specimen. He had never even addressed her.
Dr. Perez had taken her onto his lap. He had begun to talk with her
parents only after he had talked with Candy.

He had given her condition a name the Rudolphs had never

heard before: Crouzon's syndrome. They had learned that the original diagnosis, craniosynostosis, referred only to premature closing of the sutures and that Crouzon's was a broader term encompassing some of Candy's other problems. Dr. Perez had opened a book and shown them pictures. He had pointed out that Candy had a rather mild form of the disorder. He had said that Crouzon's tends to run in families and that Candy's children would have a fifty-fifty chance of being born with it.

They had asked him his opinion of a metal plate. He'd thought it unnecessary. He had surmised that the membrane covering Candy's brain was tough enough to protect her from any recoverable injury. What absolutely needed to be done for the child, Dr. Perez had told her parents, had already been done.

However, the neurosurgeon had gone on to say, if the Rudolphs wanted their daughter's appearance changed, there was a new kind of surgery that could do that. It was being done at half a dozen centers around the country, including Children's Hospital. If the Rudolphs would like, Dr. Perez would call the plastic surgeon and find out if he could see them that same afternoon.

They had waited outside Rolfe Lorimer's office for two hours. They had talked about the surgery the whole time. At one point Yvonne had burst into tears. The news given them by Dr. Perez had been earthshaking. Overjoyed to think that Candy might be made to look more normal, they had nonetheless been crushed to discover just as they'd thought the child's surgery over and done with that they might now have to start again.

Yet how could they deny Candy the happiest life possible?

They had left Dr. Lorimer's office with the date set.

They had not sought Candy's opinion. Giving a child a choice obliged a parent to abide by the outcome, Yvonne believed, and she would not have accepted a veto from Candy. This was not a choice between red and green dresses.

The surgery was actually to be done in two phases: the forehead area first, with the neurosurgeon involved, and then, several years from now, the upper jaw, a less serious operation. When the ordeal was over, Yvonne Rudolph wanted no one ever again to look at her daughter and think: *She's different.* She wanted people either to think that Candy was a cute little kid or not to notice her at all.

Anticipating Candy's birth, she and Bill had never imagined that their baby would not be perfect. Yvonne was an only child. After delivering an abnormal baby, she had been almost unable to bear giving her parents the news for fear of hurting them as much as she herself was hurting.

Her pain had not been lessened by the nurse who had come into Yvonne's room a day later to confide that she had had a baby with Down's syndrome and knew of a place where the Rudolphs could send their child and never have to see her again.

Nor had the devastation of those first few days been eased by the hospital photographer who had refused to record their daughter's arrival, saying to Yvonne's parents, "You don't want a picture of that baby." Yvonne's soft-spoken minister father had raised his voice a notch and issued an order, and the picture had been taken. But the damage had been done.

They still wondered why, she and Bill. Why Candy? Why them, when perfectly normal babies were being born to fifteen-year-old unwed mothers who seemed ready to do anything under the sun to get rid of them? She and Bill had followed all the rules. They had done everything right.

At first Yvonne had put the blame on birth control pills. But the doctors had fairly well convinced the Rudolphs that Candy's defect had not been caused by the pill or by anything else Yvonne had taken or not taken, done or not done, though what *had* caused it they couldn't say. They didn't know. Even at Children's.

In the absence of a medical explanation, Bill wavered between thinking that the answer lay simply in the laws of probability and wondering whether he and Yvonne were being tested or punished. Maybe Candy's problem was God's way of chastening them. Like his wife, Bill Rudolph had been raised in the household of a Lutheran minister. In fact he and Yvonne had met when his father became assistant pastor at her father's church.

Yvonne did not share the notion that God would tamper with a child's happiness to test adults. Instead she believed that He had chosen her and Bill as Candy's parents because He knew they would care for her and love her. As Yvonne understood Him, God would give such a situation only to people He knew could handle it.

Some days she felt she was not handling it. Most often this oc-curred when a question arose about Candy's capabilities. When the child didn't behave as Yvonne thought she should, when she ran awkwardly and bumped into things, when other kindergartners would get every single thing right on a paper and Candy wouldn't, when she had difficulty doing anything that other six-year-olds could do without difficulty, her mother both blamed herself and felt angry with the child.

She knew she shouldn't. She knew full well that poor vision undoubtedly explained many of Candy's problems. Yet Yvonne would find herself saying to her daughter, "There's something wrong with you because you're not getting it." The minute the words were out of her mouth, she would feel angry with herself and terribly guilty. "Oh, no, honey, there's nothing wrong." Deep down in the mother was a fear that tests might one day reveal some mental deficit in the child, though none of the many doctors who had examined Candy since her birth had ever given the Rudolphs reason to think there was anything wrong with the way her brain functioned.

Sometimes Yvonne thought of seeing a psychiatrist. She yearned to talk to someone who would help her get rid of the feelings she so disliked in herself. She had always considered her father the world's best communicator, yet felt this matter too personal to discuss with a parent. But psychiatrists were expensive, and Bill thought they were weird themselves.

So she turned for help to a more traditional source: her faith. She prayed to God to give her the strength to treat Candy as the child deserved, to remember that she was not a robot programmed to do everything right the first time. Yvonne further comforted herself with reminders that if her eldest sometimes seemed slow, Amy, too, had been a late walker—as had their mother, in fact—and that Candy did eventually catch up in her own time. When learning their phone number, she had invariably blanked on the middle three digits. Yvonne had finally despaired to her parents. "Let it go," they'd advised. "Drop it awhile." A month later the child had been able to reel off the number without a second's hesitation.

But her progress had never come free: not to Candy, and not to her family. Like other parents in similar situations, the Rudolphs had always tried to make the best of their lot. When talking about it, they did not complain. Asked, however, to characterize life with a youngster having all of Candy's problems, Yvonne Rudolph would reply quietly that it had been pure hell.

In principle she opposed abortion unless baby or mother was in danger of dying. Had she and Bill known in advance about Candy's defect, might Yvonne have considered aborting?

She might have.

Any child of Candy's would be as likely to be born with Crouzon's syndrome as to be born normal. If Candy should one day elicit her mother's thoughts about whether to conceive, what would Yvonne reply?

She would advise Candy to adopt.

"How can you say that when you know the problem can be corrected?" Yvonne's mother had challenged her. "Wouldn't you rather have your own child?"

Yvonne Rudolph could not imagine life without her firstborn. Candy was a warm, loving, outgoing child—a youngster who, when others her age were going through the Terrible Twos, had delighted in introducing her grandfather up and down the street to neighbors she herself had never met. She was noticeably more affectionate than her younger sister, who was unusually pretty, her parents felt, but who had never encountered adversity. Candy had a truly special warmth. She also had lot of determination. She had learned to color within the lines practicing diligently. Practice had also made her first in her kin en class to cross a piece of gym equipment hand over hand didn't see facial oddity when she looked at Candy. She sa ild she loved. The person Candy was had made all the diffic worthwhile.

But Yvonne could not contempl going through those difficulties for a hypothetical child, nor would she ever wish on her daughter the pain she herself had endured.

When the nurse had gotten the information she needed and gone off to check on another patient, the Rudolphs went down to the cafeteria as promised and bought a sandwich and a carton of milk for Candy. Upon their return they found her playing with the toddler in the next bed. After she had eaten, Candy wandered into the playroom. There she encountered a little black girl about her age who had also brought a doll to the hospital. Candy showed her Baby Diaper Rash. The two girls began skipping their dolls up and down the halls of Six Surgical.

Fifteen miles from Children's, Dr. Rolfe Lorimer worked at home on chapters he was contributing to a new plastic surgery textbook. He was dressed casually in cords and a sweater. Tall and slender, with exquisite hands and touches of white at his temples, the man at forty-two was exceptionally handsome.

His setting became him: a library furnished in antiques, original paintings, an Oriental rug in blues and browns. Orchestral sounds infused the room from a stereo in one corner. Above Lorimer's desk was a picture window overlooking lawn. Through that window in summer he could see his wife's vegetable and flower gardens and watch the children at play with the dogs. Two children now. The oldest, a boy of twelve, had died a year ago during the last and least dangerous of three operations to correct the heart disease with which he had been born. His death had intensified Rolfe Lorimer's passion for his family and his desire to help the children who came to him as patients.

He had always wanted surgery. Growing up in Texas as the sole offspring of a man who manufactured new paper from old, Lorimer had dreamed of becoming a neurosurgeon. After medical school at Tulane, he had gone to McGill University in Canada for the best training he knew of in that field. Upon finishing there, he had been drafted. Two years with a neurosurgical unit in Germany had exposed him to plastic surgery and changed the course of his life.

In retrospect he'd wondered why he hadn't thought of it earlier. He had always been interested in art and aesthetics. Artists were among his closest friends. Lorimer himself had made a hobby of watercolor painting, and he had always liked beautiful things. He had always noticed beautiful faces or bodies. While plastic surgery does not require that its practitioners be aesthetically inclined, it offers great satisfactions to those who are. Beginning his residency in the discipline that derives its name from the Greek word *plastikos*, meaning malleable or moldable, Rolfe Lorimer had found the fit amazingly natural.

He'd had no inkling that he was to become a pioneer in the field. He had finished his training in 1971 expecting to spend the rest of his professional life revising scars, repairing hands, expunging insofar as possible the record of burns from human skin, providing to aging faces and bodies the illusion of youth. He'd considered these

missions vital. It was just as important to make people happier or
more content with themselves, Lorimer still believed, as to save lives.
During his residency at the university hospital next door to Children's, he had seen many youngsters who had been born with facial
deformities. The only repairs being attempted at that time, however, were on children with cleft lip and palate.

Toward the end of his residency, Rolfe Lorimer had attended a
meeting in Montreal and heard Paul Tessier speak. A plastic surgeon from France, Tessier had come to this continent to share a
discovery: a way to make abnormal faces look more normal. He had
learned that it was possible to attack facial defects not just from
outside the skull but from within as well—by opening the cranium,
peeling down the facial tissue, and adding, subtracting, or relocat-
ing fat and bone.

Along with the rest of his colleagues, Rolfe Lorimer had listened
to Tessier in amazement. Surgeons had always assumed that facial
bone would shrink if stripped of blood-bearing tissue. The concept
of opening the head to do surgery on the face contradicted fundamental neurosurgical principles. To expose a patient's brain while
working externally through the mouth and nose was to subject the
brain to possible contamination that could kill the patient.

But Tessier had found himself using these techniques on accident victims beginning in the 1950s. Badly smashed faces had demanded extraordinary measures. At some point it had occurred to
the surgeon that these same procedures might benefit persons
whose faces had been deformed from birth. He had not trusted
himself to schedule an elective procedure until 1967. Between 1967
and 1971 he had operated on 225 people born with facial defects.
Three had died—three too many, but a very low number, the surgeons in Montreal had realized, considering the radical nature of
the operation. The inventor was calling it craniofacial reconstructive
surgery.

In 1972 Paul Tessier had returned to America to demonstrate
his techniques at five carefully selected hospitals, among them Children's. In one week there he had performed seven operations. De-
parting after the last of them, he had left behind among his
converts a junior member of the Plastic Surgery Department who
had had no doubt in his mind that Children's should offer cra-

niofacial reconstructive surgery, or that he himself should become
expert at it.

By this time Rolfe Lorimer had developed a very special interest
in faces. He had always liked sketching faces without knowing exactly why. As a cosmetic surgeon he realized that he preferred to
work on faces because he considered their function so critical. As
the first aspect of a human being to be seen, the doctor reasoned,
the face affects a person's life dramatically. These stakes challenged
Lorimer and fully engaged his aesthetic impulse. When an operation was successful and a face was improved, the patient's needs
were satisfied and so, more than in any other kind of procedure,
were Lorimer's. He found absolutely compelling the chance to try to
improve upon the futures of persons saddled from birth with gross
facial defects. In the intervening years his work in the field had
become internationally known.

He had continued to devote half his practice to cosmetic surgery.
He enjoyed the change of pace and enjoyed working on normal
anatomy. Symmetry allows for more predictable results. Working
repeatedly with structures that vary little from patient to patient
permits the surgeon to achieve a high degree of expertise in manip-
ulating those structures. Making refinements in normal faces gave
Lorimer a lot of aesthetic pleasure. In reconstructive surgery, the
anatomy is highly idiosyncratic. It sometimes confronts the surgeon
with unwelcome surprises which adversely affect results. While the
goal in every case is to make the person look more normal, and
while this goal is almost always attained, patients and surgeon alike
must often settle for a face that falls short of looking fully normal.
Compromise was frustrating to a surgeon whose standard, however
elusive, was perfection. But the artist in Rolfe Lorimer found reconstructive surgery more fun than cosmetic because it allowed him—
indeed forced him—to be more creative.

He did his major cases at Children's on Mondays. At one time he
had used Sundays to prepare. There had been many unknowns in
the early days of craniofacial reconstruction. Among the biggest
questions had been the matter of growth. If a surgeon took liberties
with the bones of a child's face, would those bones continue to grow
at a normal rate? If two-year-old cheeks were padded with fat grafts
from the child's buttocks, would the cheeks be proportionate to the
face of the eight-year-old? If only one cheek were padded, would it
grow at the same rate as the other?

It had taken time for the pioneers to learn that although some grafts fail to take for a variety of reasons, those that do take grow normally. Meanwhile the surgeons had compensated for the unknowns by laying meticulous plans. Only after doing a hundred of these operations had Rolfe Lorimer realized that he did not have to spend Sunday afternoon thinking out exactly what he was going to do on Monday.

He still did no craniofacial case lightly. He still worried about every one and planned every step. But with 260 of these procedures now behind him, Lorimer could rely much more heavily than he once had on his skills and instincts.

The operation he'd be doing tomorrow on Candy Rudolph was similar to dozens he had done in the past. Of course this case had its own peculiarities. The major challenge in Monday's surgery would be to cut free a piece of Candy's cranium comprising her lower forehead and the upper arches of her eye sockets and to advance that piece about eight millimeters. Anchored to the rest of the skull by rib grafts, the bony piece in its new position would give contour to a forehead now flat, deepen the sockets so that the child's eyes no longer bulged, and add prominence to the bridge of her nose.

Lorimer would also make some finer adjustments. He would draw up the outer corners of Candy's eyes to correct a slight droop. He would narrow the space between the inner corners by hitching together the ligaments behind them so that one pulled toward the other. Using segments of rib, he would build up the child's cheekbones and fill in the gaps across her skull left after the second craniectomy. Finally, he would straighten and elevate the patient's ears, which tilted backward.

At least these were his plans. Whether he actually carried them all out would depend on what he found once he got started. One form of trouble would be unavoidable: scar tissue from Candy's previous operations. Scarring would make it difficult for Lorimer to separate muscle and fat from bone. Scarring could also blur distinctions between structures in the interior landscape. Because the integrity of her skull had already been compromised, Candy Rudolph was not the ideal candidate for craniofacial reconstructive surgery.

Nonetheless, Rolfe Lorimer felt confident that the child stood to gain from the operation. The odd aspects of her appearance were correctable with known procedures. The corrections would almost certainly make Candy look more normal. There was a good chance that together with the surgery to be done later on the upper jaw, they could also improve her speech and breathing. Even her visual acuity could conceivably profit. While infection and death were always a danger, Lorimer himself had never had a death, and he had done well over 150 cases now without an infection.

His fee for Monday's surgery would be $3,500. Though each year he did several craniofacial reconstructions for the $150 allowed under the welfare system, Lorimer knew that the Rudolphs' insurance plan would cover what he considered a fair charge for a procedure of this complexity. He knew of plastic surgeons who would have asked $4,500 or $5,000. Lorimer thought such fees unreasonable if not unconscionable. He enjoyed having money, just as he enjoyed the acknowledgment of his peers. But Lorimer had acquired enough of both to satisfy his needs. Money was not, in his opinion, plastic surgery's highest reward.

Nor did he feel greatly rewarded now by a dramatic transformation in a given case. There is a moment of truth in any craniofacial procedure when, the repairs having been completed, the surgeon draws back over the altered architecture the flap of flesh peeled down at the beginning of the operation and provides to all present, before the distortion of swelling sets in, the first glimpse of how the new face is going to look. For the OR nurses working with Lorimer, this moment was almost always a thrill. For the doctor himself, "thrill" was no longer the word. By now Lorimer expected dramatic transformation. He expected himself to do the job well.

His greatest professional motivation these days was the desire to become the best in the world in his field. As a traditional plastic surgeon, he had started out with several thousand competitors. As an expert in craniofacial reconstructive surgery, he really had only four. Probably no one could say who was best among them. No matter. Rolfe Lorimer would know when he had achieved his full potential.

In the meantime it gave him enormous pleasure and intellectual satisfaction to do each case better than the last. For that reason he always looked forward to Mondays.

The Rudolphs had moved recently from California to Long Island, where Candy's father had taken a new job. Soon after the surgery was over on Monday afternoon, he would make the long drive back to New York by himself. He would return to work on Tuesday and rejoin his family on Friday evening.

Yvonne, meanwhile, would stay on with her parents. Bill's parents, too, lived about an hour's drive from Children's, and Candy's little sister would stay with them. After much thought about this arrangement, Yvonne had finally concluded that Amy would be happier if she did not have to watch her mother go off every morning to spend the day with Candy, and that Candy deserved under these circumstances to have her mother's undiluted attention. After all, the child was only supposed to be hospitalized a week. Having the family split for that length of time would be a hardship for everyone, but a tolerable hardship, in Yvonne's opinion.

On Sunday evening she and her husband left Children's and went out to dinner together. Yvonne's parents remained behind to entertain the patient. Candy so adored her grandfather and he her that the child scarcely noticed her parents' absence.

After supper she was playing a game with her grandparents when the nurse taking care of her on the evening shift came in to talk with Candy. The nurse wanted to be sure that the patient knew what was coming. Sitting on a chair at the bedside, the young woman began by asking Candy if she knew why she was in the hospital.

The Rudolphs had not given their daughter many details about her forthcoming operation. Candy hadn't seemed to want them. They had told her mainly that her eyes would be fixed and that she'd be a pretty little girl. Yvonne felt sure Candy knew that there would be changes made in her face, but the Rudolphs had minimized the talk of change because they hadn't wanted Candy to feel unattractive as she was. She had never once asked them about her looks. She had never asked why other kids poked fun at her. Was she aware of being different? Her parents had no idea.

For a while after her first visit to Dr. Lorimer, Candy had asked off and on when she'd be going to the hospital. Later she had gone through a period of saying she didn't want to go. More recently she'd been heard to tell Amy that she was going into the hospital because they were going to operate on her eyes, and she was going to get presents, and the nurses were going to get her glasses of apple juice and orange juice.

She told the nurse sitting beside her that the doctors were going to cut her eyes and cut her head to fix her eyes.

The nurse attempted to correct this impression. The doctors would not cut Candy's eyes, she said, but they would cut her head, and they would move some of the bone around her eyes. "But you won't feel it," the nurse assured the child, "because you'll get some medicine that will make you sleep until the operation is over." At Yvonne's request, Candy would not be told until morning that her preop medication would be administered by injection.

The nurse gave the child some details. Candy could not have anything to eat after 8:00 tonight. She could not have anything to drink after midnight except a little water with her phenobarbital. When she woke up after the operation, however, she could drink as much as she wanted.

By then she would have a big bandage over her head. It would cover her eyes. She would not be able to see. Her wrists might be tied loosely to the sides of the bed so that she couldn't touch her bandage. She would also have a bandage on her chest because the doctors were going to use one or two of her ribs to help fix her head. The ribs would grow back. Besides the bandages, she would have tubes in her arms and maybe in her chest, and she might have a tube that would help her pee.

The head bandage would probably stay on for two or three days. Although Candy wouldn't be able to see, she would not be alone. She would be in the intensive care unit on the fourth floor— "You've already seen it, remember?"—and nurses there and her family would help her whenever she needed something. If she wanted to hold toys and play with them, she would be very welcome to do that. Some children enjoyed listening to cassette tapes while their heads were bandaged. Candy could do that too.

The nurse talked of pain far less than an outsider might have expected, given the nature of the operation. Oddly enough, for reasons no one fully understands, facial manipulation causes surprisingly little pain. Rolfe Lorimer's patients were far more likely to complain that their sides hurt where their ribs had been removed, discomfort rather easily managed with morphine and aspirin.

The nurse found the child both attentive and talkative during this conversation and was pleased to note that Candy gave accurate feedback on what she'd been told. The patient's greatest concern, as best the nurse could tell, was the loss of activity and freedom involved in being restrained. Several times she asked rather fearfully about having her hands tied down. The nurse assured the child that restraints would be necessary only until she was fully awake and aware of the importance of not touching her dressings.

A short time later anesthesiology resident Susan Carlson came to talk with Candy. Carlson was petite, blond, and rosy-cheeked. She had on wrinkled OR greens, low-heeled white shoes, and a gold wedding band. In the last year of her residency at the university hospital next door, she was just beginning a three-month rotation at Children's. Next door she had assisted Rolfe Lorimer with nearly a dozen craniofacial procedures on adults. Tomorrow's would be her first on a child.

Carlson had stopped at the nurses' station to glance at Candy's chart. But as the child had been admitted just hours earlier, the chart contained little information beyond her name, age, and address. So when Carlson entered Candy's room, she made a snap judgment about her based solely on what the patient looked like.

She concluded that Candy was retarded.

Reaching for the little girl's hand, the doctor introduced herself. The moment the child began to talk, Carlson saw that her snap judgment had been wrong. At that same instant the anesthesiologist realized that she was patting Candy's hand as if it were a dog's paw.

Carlson recovered enough to conduct her business with a patient she found to be amiable, loving, giving, and not at all self-centered or self-conscious. But the doctor left the room knowing that whatever happened in the operating room on Monday, she had already learned the most important lesson this case was likely to teach her.

Ø

Children's Hospital stands beside a busy boulevard in a major American city. Its nearest neighbors are a massive civic center, a high-rise hotel, and the medical school and hospital of a distinguished university. For decades Children's was housed in a turn-of-the-century edifice of red brick which had grown dingier and more cramped with every passing year. The new facility is a classy, modern, energy-efficient structure of gleaming brown, striped horizontally by brown-tinted windows, with three times the square footage of the old building and space for twice the number of intensive care beds. Its defining characteristic is a one-million-cubic-foot atrium which rises from the lobby through all nine floors and lets in the sky through a stepped glass roof. The new Children's was designed to please children and to allay their fears. To a visitor, the dominant impressions are of openness, color, and natural light.

It is light that first strikes a person coming into the hospital in the daytime. One has passed through an entrance, one is definitely inside, yet the light makes the lobby feel out-of-doors. As if drawn by pulleys, the visitor's eye climbs the nine stories to the source. Only when the light has been accounted for does one look around at ground level and begin to appreciate the lobby itself.

It's enormous. It compares favorably in size with the multipurpose lobbies of the newest hotels. Like many hotel lobbies, the lobby at Children's features live trees and a working fountain. Wooden planters, a quarry tile floor, and molded plastic benches in orange and yellow contribute further to the visitor's sense of being in a park.

But in common with few if any hotels, the Children's lobby is occupied on one side by a McDonald's restaurant. Seating is arranged in the manner of a sidewalk café. Across the floor from McDonald's is a carpeted play pit where a child who feels well enough may roughhouse with siblings in reasonable safety, or a patient in a wheelchair may picnic quietly with parents. At some remove from the pit and right next to the main entrance stands a distorting mirror that could have come straight from a fun house.

The rear of the ground floor is occupied by the hospital cafeteria. Beneath the cafeteria and lobby is a two-level parking garage. The floor below that is the province of computers, equipment, and building engineers. Short wings off the lobby house the Emergency Room, a small chapel, the day surgery unit, and a branch bank as well as the Admissions Office. Floors One through Three are for offices and outpatient clinics.

Four is given over to the operating room complex and four intensive care units. Five and Six are likewise for inpatients. On each of these floors the choicest space has been designated for the children. Head nurses' offices do not have windows at Children's, nor do many doctors' offices. But half of one wall in every patient room is a large window overlooking either the city or the center court. Each wall opposite contains a window through which patients may see into the hall. Every playroom at Children's has huge windows. Some playrooms actually jut out into the court like enclosed balconies with windows on three sides.

Halls play an important role on the first six floors at Children's. The major hallways all overlook the court through tempered glass partitions. From a distance that honors privacy, these halls afford a look into patient rooms, playrooms, clinic waiting rooms, and offices around the court from lobby to skylight. This view diminishes the mystery one usually associates with hospitals. To a parent or child immersed in private misery, the view also offers perspective. Other children are sick enough to be in here too, it says. Some may be worse off. Some are getting well. The view provides a glimpse of institutional business-as-usual which can serve as a reminder that while one's personal world may have stopped, the larger world goes on as dependably as the tides. At night someone standing in a main hallway at Children's can look up through the skylight and see stars.

The tops of the tempered glass partitions do not meet the hall ceilings. For this reason and because planners sought to isolate sick children as little as possible from life around them, sounds of the hospital reach the hallways from many parts of the building. Somewhere a baby cries. Somewhere a toddler laughs. Somewhere a mother reprimands a clinic patient springing for the elevator. "Anthony! You get back here!"

Somewhere a child demands a milkshake *and* French fries. The fall of water from the lobby fountain reaches the sixth floor. So does the aggregate of voices from the lobby—a hum of many people with many different missions, much like the buzz one hears in a shopping mall on a weekday afternoon. Together the sounds impart an air of informality and normalcy.

Varnished benches of light wood run along the low walls supporting the glass partitions. Though most units have small waiting rooms off the halls, the benches get heavier use. Patients come out to sit on them for a change of scene. Parents give themselves moments alone on the benches. Aunts and uncles and grandparents spread out on them while waiting their turn to visit a child. Doctors or social workers or the chaplain join families on the benches to talk. Secretaries relax on the benches with sandwiches or yogurt. Parents wait out surgery there.

As hours pass, or days, the groups in the halls become small cultures. Each has its own habits, its own personality, its own pitch. Cigarette stubs and ashes build up in disposable silvery ashtrays. People stretch out and nap. Group weather brightens or darkens with news. When the news is grave, the sorrow touches anyone who passes. But the halls are long. The benches are long. No one culture can dominate. Traffic continues to go by. Nurses and doctors talk to each other in ordinary voices. Usually in the hallways at Children's, and often in the units themselves, there is notable absence of hush.

Color abounds on the first six floors. In some rooms painters made big orange circles on ceilings. They stenciled big yellow C's and D's on clean and dirty linen bins. Floor experts laid red and blue paths of linoleum tiles in the halls and added red and blue baseboards to match. For clinic waiting areas Purchasing ordered child-sized tables and chairs in orange and green. The color is meant to lift heavy spirits, as is the lilt of popular music which permeates the hospital day and night so unobtrusively as to escape conscious notice.

For all the resemblance they bear in mood to the floors below, the top three floors of Children's might as well be in another city. Floors seven through nine are for research. They are not for patients but for scientists, not for parents but for technicians. On these floors decorators bothered little with color. The rooms are white. The halls are white. The linoleum is gray with white flecks. Hospital sounds seem remote. One imagines bacteria shushing each other in saucers. On three floors of odoriferous laboratories, small and large medical questions are being addressed with such aids as microscopes, scalpels, chemical solutions, government grants, dogs, cats, mice, rabbits, petri dishes, and equations that only scientists comprehend. For all this activity, the atmosphere of these floors feels quiet and white, as after heavy snow.

Hospitals for children evolved over more than a millennium from institutions devoted to the care of children who had been orphaned or abandoned.

The early Christian church established foundling asylums in the sixth century. In the next twelve hundred years facilities of this nature were erected throughout Western Europe and in Scandinavia, Russia, and Great Britain. After the Reformation many were run by the Protestant church under the name of orphanages. Historians surmise that these charities were intended purely for refuge, not for the treatment of ailments.

But children who were sick and crippled received such ministrations as could be provided by nuns and other women whose primary vocation was religion. Beginning in the seventeenth century with the formation by St. Vincent de Paul of the Sisters of Charity, foundlings in Catholic asylums were cared for by nuns trained in nursing. Also in this period links were forged between foundling homes and medical schools, particularly in Paris, In 1802 a Parisian foundling asylum called La Maison de l'Enfant Jésus was transformed into L'Hôpital des Enfants Malades, thus becoming the first hospital in the world meant solely for children.

The first in the English-speaking world was in London. The Hospital for Sick Children in Great Ormond Street began receiving patients on St. Valentine's Day in 1852. Three years and nine months later, on November 23, 1855, Children's Hospital of Philadelphia opened its doors as the first permanent institution of its kind in North America. It was chartered "for the treatment and cure of sick children." It had just twelve beds. Like its predecessor in London, CHOP was a charity, an alternative to almshouses for children who were sick and destitute and who were also between the ages of two and twelve. Prevailing wisdom held that separation from parents and the possibility of incurring fatal infections made hospitals too dangerous for infants.

In fact, at that time such institutions were deemed dangerous for persons of any age. Patients in hospitals contracted typhus and died from it. Almost all who underwent surgery died from wound infection. Most sick people were cared for by their families at home. Sick children in particular were thought to belong at home with their mothers except when desperate circumstances made hospitalization unavoidable.

But infant mortality rates in this period were alarmingly high. Seventeen percent of all Americans whose deaths were recorded in 1850 were babies. Many little ones died before they had lived five years. Always the poorest were the most vulnerable. By this time doctors had begun to realize that children were not, physiologically speaking, adults in miniature. Children's hospitals were seen as a logical setting in which to investigate the differences. For these reasons and many others, institutions such as Children's of Philadelphia were to proliferate in North America as they had begun to proliferate in Europe.

The second on this continent was Boston Children's, which opened in 1869. By the beginning of the twentieth century there were more than two dozen hospitals in this country dedicated exclusively to the care of sick and injured youngsters. Today there are 128. Seventy-six of them, including nineteen orthopedic hospitals and three burn units run by Shriners, specialize in a single area such as rehabilitation or psychiatry or cardiac care. The remaining fifty-two are general hospitals offering a full range of services to children with medical problems of every description. They do not, however, offer birthing facilities. Virtually without exception the newborns treated in children's hospitals have all been delivered elsewhere. While not every state has a full-service pediatric hospital, all major metropolitan centers have at least one. Certainly in principle, each of the fifty-two institutions attempts to be accessible to all children in the surrounding region. In fact these institutions depend for most of their patients on referrals from pediatricians and other physicians practicing in the surrounding region.

Among the fifty-two, the hospital in which Mark Price and Candy Rudolph were patients is one of the oldest and largest in the nation. Autonomous and freestanding, it also has the closest possible ties to academic medicine. Children's serves as the pediatrics department for the university medical school next door. Doctors at Children's all have teaching appointments at the university. This affiliation endows the hospital with broader responsibilities than it would have without such a connection. Roughly equal in emphasis, these responsibilities include patient care, research, and the training of young physicians. As the medical school is also recognized as one of the finest in the world, as it attracts an outstanding faculty, men and women at the forefront of their professions, state-of-the-art medicine is practiced at Children's Hospital, and the research and teaching conducted there are pursued with a zeal and a brilliance that leave no stone unturned, no pertinent question unexplored.

Most children grow up without ever being admitted to a hospital of any kind. Serious illnesses and accidents are uncommon in the pediatric population. Hospitalization is so traumatic for children that most physicians do everything possible to avoid admissions for the youngsters in their care. This explains in part why children's hospitals treat so many more patients through clinic visits than do adult hospitals, and why day surgery units in pediatric hospitals have met with such community enthusiasm. The unit at Children's functions close to capacity year-round. Though a tonsillectomy still requires an overnight stay, patients with inner ear infections, minor eye problems, hernias, small growths, or undescended testicles can have these conditions corrected in a matter of hours.

Children who do become inpatients confront hospital staff members with challenges never encountered in the care of adults. Grown-up patients receive standard doses of most medications. For children nearly every dose of nearly every medicine must be individually calculated in relation to the patient's body weight. Placement of an arterial or intravenous line in an adult takes a moment so long as the blood vessels have not been scarred by prolonged IV therapy. In an infant, whose vessels are minuscule, placement of an A-line may take as long as an hour.

Fully half the youngsters admitted to Children's each year are thirty months old or less. Those who haven't yet learned to talk can't contribute information about themselves to anyone involved in their care. Some physicians count this an advantage, believing that a young child's reporting, which might be misleading for any number of reasons, needlessly compounds the picture of the patient developed by tests, x-rays, and close observation. Other doctors find it a frustrating aspect of pediatrics that they must try to divine where a young child hurts without help from the child. Some days these doctors go home feeling a lot in common with veterinarians. Illness increases anyone's dependency on others, but while many sick adults continue to feed, wash, and entertain themselves, patients one or two years old need assistance with almost everything. Newborns, of course, are totally dependent beings.

Patient fear makes huge demands on staffs of pediatric hospitals. Adults fear hospitals too. But adults understand that hospitalization can be beneficial even when treatments are unpleasant or painful. Young children know only that they are confined in a strange place and surrounded by strangers who can exert their will by simply picking a patient up and carrying him or her to a destination dictated least of all by the patient's own wishes. In these circumstances a child's fearfulness may precede any experience of pain. Youngsters new to Children's have been known to cry while being weighed.

Patients old enough to understand why they're in the hospital are not necessarily less frightened. Actually the reverse may be true. Adolescents appreciate that serious illness or injury may have serious implications; yet while fear of implications is more sophisticated than fear of being hurt and might be supposed to supplant it, in fact the older child appears to suffer both.

Teenagers are every bit as afraid of needles as are the little kids, Children's staff members say. While the teenagers don't admit it, they show it physiologically. The veins of an adolescent about to be stuck with an IV needle may constrict and disappear in what the nurses call a classic flight reflex. Nineteen- or twenty-year-olds hyperventilate or breathe so shallowly that every so often one faints. Children's IV nurses try to forestall these reactions by leading older teens in the controlled breathing exercises familiar to many adults from Lamaze childbirth classes.

Fear is addressed in a variety of ways at Children's. Except in the Infant Intensive Care Unit and the Operating Room, nurses throughout the hospital work in street clothes. So do most other staff members, though some physicians wear lab coats as well. Tiny teddy bears or grinning Smurfs climb many of the stethoscopes hanging from staff necks.

Every effort is made to place children in rooms with their contemporaries. Every effort is made to assign a patient's day-to-day care to nurses the youngster knows and likes. Nothing is done to a patient at Children's that is not first explained to the child in terms he or she can understand. Tours such as that given Candy Rudolph preoperatively are offered all youngsters headed for surgery. Recreation therapists lead patients in doctor or nurse play simulating real procedures, sometimes with real equipment, to demystify those procedures and that equipment.

The most significant step ever taken toward reducing patient fear at Children's was the lifting of all restrictions on parental visiting. Today the benefits seem obvious. Yet historically parents were not welcome in pediatric hospitals or wards. Their presence, it was

thought, would contribute to the spread of infection and to the de-
moralization, according to someone writing in 1907, of "the discipline of the hospital and the other children." Mothers who insisted
on remaining at their sick children's bedsides were sometimes
viewed with irritation. Hospital staff members of the period, noting
that patients shed tears when their parents left, concluded that visits
from parents made children unhappy.

Antibiotics and vaccines helped invalidate one of these arguments. The others died hard. Though in the 1940s a physician in
England broke new ground by actually admitting mothers to the
hospital along with their very young children, policy at Children's at
the beginning of that decade permitted parents to visit only once a
month. By 1947 they were allowed in weekly, but only on Sundays.
A nurse who worked there at the time recalls that she and her colleagues spent the rest of the week "mopping up after kids crying."
Eventually rules were relaxed to permit visiting on Tuesdays and
Thursdays as well as Sundays and then daily from 2:00 P.M. to 6:00
P.M.

In 1951, meanwhile, the World Health Organization had published landmark studies revealing the ill effects on institutionalized
children of maternal deprivation. These findings were subsequently
buttressed by a growing literature on growth and development. In a
1958 book entitled *Young Children in Hospitals,* author James Robertson championed unrestricted visiting on the grounds that anything less did young patients a great disservice. In the early 1960s,
play therapists at Children's, along with others on staff who shared
their viewpoint, began to press for a policy of open visiting twenty-
four hours a day every day.

The proposal met resistance. Those opposed argued that open
visiting would increase traffic within quarters already cramped, that
parents might see something go wrong and sue, that the presence of
parents would interfere with the child's care.

But pressure for change continued to build. Keeping parents at
bay precisely when children needed them most was the antithesis of
good child care, proponents argued. Eventually the fears of the
children were allowed to prevail over the fears of the staff. Open
visiting became a fact of life on general floors at Children's in the
mid-1960s and in the intensive care units in 1975, though parents
are still asked to check with a nurse before entering an ICU. By

lifting the restrictions, hospital administrators in essence acknowledged that children even as patients belong first and foremost to
their mothers and fathers.

Parents are also freer now to stay overnight at Children's. In the
old hospital only mothers could stay, and only those mothers who
could afford one of the handful of private rooms available for the
purpose. This practice was common in similar institutions throughout the country well into the 1970s. These days it's unusual for a
pediatric hospital to have no overnight facilities for parents, though
shortage of space in older buildings may still preclude lodging for
fathers. The goal of such arrangements is not to run a hotel for
parents but to accord sick children easy access to the parental support now seen as vital to their emotional well-being.

Today parents may also stay at the Ronald McDonald House a
few blocks from the hospital. With funds donated or raised by the
McDonald's fast-food chain, the city's professional football team,
and families of children with cancer, a huge old residence near
Children's was converted in 1974 into a home away from home for
children needing extensive cancer therapy as outpatients and for
parents accompanying them. The idea was to provide inexpensive
and comfortable lodgings for families coming great distances for a
child's treatment. A family able to afford it pays ten dollars a night.
Poorer families pay nothing. While preference is given to children
with cancer, empty beds may be claimed by the parent of any seriously ill child when the family lives far from the hospital.

Visiting facilities within Children's remain far short of optimal.
Opened in 1974, the new building was planned before the 1950s
research bearing on the needs of children in hospitals had gained
wide acceptance. Thus policy welcomes parents much more warmly
than does the physical structure. Most "lounges" are alcoves far too
small to separate smokers from nonsmokers, to provide frazzled
adults a comfortable place to stretch out for a nap, or even to accommodate a television set. Many patient rooms at Children's are
set up for six patients. If even three cots are moved in at night for
parents, a six-bed room becomes crowded. Everybody's rest may
suffer. Parents are asked to have their cots put away by 7:30 A.M.
when the day-shift nurses begin their tasks. Showers must be taken
only during certain hours. At other times the shower rooms might
be occupied by residents for whose exclusive use they were originally intended.

For parents of children in intensive care, the visiting situation is even less ideal. On general floors there's at least one chair beside every bed. The ICUs don't have the space for more than a few per unit. Almost whenever a parent comes in, a chair must be located. Mothers or fathers who sit for long periods may feel, and may be, in the staff's way. Those wishing to spend the night cannot sleep beside their children but must go to a Parents' Hospitality Suite adjoining none of the ICUs, thereby being of no more support to their offspring than they would be across the street in a hotel room or home in their own beds.

The designs of newer pediatric hospitals have resolved many of these problems. At Children's, because the building is new yet not quite new enough, families and staff must live with its limitations in an era when parental participation in the care of sick children is deemed critical to the youngsters' welfare.

One issue currently seeking solution has to do with patients' siblings. Visitors under fourteen are not ordinarily permitted on patient floors at Children's. So what happens to little brothers and sisters when Daddy has to work, or there is no Daddy, and Mommy has to visit Joey who's sick? Baby-sitters can be hard to find. Some parents can't afford them.

Newer hospitals have day care facilities. At Children's some parents have shown themselves increasingly less willing to leave young family members at home. Healthy siblings come along with Mommy and hide out in bathrooms or stairwells. Clearly this arrangement is ideal for no one. Staff is all too well aware how much stress is placed upon a family when parents feel torn for long periods between the child in the hospital and the siblings at home. An administrator at Children's has been moved to wonder whether whole families might one day be admitted to the hospital with a sick child, much as happens informally in tribal societies of the Third World.

Beyond the factors of size, age, and fear that distinguish young people as patients, hospitalized children differ from adults in one other extremely important respect. They are growing and developing. Day by day, week by week, they are working their way toward grown-up, independent lives. Serious illness or injury can slow the process. A cardinal principle at Children's is that to whatever extent is possible under the circumstances, growth and development must continue while a child is hospitalized. Circumstances sometimes don't allow very much. But staff works hard to assure that at least those youngsters are not discharged having lost ground at Children's.

This means time, and it means teamwork. It means not only doctors and nurses but specialists in nutrition, in play, physical, occupational, and speech therapy, and in social work. A fundamental goal of social workers at Children's is to keep a family operating as a unit during the transition in their lives that is the child's hospitalization and to help the family identify resources within and without that will help members meet their own needs and those of the child. Workers see any number of parents having little or no sense of how growth and development should normally proceed. Many are just teenagers themselves. The social workers look for ways of enabling these parents to learn more about their children and about their own role in a child's progress in and out of the hospital.

Therapists in pediatric hospitals have a somewhat broader role than do their counterparts in adult hospitals. In the latter setting, an occupational therapist, for example, is primarily concerned with helping patients return to a state of function they had previously enjoyed: to walk, to feed and dress themselves, to work, to run homes, to utilize leisure. The OTs at Children's have this responsibility and one other: to teach routine functions of living to people too young ever to have learned them.

Considering all that is and must be done for patients in pediatric hospitals, it is not surprising that many more people are required to take care of them than are needed for hospitalized adults. The average community hospital has 2.5 staff members per patient bed. Institutions that devote themselves exclusively to the care of sick children have at least twice as many employees as do community hospitals, which largely explains why the cost of being a patient in a children's hospital is just about twice as high.

Pediatricians in communities throughout the land treat a population of youngsters who are all or almost all essentially healthy. A third to half of these doctors' time is spent on well babies. The time remaining goes to the treatment of colds, rashes, ear and upper respiratory infections, and minor traumas in children who, with occasional exceptions, have nothing else wrong with them. Medically speaking, the practice of community pediatrics is so routine that practitioners who fail to become interested or involved in their patients' growth and development may get bored "sticking kids in the bottom all day," as one doctor puts it, and turn to other work. A layperson could sit in a pediatrician's office for weeks on end and see nothing more upsetting than a broken leg or a nasty cut.

One could not sit long at Children's Hospital.

One can rarely walk through the lobby at Children's without being stopped in one's tracks figuratively if not literally by children to whom fate has been breathtakingly cruel.

A child with both legs withered and braced swings across the floor on crutches. A pale child with a healing incision in the back of her shaved scalp stares as if dreaming from the wheelchair being pushed slowly around the court by her mother. In a wheelchair next to a table at McDonald's a child slumps, drooling, and attempts to control his spasticity long enough to get pieces of a hamburger into his mouth. On a litter near the play pit lies a child with both legs casted. He is observed by a child whose hair has vanished from chemotherapy.

Children's Hospital offers such youngsters a whole array of experts in the care of sick children—not just doctors who have made international reputations in pediatric medicine, as many have, but also nurses, social workers, nutritionists, and therapists of all kinds who have specialized in work with children and who together with the doctors continue to refine their skills and their professional judgment as their experience with children deepens and broadens daily.

This in fact is a primary function served by pediatric hospitals. By concentrating resources in one facility, they attract patients in numbers great enough that lessons may be drawn from them which in turn improve the resources for the benefit of patients to follow. From a technical standpoint the care given in these institutions is the best available to children anywhere in the world. Patients at a place like Children's get the benefits of the latest research months or years before the innovations based on research findings become accepted practice. Treatment is pursued aggressively and even doggedly as the experts exhaust their ingenuity in the effort to salvage life or limb.

To a considerable extent the aggressiveness of these hospitals is a natural outgrowth of their commitment to research and physician education. Staff tries hard to learn from each patient whatever that patient can teach. This does not mean that patients are looked upon merely as guinea pigs. They are admitted for treatment. They get the best treatment the experts know how to give them.

But when known therapies fail, the experts try others. Though these approaches are based on educated guesswork, not pulled from hats, the chances of their being successful may sometimes be slim. Experimental treatment is often less likely to solve a particular problem in a particular patient than to yield information that may benefit patients down the line. Of course the experts are glad when a particular child is helped by the therapy. If the child is not helped, science gains nonetheless.

"There's no doubt," according to a man once president of Children's Hospital, "that in a place like this, certain things would be done which would not be done elsewhere. Certain efforts would be made which would not be made elsewhere. Because how else do you advance medical knowledge? You can't do it in the abstract."

Almost certainly the aggressiveness is also inspired in part by the patients themselves. Few human beings are more defenseless or more guileless than a child; no human being has more to lose or to gain. As one physician puts it, "We're playing at the high-stakes table." The temptation to go all out for a child is exceedingly strong among staff members at Children's, as is the reluctance to give up on a child. Children are not supposed to die. The whole world knows that.

There are people in and out of Children's Hospital who believe that this particular institution is even more aggressive than others of its kind. In the words of a senior neurosurgical resident working with Guillermo Perez at the time of Candy Rudolph's surgery, "They're very gung-ho at Children's. I haven't worked in another hospital that has as much of a gung-ho attitude as they do here. About anything—malignant brain tumors, terrible cancers, bad injuries, you name it. It's just a kind of personality of the hospital that everything is done that can possibly be done until either the child is not salvageable anymore or it becomes clear that what you're doing is not prolonging a good quality of life."

Or, as one nurse administrator puts it to nurses starting orientation at Children's, "We try till the bitter end for most patients. If you're uncomfortable with that, you don't want to work here."

Those who believe Children's to be unusual in this regard tend to believe also that the difference owes much to the philosophy of Dr. Pierce Lynd. A devout Christian with a fundamentalist creed, Lynd retired from Children's in the early 1980s after serving there as surgeon in chief for thirty-five years. He was a pioneer in pediatric surgery and a virtuoso at the operating table with worldwide stature in his field. As time passed, and especially after the accidental death at twenty of a son, Lynd had become an increasingly passionate advocate of pro-life principles.

How much he actually shaped institutional philosophy can only be conjectured. Some say that while the surgeon in chief may well have influenced other surgeons, his views had limited impact outside that realm. But he was a potent personality in an important position, and he was there a long time. That the philosophy of treatment at Children's is consistent with Lynd's own philosophy is beyond dispute.

Whatever the reasons for it, the effects of the aggressive posture at Children's can be most sobering. Some patients are saved to lead severely compromised lives. A number of them become regular visitors to the hospital's Rehabilitation Department. There multidisciplinary teams attempt to help them and their families cope with medical, social, and psychological problems so enormous as to seem nearly overwhelming sometimes even to the professionals. Other pediatric hospitals with aspirations similar to those at Children's are reaping similar harvests, according to the Children's rehab director, and he adds, sadly, "These great institutions are both monsters and white hopes."

A colleague elaborates, anesthesiologist and intensive care specialist Peter Crossin. When no one else wanted to, Crossin assumed responsibility at Children's for the care of youngsters alive thanks to modern technology who, technology notwithstanding, are so far unable to breathe in and out on their own. "Many moving, exciting things are going on in this building," Crossin says with pride, yet he frowns as he says it. "Emotions are high. First-class clinical physiology is being practiced here. But everybody pays a price for being on the cutting edge."

There are those who feel that the price is too high, that aggressiveness is carried to extremes at Children's Hospital, that prodigious efforts are being exerted on behalf of patients better left in nature's hands.

Mostly one hears these criticisms from residents and others on staff temporarily. Permanent staff members who find themselves strongly opposed to the general philosophy tend to move on. One who did had been a well-respected head nurse in the unit for which Peter Crossin was medical director. Among her several reasons for resigning, the nurse had developed grave reservations about the "extreme interventions" undertaken to prolong life in certain cases, feeling that in their attempts to give the best medical care, the best nursing care, the best social work they were capable of, the experts at Children's tended to get caught up in pride, in technical achievement, and to forget the larger implications of that achievement for the children themselves.

An informed outsider has observed of this institution that its philosophy of going flat out for all but the most hopeless patients makes Children's in some ways "a harsh place." The observer is a veteran local newspaper journalist who has won a dozen national awards for medical reporting and who believes it would be "criminal" if every hospital in America took the approach espoused at Children's.

Yet he supports that approach. Though it galls him to think some youngsters might be suffering because of one man's religious beliefs, the reporter can name doctors at Children's with views similar to Pierce Lynd's grounded not in religion but in medicine, a discipline which exists, after all, to save life, and he points out that extending the boundaries of medical knowledge involves a transition period during which patients unavoidably suffer. He believes that the price of medical progress must be paid—not everywhere, but somewhere.

"I personally feel that there ought to be hospitals where kids are pushed to the breaking point," the journalist says. "In a country this size, perhaps twelve." He is referring to what he calls centers of excellence, Children's among them, institutions in which the medicine practiced is topnotch and the lessons of experience are scrupulously recorded and distilled. The crime, the reporter observes, would be to push the kids without drawing the lessons.

Society's need for such information, of course, may diverge from the needs of an individual sick child. The wishes of individual parents will not always coincide with the mandate of an institution invested heavily in research. Children's Hospital may not be ideal for every patient or every situation.

Yet patients are cured at Children's who once might have died, or who might even today have died in another hospital. Youngsters with terrible diseases or massive injuries or birth defects that could easily kill them get better at Children's. Untold numbers of these youngsters get much better. Evidence can be found in classrooms, on playgrounds and athletic fields, at school dances, in church choirs, on bicycles, trampolines, skateboards, ski slopes, in the driver's seats of family cars, at the altar, in the delivery room, in every walk of life. Kids arrive at Children's on stretchers and leave skipping. They come in comatose and go home to squabble with their siblings over toys. Infants brought in with gross deformities are discharged with neat scars and excellent prospects. There are miracles. Not every child improves who is treated, but the patient who cannot be cured at Children's is most unlikely to be cured anywhere else.

"This is the hospital of last resort, really," says a surgeon who has worked there for more than a quarter of a century. "The child who comes here has reached the pinnacle. Children who come to this institution have reached a place from which there is nowhere else to go."

Not every sick child can be cured. But if a child has a chance in the world to get well, he or she will be given that chance at Children's Hospital.

Monday, December 3

At 6:30 A.M. Dr. Daniel Earnshaw left his house by the back door and walked in virtual darkness to the garage. He lived with his wife in a neighborhood of comfortable old stone dwellings at the edge of the city. On nice mornings he took a train to work. His constitution appreciated the walk from the station to the hospital. Father of two grown daughters, Earnshaw was fifty-six and fit, a tall, handsome man with light brown skin and thick hair turning dark-and-light silver.

He backed his car down the long driveway and moments later turned east onto a major thoroughfare. Mist-fine rain covered his windshield. Earnshaw switched on the wipers, the heat, his classical music station. He drove toward Children's thinking about what had happened to Mark Price over the weekend and recalling all too clearly what had happened to his last patient who had developed a spontaneous pneumothorax.

The case had been unusual in several respects. For one thing, though cystic fibrosis almost always affects white children, Perry Smith was black.

His lung collapse in itself had been unusual. Until past the middle of this century, pneumothorax was all but unheard of in cystic fibrosis patients. The children almost never lived long enough to develop that particular complication. Even now it remains rather rare. In twenty-three years of treating the disease, Earnshaw had seen fewer than half a dozen cases.

Sooner or later all but one of these children had responded to chest tube therapy. Perry had not. His lung had failed to stay up even after a second chest tube had been inserted.

A healthy person in this situation is sent to the operating room for a pleural abrasion. Surgeons open the person's chest and rub the outer surface of the lung and the inner surface of the chest wall with gauze pads. This irritation causes the tissues to mount an inflammatory reaction. Postoperatively, while a chest tube attached to suction keeps the lung fully expanded and in direct contact with the chest wall, the inflamed surfaces recover by healing into a scar which fuses them, a process called pleurodesis. The operation solves the immediate problem and almost always prevents further lung collapse.

But pleural abrasion must be done under general anesthesia, which can kill a patient with bad lungs. Though Daniel Earnshaw knew of respected doctors in his field who believed the risks worth taking in such circumstances, he himself had been unwilling to take them with Perry.

Yet he knew he had to do something. CF children have little reserve to spare for complications of any kind. The chief complication of spontaneous pneumothorax is recurrence. While one lung collapse may not make a cystic much sicker, recurrent pneumothorax debilitates these children and accelerates their downhill course. This had happened with Perry Smith. His condition had worsened and begun to sabotage his will to fight.

So Earnshaw had turned to the literature on sclerosing agents, a treatment similar in principle to surgery but much less hazardous. Inflammation was induced by an irritant blown or poured down the chest tube. Since no one knew exactly how long scarring took in these cases, the procedure was considered useless as a short-term remedy but promising as a preventive.

Sclerosing agents are used most commonly in cancer patients to forestall the accumulation of fluid that may accompany chest or lung malignancies. Their use with pneumothorax was reported in medical literature as early as 1939. In subsequent years, individual physicians had experimented with a variety of agents and eventually abandoned all of them. Some caused too little scarring, some too much, and some were toxic, causing systemic reactions that were occasionally severe.

However, when spontaneous pneumothorax began to develop with increasing frequency in CF children, their doctors had resorted in desperation to a number of sclerosing agents that hadn't been tried before. By the late 1970s, at least half a dozen papers had been published on these experiments. No consensus had emerged. But reviewing these papers for direction in the predicament of Perry Smith, Earnshaw had felt bound to consider tetracycline, an antibiotic that had been tried here and there and was said to produce good scarring in some instances without triggering adverse systemic reactions.

However, Earnshaw had heard at CF meetings that tetracycline used in this fashion was exceedingly painful to the patient.

For this reason he had finally rejected tetracycline for Perry Smith. Or, as Earnshaw thought of it now, he had chickened out. He had not even given Perry the option.

And the boy had died. Of course he would have died anyway. But he had died *then* of giving up.

Earnshaw had made himself a promise when Perry died. He had promised himself that the next time he had a patient who blew a lung, he would muster his courage.

He was on the expressway now. Sleet came against the windshield like mush. He was grateful for the warmth inside the car, for the warmth of Bach on harpsichord. Earnshaw played fiddle in some of his spare time. Yesterday he had made music with friends who also gathered annually in January to celebrate Mozart's birthday. On Saturday he and his wife had puttered all day in the kitchen. They had been happily married some thirty years. These days she divided her professional energies between the university museum and the city's black cultural museum, where she was assistant to the curator.

Earnshaw headed the Division of Respiratory Disease at Children's. Of his chronic patients, the largest group by far was the hundred or so children who came to the hospital to be treated for cystic fibrosis. Earnshaw and Bruce Griffin took care of these patients in tandem, to some extent. Certain children and parents preferred to see the older, taller doctor with the gray hair. Others gravitated more naturally toward Earnshaw's bearded associate, who was twenty years younger and a passionate skier and birdwatcher. Each had other responsibilities. But whenever a cystic was hospitalized, both doctors saw that patient on rounds, though not necessarily every day.

Daniel Earnshaw had become a doctor intending to follow in his father's footsteps. Sole surviving offspring of a railroad company messenger and his wife, Earnshaw's father had received the best education his parents could give him that segregation would allow and had become a doctor, a general practitioner with a special interest in obstetrics. He had set up a private practice in his own neighborhood. Earnshaw had graduated from an Ivy League medical school determined to become a community physician like his father, though with a different specialty.

His own particular interest was—still was—tuberculosis. Along with general pediatrics, he had hoped to develop a small TB service. Streptomycin had eviscerated this plan. At the time it was issued, Earnshaw was a first-year intern at Harlem Hospital in New York City. In his first months at Harlem, the TB wards had been full to overflowing. Patients had lain on cots and beds in the hallways. Streptomycin had cleared out the hallways within a year. Several years later, just as Earnshaw was finishing his training, another drug had come out, isoniazid, which was even better for treating TB than streptomycin. Wards and sanatoriums had begun closing all over the country.

With his residency and his military obligation behind him, Daniel Earnshaw had become his father's first associate. He had practiced community pediatrics for eleven years and found in it many rewards. But as time passed, he had grown increasingly restless with the repetition of problems and too busy to manage without help. Yet he'd had reservations about a pediatrics partnership. He'd been ripe, then, when a friend from med school days, knowing of Earnshaw's interest in chest disorders, had invited him to come to Children's Hospital to take care of children with cystic fibrosis. It had never occurred to Daniel Earnshaw that he might be working in CF for the remainder of his professional life.

"I'm shifting from a disease for which the answer has been found to a disease for which the answer is still being sought but will ultimately come along," he would tell parents in his early months at Children's. Twenty-three years later the critical clue remained elusive.

Earnshaw drove the last few blocks to the hospital resolved to give Mark Price the chance he had failed to give Perry Smith. This morning he would call Neil Martinson, a cardiothoracic surgeon at Children's who not only was an expert on lungs and lung problems but also, as it happened, was studying the effectiveness of tetracycline as a sclerosing agent in rabbits with pneumothorax. Martinson would surely have thoughts on the best way to proceed with Mark.

Earnshaw did not feel greatly worried about the pneumothorax. Mark was a long way from being as sick as Perry Smith had been. Mark would have tetracycline right away, before he got into the kind of trouble Perry had gotten into, and he'd be okay for a good while longer. In recent years, as treatment had improved, Earnshaw had realized that more and more his goal with the CF children was to get them through high school. Despite what had happened over the weekend, doubts about Mark's graduating had not entered the doctor's mind.

He eased his car down a steep spiral ramp into the vast, dim shelter of the hospital's underground garage. Another Monday. Another problem. Throughout his long career at Children's, Earnshaw had been asked by any number of people how he tolerated his job. Sometimes he replied that he didn't tolerate it very well. In fact, he had left it once to work as health director for the city school system. One factor in that decision had been a large population of aging cystics who were about to start dying. The school job had offered an escape from a long season of trauma. He had taken it as a change, fully intending to return to Children's within five years. He had returned in four to find that some of the children had waited for him.

He tolerated his job by defining it carefully. Cure was out of the question, so cure was not the aim. Rather Earnshaw strove to look after his patients as best he could for as long as they lived. As best he could, he orchestrated good deaths for them so that they and their families got something positive out of the experience and did not fall apart. He viewed the children's lives as poems. A poem could be short or long. Its merit did not correlate with its length. Virtually always, the life of a child with cystic fibrosis was a short poem. Daniel Earnshaw saw his role as helping to make that short poem work.

Ø

9:45 A.M. Bathed in light on a narrow, padded stainless-steel table in the center of Operating Room 10, Candy Rudolph lay ready for surgery. From her upper lip down she was covered by green cotton drapes. All that showed of her body was a small patch of chest below the right nipple. Most of her hair had been shaved from her head. Only a long fringe around the back of her neck had been spared. Across the top of her head could now be seen the thick band of old scar. Hidden by the drapes were the endotracheal tube connecting Candy to a respirator, the catheter draining her bladder, and half a dozen monitoring devices including a blue denim blood pressure cuff printed colorfully with Raggedy Anns. Deep sleep had brought sweet relaxation to the odd little face.

Around her in the big, beige-walled room, adults in gowns and masks and caps of green made final preparations. One was anesthesiology resident Susan Carlson, who had come in at the crack of dawn to begin the long process of setting up and checking out equipment. Carlson felt tense. Craniofacial cases make rigorous demands on anesthesiologists. Because the respirator connections are beneath the drapes, and because the drapes are constantly being rustled by the surgeons, the doctor may have difficulty distinguishing the patient's breath sounds from the surrounding hubbub. If a monitor fails, the oxygen supply can actually disconnect accidentally without the anesthesiologist realizing it until the patient is in cardiac arrest. Strict concentration is required.

Furthermore, the scalp and face are well supplied with blood through countless tiny vessels that during this kind of operation ooze for hours. Blood loss is subtle in these cases. The stuff builds up on sponges. It drips onto the floor. Pressure drops steadily and must be watched very closely, especially in a child, whose total blood volume is much less than an adult's and who can be fine one minute and the next have no blood pressure whatsoever. Except for a brief lunch break, when she would be spelled by a colleague, Susan Carlson anticipated no tranquil moments until she had delivered Candy Rudolph safely to the Acute Intensive Care Unit.

OR nurse Constance Mitchell stood at a small draped cart double-checking all the instruments she had laid out earlier in the order in which they were likely to be used. The basic set for craniofacial procedures at Children's numbers 125 pieces. Included in it are scalpels, skin hooks, saws, drills, brain retractors, plastic scissors, and holders for needles and wires. All are of standard size except the retractors, called Tessiers. These depend on the size of the child. In only two other kinds of surgery is the instrumentation as complicated: open-heart cases and the insertion of Harrington rods into youngsters with severe curvature of the spine.

Mitch was far too experienced to feel tense going into an operation. She had worked at Children's for twenty-seven years, seventeen of them in the OR. Assigned to assist Paul Tessier when he'd come to demonstrate his techniques in 1972, Mitch now scrubbed for nearly every craniofacial case done at Children's and was highly respected by Rolfe Lorimer for her dedication and steadiness. She found these procedures fascinating. The only time she became anxious during the surgery was when the doctors were working around the brain. Sometimes the residents would lean a little too hard on the retractors. Mitch would have to remind them to lighten up.

Also in Operating Room 10 were two young surgeons who would be assisting Rolfe Lorimer. Kevin McCoy was a dapper Canadian who had recently finished plastic surgery training in British Columbia and was doing a six-month fellowship with Lorimer to learn more about craniofacial procedures. Dean Whitehill was a dimpled, broad-shouldered Kansan serving this year as the university's chief resident in plastic surgery. While McCoy worked side by side with Lorimer on Candy's head, Whitehill would harvest the ribs to be used in the reconstruction.

As nurses put gloves on his two assistants, Lorimer himself, scrubbed and eager to get going, took a last look at photographs of Candy he had spread out on a table. For this kind of surgery, photographs are far more important than x-rays. The world does not see a face as an x-ray machine sees it. Lorimer glanced at the photos for the freshest possible reminder of Candy's face in an upright position. Contours change subtly when the patient is lying down.

At three minutes of ten, Rolfe Lorimer stepped to the operating table. He focused the big blue lights above his head. The sounds in the room were soft—the whir of an air filter, the low voice of a visiting plastic surgeon commenting into a tiny tape recorder—but the atmosphere had tightened noticeably.

As Dean Whitehill swabbed the exposed patch of Candy's chest with a brown antiseptic called Betadine, Lorimer painted her scalp with the same substance and attached a blue towel to the back of her head with sutures. He began to shoot epinephrine into her cheeks and the flesh along the incision line to help control bleeding, jabbing until the patient's head was blanched and bumpy from the fluid. He cleaned off the bloody rivulets with a gauze pad.

As Whitehill began his incision in Candy's chest, Mitch handed Lorimer a scalpel. For the briefest moment he held it poised. He'd be cutting along the scar. To make a new incision would compromise the blood supply between that cut and the old one. He examined the scar. In earlier days Lorimer had felt considerable tension at the beginning of a craniofacial case. He still felt some, though not nearly as much. He cut into Candy's head.

Her bare skull parted slightly behind the knife. Kevin McCoy applied an electrocoagulator to severed vessels and suctioned out the blood. Often surgeons can forestall heavy bleeding in these cases by running a line of stitches along either side of the incision line before the incision is made. Because Candy's skull had never closed, Lorimer didn't want to risk inserting needles until he could see where they were going. With the knife he had had no choice. As soon as the scalp had been opened ear to ear, however, he and McCoy working together put a suture line along the edge of each flap of flesh, front and back. Eight minutes into the operation the towel attached to the back of Candy's head was soaked dark from blood.

Lorimer began to peel the face from the bone. He used blunt

instruments resembling miniature garden tools. Usually the stripping phase of reconstructive surgery serves as a kind of warm-up
exercise which relieves the surgeon's tension. In this case, as anticipated, scarring hampered the separation of flesh from bony tissue.
Albeit with exceeding care, Lorimer had to dig and push hard. He
had not anticipated the gap in the child's cranium to be as wide or
long as it was. Between the bones split twice in Candy's infancy,
blood-smeared scar tissue glistened broad as a hair ribbon, its
patchiness exposing here and there the dura, the tough gray-white
covering of the brain.

This initial phase of the operation was to take Lorimer almost
exactly an hour. Toward the end of that period, working to separate the tissue above Candy's left ear from the dura directly beneath
it, the surgeon saw the tip of his implement washed clean by a small
amount of clear cerebrospinal fluid, the brain's lubricant. The two
surfaces had bonded so tightly that in pulling up flesh, Lorimer had
put a small tear in the membrane. This almost never happens in
virgin cases. When scarring is present, however, dural tears are not
uncommon. Potentially a source of infection, they must be repaired
as they occur, though the most minuscule may not be obvious and
may repair themselves spontaneously. Lorimer closed the tear in
Candy's dura with a suture.

Dean Whitehill announced that he had taken sections from three
of Candy's ribs and was starting to close the incision. By now
Lorimer had freed from the patient's cranium all the flesh from the
top of her head to her nose. When he had loosened on either side
of the jaw the muscles that become noticeable when the teeth are
clenched, he peeled back the flap of the upper face to the top of the
eyes and laid it over the drape covering the lower face, revealing the
contours of the skull. The back of the flap was whitish, spotted
darkly in places like the deeps of a stream, and bloody. The child's
face had disappeared.

In a sense the child had disappeared. Even the fringe of hair at
the back of her head was now concealed by bloody towels. All that
met the surgeon's eye was a surgical problem waiting to be solved.
Only Susan Carlson could actually bear witness to the presence of a
child in Operating Room 10. From where she sat, the anesthesiologist could see beneath a drape a little girl's hand.

"Okay," Lorimer said to the circulating nurse standing near him. "Tell Dr. Perez we're ready for him anytime he's ready for us."

Some minutes later, with a hand drill very similar to those used centuries earlier by Incas, Mayans, and Egyptians for exactly the same purpose, neurosurgeon Guillermo Perez bored a hole half an inch wide into Candy Rudolph's skull.

He stopped just short of the dura. Bone shavings pale as grated Parmesan built up around the drill bit. In no time Perez had added three more holes: the corners of a rectangular plug approximately two inches wide by three inches long that the neurosurgeon would eventually remove from the patient's upper forehead.

This task was to take him a full hour. Ordinarily a plug once isolated with drill and saw can simply be lifted off the dura. In Candy's case, because of the two previous craniectomies, the bone stuck to the membrane in peaks and valleys. To avoid tears in the dura, the plate had to be extricated with painstaking care. Perez, a wavy-haired and humorous Argentinian who preferred to work like a madman, as he put it, controlled his impatience by kibitzing.

"Boy, you've got a thick skull here.

"The main principle of neurosurgery is to concentrate the glory and divide the blame.

"The problem is that this vein under here accounts for twenty percent of the blood supply to the heart, so if we hit it, we're going to say, 'Oh, my.'

"No, I'm talking to myself, I'm sorry. I have a strong tendency to do that, since I'm the only one who listens.

"Now is the time to start complaining that I should have been a dentist.

"That's better. Or, as we say in neurosurgical circles, more better."

At last the plug came free. Perez handed it to Mitch, who put it in a small basin of Betadine next to another small basin of Betadine containing the three lengths of rib. Next the neurosurgeon covered the rectangle of exposed dura with several layers of gauze made from a synthetic material that would absorb blood without sticking. The gauze would also help protect the membrane. Until surgery was over, the patient would continue to receive a drug that would rid her body of excess fluid. This would shrink her brain slightly and make room within her cranium for the plastic surgeon's tools.

Having recharged his energies with a sandwich in a small lounge within the OR complex, Rolfe Lorimer was standing by now in Operating Room 10, freshly scrubbed and gowned. Perez stepped back from the table. "Okay, doctor," he said dryly, "the brain is very nicely retracted. Now if you can only do the operation, we can all go home."

Lorimer glanced around the operating field, over at the small cart where the ribs and plug lay soaking, then at Mitch. "Guillermo didn't save any bone dust? We need all we can get."

For answer she handed him an instrument. He scooped up tiny heaps of blood-soaked particles from the towels and the surface of Candy's skull and deposited them in a small stainless cup which Mitch held out to him. Bone fragments are useful in all craniofacial procedures. Along with pieces of rib, they can be laid into gaps resulting from the surgery and will eventually unite to bridge those gaps. They were especially precious today because Lorimer hoped to fill in as well at least part of the breach left from Candy's earlier surgeries.

The crux of the operation would take place over the next two hours and ten minutes. This was the period in which Lorimer would execute his careful plans as best he could given the anatomical realities now apparent. Even without contingencies this phase of the operation would be highly demanding of the surgeon's concentration. In dismantling existing structures he would work around the child's brain and eyes with tools that could kill, blind, or maim her. Reassembling the face would require aesthetic judgment as well as technical skill. No guidelines exist that tell a plastic surgeon how high to build cheekbones.

"How do you know how far to advance the forehead?" Lorimer had asked Paul Tessier back at the beginning, to which the master had replied, "I just know." Lacking Tessier's experience, the young surgeon had delved into physical anthropology, trying to pin down the elements that characterize a normal human face. He had come up with some useful principles about the relationships of facial features and a reminder that principles have limitations. Going by measurements, the eyes of Jacqueline Kennedy Onassis are too widely set, yet who would deny her beauty? Though mindful of ideal relationships when reconstructing a face, Lorimer nonetheless had to make decisions appropriate to individual circumstances. The final touches were always hard: the details people would see.

He had enough experience now to feel confident that he could dig out of just about any hole in which he might find himself as he began the most critical part of a craniofacial procedure. But it was not a time for the small talk he could enjoy while stripping tissue. For most of the two hours and ten minutes in which he strove to make Candy Rudolph look more normal, Rolfe Lorimer went about the job in silence.

He worked hardest and longest on the forehead advancement. As Kevin McCoy held the brain out of the way with flat stainless retractors and occasionally suctioned, as Mitch irrigated with dilute Betadine, Lorimer first applied a high-powered saw which sent up clouds of bone dust as it tore through Candy's skull and then a slender wedge. This he positioned against the cranium from the inside and tapped with a hammer. Now and again he tapped with real force. The patient's head jerked with each blow. Bits of bone flew onto the bloody flap that was the back of Candy's upper face. Her whole skull was bloody. By the time Lorimer had managed to cut loose the ridge he intended to move, his gown sleeves were heavily flecked to the elbow with blood and Betadine.

He had trouble with the placement of the ridge. It was not symmetrical, for one thing. The left edge was slightly misshapen, meaning that Lorimer could not get a smooth plane on the left temple. In an infant he could simply have bent the bone into a normal curve. Older bones break when bent.

The other problem was that because the patient's skull had long since been divided ear to ear, it did not prove a particularly stable foundation for the piece Lorimer had moved forward. The first time he tried anchoring ridge to skull using wires and a length of rib as a strut, the ridge sagged on the left side like eyeglasses slipping down a nose. Lorimer did finally succeed in getting the ridge to stay put, but he would have felt greater security about the forehead advancement had the patient's skull been intact.

He was forced to make two further compromises before he was through. Because the split in Candy's cranium went so far down her head on either side, he was unable to realign her ears. He had nothing solid to attach them to. Because the split was wide as well as long, he was able to fill in very little of it. He needed most of his leftover bone fragments for the spaces he himself had left in Candy's cranium.

The tasks remaining went without a hitch. Using fine wires, he produced an upward tilt to the outer corners of the patient's eyes and brought the inner corners closer together. He also rounded Candy's cheeks with rib grafts fashioned by Kevin McCoy, each a short segment of rib split lengthwise with a shorter segment affixed on top of it to provide a tapering effect. At each step Lorimer overcorrected by a few millimeters to compensate for the inevitable slippage when tissue settled.

"Okay," Lorimer said finally, four hours and eight minutes into the operation, "let me have a scalpel."

Swiftly he began to remove the sutures put in at the beginning to hinder blood flow along the edges of the incision. Blood ran onto Lorimer's gloves. He tried the upper face briefly over the structures he had just modified, then folded it back again while he fiddled with a rib graft.

"You'd better be careful when you close this, Kevin," Lorimer warned. "The forehead's out so far that you'll really have to pull to make the edges of the incision meet. Okay, are we ready?"

He took a few seconds to survey the whole of his handiwork. Seeing nothing left undone, he lifted the face flap in both hands, fitted it over its new framework, smoothed it out quickly, pulled it tight with effort, and reattached it to the rear flap with a single stitch at the top of the head.

Given the difficulties posed by the patient's abnormal anatomy, the surgeon felt generally satisfied with the way the operation had gone. But the aesthete's eye went straight for the imperfections. Rolfe Lorimer touched the slight protrusion at the child's left temple. "That's the end of that bone," he mused, "which we can't do anything about. We'll just have to leave it." He consoled himself that Candy's bangs would cover the bump.

Those around Lorimer saw the bump in context. Before them lay a child who had entered the operating room with bulging eyes and a flattened midface marked by features that seemed afraid to venture forth and be seen. It some ways this child now looked much worse. Her whole crown was shorn. Across it was a gaping, bleeding slash. The hair at the back of the patient's neck was matted and black with blood. Her lips and face were very pale. The skin was stained yellow from Betadine and patched with the dark crust of dried blood. By the time the blood and Betadine were cleaned off, the swelling would begin. The forces of healing are unpredictable and slow. A year would pass before Candy Rudolph's new face came into its own. More surgery would be necessary to advance her upper jaw.

But the improvement was undeniable. The little girl's eyes snuggled into their sockets as if they had never bulged. The child now had full cheeks, a bridge at the top of her nose, and an appropriately prominent forehead. Though very subtly, the lift of her eyes at the outer corners suggested a person with reason to smile.

"It's beautiful," breathed an older nurse who had come into Operating Room 10 to get an update for the patient's mother and father. "Boy, that forehead is beautiful!"

Rolfe Lorimer stepped away from the table at 2:24 P.M. He pulled off his gloves. After dialing his secretary and dictating his report on the operation, he removed his gown and hurried off in his scrub suit to find Candy Rudolph's parents.

Ø

Upstairs on Adolescent, Mark read aloud from the drug index Kate had brought him. The chest tube showing below his pajama top was continuing to drain blood-tinged fluid into the clear bulb of the suction device that dangled from his mattress.

"'Codeine. A narcotic, analgesic, and antitussive . . .' What does that mean?"

"Anti-cough," Kate said. She was tending Mark's roommate, a youngster who had fallen headfirst out of a tree. The boy was probably going to live, but no one knew when or if he'd come out of his coma. In essence Mark had the room to himself.

"Oh, yeah. 'A narcotic . . .'" He grinned. "Like percussion would be pro-cough!"

"That's us," Ellen said from the armchair at his bedside. "Pro-cough!"

"Geez, Mom, I always thought you were antitussive."

"Well, Mark, how little you've learned about your mother in fifteen years!"

His laugh was a short, soft line of rapid-fire dashes, the cute giggle of a much younger boy. A way to conserve air.

"'A narcotic, analgesic, and antitussive which resembles morphine pharmacol . . . phar-ma-col-ogically but with milder actions,
less sedation . . .'"

He had asked for the drug index because he had never taken
codeine before. His desire to learn all about his new medicine was
reassuring to Kate, who saw Mark today as a different person from
the frightened youngster who had huddled against her on Saturday
night. When feeling comfortable, he was actually in good spirits.

He was getting codeine and Tylenol once or twice a shift. When
the drugs wore off, he had pain which coughing made sharp. Kate
had taught his mother how to splint his chest with a pillow when he
coughed to reduce the pull on sore tissue. Percussion also hurt him.
The doctors had let him skip it yesterday, but it was critical to his
lung hygiene and had been resumed. Though his lung was ninety
percent reexpanded, Mark still had decreased breath sounds on
that side. On Sunday he had used oxygen a few times. His appetite
today was only fair. He couldn't wait to get the chest tube out so he
could get up and move around.

He was more himself, and yet in one very important way he was
not himself: he did not want his mother out of his sight. On all his
other admissions he had been very independent of everyone. Now
his mother could not go down the hall for a cigarette without Mark
sending somebody after her to find out where she was and when
she would be back. Until the pneumothorax, Ellen had never spent
a single night at Children's. Now Mark had made it clear that he
wanted her to stay. Bob would be coming this evening to bring her
some fresh clothes.

Mark finished the ice cream on his supper tray and began to
cough. Anyone who has observed it does not soon forget the sound
or sight of a cystic child coughing. Like a smoker's cough, the sound
is loose and junky. But a CF cough is more wrenching, and it goes
on and on. The child's whole body is seized by paroxysms for minutes at a time. Or perhaps the coughing just seems overpowering
because the children are so thin. The rhythm is that of a weak automobile battery turning over and over and over. The coughing
grows more frequent as the disease progresses. Of course the kids
want to cough. They work hard at bringing up mucus. Often the
effort causes gagging. Mark could not receive percussion after a

meal now because too often it made him vomit what he had eaten. The pain of coughing with the chest tube in brought tears to his eyes.

He spit into his stainless-steel sputum basin. The blob was greenish-tan, malodorous, and streaked with blood, a sign of broken vessels in his lungs. He knew from the hemoptysis meeting he had attended that such bleeding usually stops itself.

He bowed over the pillows he'd been hugging in front of him and felt the codeine and Tylenol begin to take the edge off the burning in his chest. He closed his eyes. The drugs made him sleepy. Before she had gone down to the cafeteria for supper, he had asked his mother to turn off the overhead lights and draw the curtain around his bed. He wanted to sleep.

She had seemed nervous about leaving. He knew this was because the pneumothorax was such a new thing for her. He told himself that that was why she had been staying overnight.

It was a new thing for him too, and more serious than he had realized at first. It turned out that when a lung collapsed, the odds were high that it would collapse again. Only one or two kids out of a hundred with cystic fibrosis ever have a pneumothorax, Mark had been told, but after they have the first, one of every three kids will have another. So the odds for him now were thirty-three percent.

He refused to fall apart over that possibility. When one had a bad disease, one simply had to become strong. Mark knew a girl with CF whose brother had died of it. Though she always said she was scared to death, she enjoyed going to parties and drinking beer and seemed to be living a happy life. To Mark she seemed strong. He wondered if she realized how scared *everybody* was. Whenever he was in the hospital, he'd see kids with cancer who had lost their hair from chemotherapy. He knew those kids had to be pretty scared. Yet they weren't falling apart any more than the CF kids were. Each person just learned to become strong.

In a way, Mark felt lucky. He had had years to develop his strength. He had never known what it was like to be perfectly healthy. For somebody perfectly healthy to suddenly learn that he had leukemia—Mark thought this would overwhelm a person. He himself had realized gradually what his disease meant. He had built strength as he went along. For most of his life he had been happy.

He certainly felt overwhelmed at times. This usually happened when he wasn't feeling well, and it almost always happened at home. He got weird thoughts. He never got them when he was with people. More often he got them at night in his bed. Hunched over his pillows, looking through his window at the stars glittering in the country darkness, he would realize the full impact of living only twenty years. Average age for a male, he knew, was around seventy. How much longer that fifty years was! His life, the life he would have only once, would be gone so much quicker. In a few short years he was not going to be here. He could not fathom how a person could be here and then not be here. All he had ever known was life. How could something live be without life? Where was he going to be when he was gone forever from this world?

He coped with these thoughts by shaking his head hard and turning on his radio. The radio usually helped. Sometimes even with the radio he found it difficult to get rid of his dread. But he always found some way to get his mind off it. Eventually it always wore off.

Since he was going to be on earth such a short time, he naturally hoped there would be something for him afterward. But he had problems believing in life after death. He figured that every Christian had problems believing in it, which was why people went to church. Anybody could *say* they believed. Really believing was hard. Mark went on trying so as to give himself some type of hope.

He had been comforted by a book called *Life After Life* about people who were saved after they had actually been medically dead. Most said they had experienced death as a light calling them. As they went toward the light, they had felt their bodies calling them back, and they had felt so good that they hadn't wanted to come back! They hadn't wanted to see their parents again! Mark found it hard to believe that death could seem that desirable. But that's what the people had said.

In very recent times he had sought comfort by reading his Bible every night. He had never done that before. Until his mother had remarried, religion had not really been part of their lives. But Bob read his Bible and went to church regularly, and the whole family now went to church together every Sunday.

Bob's influence had started Mark thinking. Then at Children's in October he had gotten a roommate who'd had a Bible with him.

Being halfway religious, Mark had thought a Bible might do him good in the hospital too, just in case he got scared.

Back home he had started himself on a program: a chapter of the New Testament, a chapter of the Old Testament, and a Psalm every night. Somebody had told him that the book of John contained a lot about life everlasting, so he had started with John in the New Testament and with Genesis in the Old. He used a copy of the King James version. He dated his readings in pen. When his grandfather had learned what he was doing, he had given Mark a Beck Bible, a modernized text, telling him it would be easier to understand. This was the Bible he had brought back with him to Children's on Thursday. He depended on the Scripture now. He never skipped a day's readings for any reason.

He opened his eyes and glanced at his watch—his new watch, a digital, identical to Bob's, which timed to the hundredth of a second. He had asked for it for Christmas. His parents had given it to him early, thinking he might enjoy having it in the hospital.

Six-fifteen. He wondered when his mother would get back.

He was very groggy, but his pain had eased.

Mark prayed. He asked God to let his lung stay up. He asked to gain weight. He asked for his lungs to get better. As he asked this every night of his life, he told God he hoped he wasn't being too greedy in asking one more time.

Tuesday, December 4

The sun ascending red over the city sent light through the windows of the Acute Unit which filtered in around equipment and fell across the sleeping form of Candy Rudolph in geometric figures.

Her head was swathed to the tip of her nose in a thick turban of gauze. What could be seen of her lower face under a clear green plastic oxygen mask was colorless and puffy as risen dough. The child's body seemed disproportionately small. She wore only the bottoms of a pair of blue pajamas. In the back of her right hand was an IV line; in the left wrist, an arterial line for monitoring blood pressure; on her chest, a round adhesive lead by which her respirations were being monitored. Bandages concealed her chest incision. A smaller dressing covered the point of entry of a chest tube. During the harvesting of the third rib in the OR on Monday, the patient's lung had partially collapsed. The drainage in the tube was bloody.

Less than twenty-four hours had passed since Dr. Lorimer had opened Candy's skull. She slept, aided by morphine, fitfully. Her limbs twitched. When monitor buzzers went off nearby, her fingers stiffened momentarily. One arm came off the bed. It seemed mid-gesture to forget its purpose and dropped back. She stirred, whimpered, appeared about to cry, and was suddenly recaptured by slumber. At her feet lay Baby Diaper Rash in a flannel nightie.

Candy was to remain in the Acute Intensive Care Unit for two or three days. Set up to provide maximum surveillance to critically ill children over the age of three months, Acute is a twelve-bed unit on the south wing of the hospital's fourth floor—a big, light, open room with a panoramic view of city neighborhoods through big windows across one long wall and, against the wall opposite, a nurses' station next to double doors leading into the hallway. Further along that hallway was the ten-bed Intermediate ICU where little Jody Robinson now lay sleeping with his red telephone receiver clutched in one hand.

A nurse came to Candy's bedside to check her patient's vital signs. The child had been stable since arriving in Acute. Among the youngsters currently in residence, she was one of the least worrisome. From a technical standpoint, her care was more or less routine. Nevertheless, it would challenge the staff. Some Acute nurses prefer not to take craniofacial cases. The kids are not pleasant to look at. Those who can't see are often very frightened. Those whose jaws are wired can't talk, often don't feel well enough to write, and sometimes bang on the bed out of sheer frustration at not being able to communicate. Tending such children is very demanding psychologically.

Working with their mothers and fathers is almost more difficult, nurses find. Some parents seem well prepared for the surgery and have realistic expectations about the results. But few, the nurses believe, are truly ready for how their children look postoperatively. Many parents need a lot of support at this point. Those attempting to provide it do so in the knowledge that from a social standpoint, these families have led rather traumatic lives. Therefore the Acute nurses who care for children recovering from craniofacial procedures go out of their way to be accepting of those children's deformities.

Yvonne Rudolph and her father entered the unit about 9:30 and approached Candy's bedside. Pastor Brandt—his granddaughters called him Poppa—wore his clergyman's black suit with a stiff white collar. He was short and silver-haired and had a ruddy, kindly face.

The moment she heard his voice beside her, the child grew agitated and began to whimper.

"It's all right, honey. It's all right, Candy." His words brimmed with love. He stroked her arm. "No, I can't hold you, but I have my hand on you right here. Do you feel my hand? Candy, I know you don't feel well, but try not to move around because it would just be harder if these things got pulled out . . ."

She cut him off with a wail of utter misery. "My head hurts!"

Ø

A patient's bed is sacrosanct at Children's. Policymakers believe that a child who is sick or injured, away from home, family, school, friends, pets, and his or her own bed, cared for by strangers who may cause a child to cry deserves, is owed, and must have one place he or she may consider safe. That place is bed. Unless it cannot be avoided, nothing that will hurt is done to a child in his or her bed.

So it was in the Adolescent treatment room, the place where his life had been saved so dramatically on Saturday, that Mark Price got his insides washed with tetracycline. Pain was anticipated.

The procedure was not done until 11:00 P.M. It was performed by Dr. Drew Cipriani, a second-year resident in general surgery at the university hospital next door who, as preparation for a cardiothoracic specialty, was spending three months as a CT resident at Children's. Hours later Mark's mother would wonder what had possessed Dr. Cipriani to administer the tetracycline when the boy was least rested.

The reason lay partly in priorities. The main business of cardiothoracic surgeons is to operate on hearts. This requires long hours in the operating room and close bedside monitoring afterward, often late into the evening. Dropping something down a chest tube is simply less important than stabilizing heart patients.

But it was also true that Neil Martinson, whose expert consultation Daniel Earnshaw had sought on Monday, did not expect Mark to have as much pain from the procedure as he had. All of Martinson's experience with tetracycline in humans had been with the fluid in the chest cavity that may accompany chest or lung malignancies. None of those patients had complained of severe pain. One youngster had appeared to experience severe pain, but as the child had had Down's syndrome and cried easily, it had been difficult for the resident involved to gauge her pain with any accuracy.

Furthermore, nothing Martinson had read on the subject while preparing to do his rabbit study had alerted him to expect that Mark might experience severe pain from the procedure. Daniel Earnshaw knew about the pain from word of mouth in CF circles and from talks at CF meetings. Outside those circles that knowledge was not common.

In fact, it had been the very dearth of information available on tetracycline and pneumothorax that had persuaded Martinson to go ahead with a small research project. The idea had actually originated with a pneumothorax patient of his at the university hospital who had asked whether something couldn't be put down his chest tube to make his lung stick to his chest wall. Martinson had begun to ponder tetracycline. Finding no evidence that it had been tested systematically in either animals or humans with pneumothorax, he had decided to study the problem in rabbits.

In their conversation on the phone, Martinson had told Earnshaw that while the study was several months short of completion, preliminary findings were promising. Earnshaw had asked Martinson how he would manage Mark's pain. The surgeon had replied that in view of his experience with the Down's child, the resident would take extra precautions with Mark. He would premedicate him with morphine and if necessary give him Demerol afterward. This exchange had given Martinson no new information and Earnshaw no reason to doubt that Martinson knew what in fact he would not learn for some months, after he had used tetracycline in half a dozen of his pneumothorax patients: that almost always in these patients, tetracycline down the chest tube caused excruciating pain.

Why should this happen with pneumothorax and not with fluid accumulation? Doctors speculate that although a physician always drains the fluid through a chest tube before putting tetracycline in, enough fluid remains to dilute the irritant. Further, cancer thickens and toughens tissue and perhaps makes it somewhat oblivious to painful stimulation.

Whatever the explanation, reports that would eventually reach Martinson from colleagues in other centers would reveal amazing uniformity in the way pneumothorax patients reacted to tetracycline, a uniformity extending even to the phrase these patients would use to describe their ordeal. They'd say it was like having scalding water poured into their bodies.

Except for the soft background of piped-in music, the Adolescent Unit was silent. The halls were lit as usual. Most of the rooms had been darkened for sleep. Two of three nurses on the night shift moved quietly about the floor taking vital signs, checking IV setups, tending to all but one of the few patients still awake, leaving their colleague as free as possible to be with the fifteen-year-old cystic in Room 610.

In that dim room, secluded in a chamber of light by the yellow curtain drawn around the patient's bed, three people sat in pathetic tableau. Two were women. One was the patient's mother. The other was nurse Julie Wixted, a short, somewhat stocky woman of twenty-three with a perfect complexion and fine brown hair in a blow-dry cut. Leaning from chairs on either side of his bed, the two women tried to comfort the boy, at times holding his hands, at times caressing his thin legs or shoulders, reassuring him of something they did not know themselves: that his pain would end.

The top third of Mark's bed had been cranked upright to provide him maximum support for breathing. He sat cross-legged against it, head bent low, the inside of his chest burning with pain worse than any he'd ever known. He was also having trouble breathing. Ever since the tetracycline had been put in, he'd been getting oxygen through the nasal prongs.

He felt tears starting up again. He lacked the energy to even try to hold them back.

"It's like fire," he said. He shook his bowed head slowly. "It's just like a fire in my chest."

Julie stood and bent over him, dabbing his cheeks with fresh tissues. He took the tissues from her and blew his nose. "Julie?"

"Yes?"

"Do you think you could rub my back?"

"Oh, Mark, of course." She carefully massaged him, feeling glad to do anything at all that might ease his misery.

She was very upset with the doctors. They had told Mark there would be pain. But if this was the kind of pain they had expected, why hadn't the CT resident done the procedure during the day? Then Mark could have gotten maximum doses of pain medication because there would have been lots of doctors around to monitor his responses. The morphine and Demerol given at the time of the procedure had long since worn off. Knowing it wouldn't be good to overload the patient, Julie had nonetheless paged Darryl Barth a little while ago and begged him to ask the CT resident if there wasn't something Mark could have that would help him.

"What time is it?" The boy's voice was dull. His own watch displayed the hour and the second on his wrist.

"It's two o'clock, honey," his mother answered. She added heatedly, "It's been three hours."

Julie knew she'd feel angry in Ellen's shoes. "I'm sure Dr. Barth will be calling soon to order something," the nurse could say with certainty. Darryl had been up to see Mark. He knew how badly he needed relief.

As she stopped her massage to check the patient's IV infusion, he grabbed her hand.

"I like you so much, Julie. You nurses are really great. Thanks so much for helping me when I need you."

At 2:15 A.M. Dr. Barth called to say that Mark could have chloral hydrate, a sleep medication.

The chloral hydrate did not make him sleep and did not diminish his pain. At 3:00 Julie paged Darryl to inform him.

At 3:15 Darryl called back to say that Dr. Cipriani had okayed codeine and Tylenol.

When Julie went in to give it to him, Mark was alone and barely able to talk.

"I think my mom went into the rec room. Could you ask her to come back?"

The lounge was dark. From the doorway, Julie saw Ellen silhouetted against the window overlooking the court. She was weeping softly.

The nurse felt reluctant to intrude. A number of times in recent months Mark's mother had said to various nurses in Adolescent that she wished her son would die so he could be at rest. Tonight she seemed very much afraid of his dying.

Ellen turned. "Oh, Julie. Hi. I just had to get out of there for a few minutes."

"I know exactly what you mean."

"It's so hard not to be able to help this babe in any way, shape, or form."

Julie nodded, swallowing.

"Was Darryl able to order anything?"

"Codeine and Tylenol. I just took it in now." Then she added, "Mark would like you to come back."

Ellen tried to laugh. "I guess it's nice to be wanted, anyway!"

In the doorway, both in tears, the two women embraced.

"Never again," Ellen whispered. "Never again will they touch my son."

Eyes closed, head resting on the back of the chair, she sat by his bedside in the dark. Taking slow, deep breaths, she tried to make herself relax. A few feet away, her younger son shifted about on his mattress in search of a position he could sleep in, slapping pillows, rearranging sheets, panting for breath, gasping in pain or exasperation, coughing. For this she had brought him into the world.

At 3:45 he spoke. "If I'd known it was going to be this bad, I would have wanted Bob to be here."

"If I'd known it was going to be this bad, I'd never have let them do it."

"Well, if it keeps my lung up, it'll be worth it."

Ellen marveled bitterly at his willingness to pay so dear a price for the little bit of difficult life that remained to him.

In a voice hoarse with grief and guilt and rage, she apologized to her son. "Sometimes I wish I'd never given birth to you."

"No!" He said it with such vehemence that her eyes flew open, and she jumped. "Don't ever say that again!"

About 4:00 he quieted and seemed to fall asleep. Ellen dozed. When he began to talk, she thought at first that she must be dreaming. He was thrashing and very restless, obviously still in pain, but talking, and Ellen realized immediately that he was not talking to her.

"I'll be kinder to her," he was saying. "I know she's my sister, and really, I do love her. I'll be better to her. I'll . . ."

Ellen was amazed. Mark's relationship with Denise, now twelve, was the one area in which her middle child had disappointed his parents. He ignored Denise. Or he used her. When he couldn't go up and down the steps to get things, he sent his little sister on his errands. He asked her nicely, but he never thanked her. If he disapproved of her behavior, he was quick to let her know. He could never bring himself to acknowledge her accomplishments. He made it obvious that he did not appreciate her company either at home or in the hospital. He was also jealous of her relationship with Bob.

The reason for his nastiness to his sister Ellen could only guess at. She suspected that he simply needed to feel power over something and so tried to exercise it over the only person he knew who was weaker than he was. Every aspect of his life was admirable to his mother except for that one. Mark's treatment of Denise reminded Ellen that he was not a saint.

As she listened transfixed from her chair by his bedside, he continued to talk about Denise for several minutes. Then suddenly he changed the subject. "No, I can't go to sleep yet. I haven't read my Bible."

"Mark," Ellen said softly, "would it be okay if Mom read to you?"

She had no idea whether her words would register on him. But when he answered yes, she turned on his light, brought her chair as close to his bed as possible, and read to him wearily but with emphasis the great reassurances, the great promises of deliverance to be found in the Ninety-first Psalm, feeling that if God did exist and if He were truly good, He would spare her child any more pain tonight and let him get some rest.

Wednesday, December 5

At 7:30 A.M., walking down the hall toward the parents' shower room with fresh clothes and a towel over one arm, Ellen Price ran into Daniel Earnshaw and planted herself in his path.

He stood at least a head taller. Ellen had known him too long to be intimidated by his height, his white lab coat, or anything else about him.

"I will never let you or anybody else do this to Mark again."

His gears shifted automatically. "Tell me about it."

She told him. He had never seen her as distressed or as noticeably exhausted. She was a very articulate person, in Earnshaw's opinion, and also an emotional and dramatic person. He worried about what would happen to Ellen Price when Mark died. The boy mimicked her, to some extent; he, too, was often somewhat dramatic. On occasion Earnshaw took what Mark and his mother said to him with a small grain of salt. Yet he thought the Prices a good, stable family and appreciated the fact that he and the boy's parents talked well together. Ellen Price said everything that was on her mind. She did not ask or want to be protected from hard truths.

"What I just can't understand is why we weren't told in advance how bad this was going to be." Her voice shook. "I specifically asked the CT resident how much pain would be involved, and he minimized it, and Mark had a hell of a time." She blew her nose, then looked him straight in the eye. "I don't think you should ever give that stuff to a patient again. Not to Mark, not to any child."

Earnshaw was sure he had warned them himself when seeking their consent for the treatment that there would be severe pain. But even he had not anticipated pain so severe as to inspire this reaction in the patient's mother. It was not like Ellen to condemn a treatment before she found out whether it would work.

"I'll go see him. Is he awake?"

"He's awake." Touched by the concern on Earnshaw's face, she added softly, "I'm sure he'll be glad to see you."

He felt closer to Mark than to any other patient still living. Two he had loved as much were gone now: Perry and Nicole, an extraordinary personality who, though she had lived just twelve years, had made an indelible impression at Children's.

The closeness he felt with Mark was increasingly a bond between friends. Earnshaw looked forward to seeing the boy on rounds. Mark was usually very cheerful and doing or thinking about something interesting, and he had an impressive curiosity, in his doctor's opinion. While many CF patients become knowledgeable about their disease, no others in Earnshaw's experience had ever asked to attend a conference about it. The meeting on hemoptysis had turned out to be a rather rough introduction to lung hemorrhage. The visiting physician had talked at length about a young man with massive bleeding who had not been helped by multiple transfusions. Later Earnshaw had emphasized to Mark that this had been an extreme case. But the boy had not appeared frightened. His response to the reassurance had been to say that he just wanted to learn as much as he could about CF.

Over the years the two had had many conversations on a wide variety of subjects. Yet despite the affinity between them, the doctor recognized a limit to the depth of their exchange. One reason, he thought, was that Mark guarded his privacy. But Earnshaw believed the main reason to be his own inability to communicate well with the teenagers about the matter uppermost in their minds: dying.

With younger patients he felt he communicated very well. But the adolescents, separating from their parents, had made it clear to Earnshaw that they preferred to do business with his younger associate, Bruce Griffin, a preference the senior man found understandable. Still, it bothered him that the kids didn't want to talk to him and that he lacked the skill to get through to them.

He had tried. Most recently he had tried using books as a stimulus to discussion with Mark and one other patient. Last year Mark had come in for a tune-up bringing *Watership Down,* a book he'd been assigned to report on. Earnshaw had loved the book. "If you liked that," he'd said to Mark, "I have another I think you'd enjoy," and he had brought in the first book of Tolkien's *Fellowship of the Ring* trilogy. His underlying idea had been to acquaint Mark with the main character, Frodo, the little Hobbit who finally triumphs despite great obstacles and his diminutive size. Thinking that Mark might be able to identify with Frodo, Earnshaw had hoped that a conversation about the Hobbit might deepen the level of their communication.

Mark had passed the book on to his brother without ever giving any indication of having read it himself. Earnshaw had concluded that with these youngsters one probably needed to be more direct than he knew how to be. He was grateful for the other people at Children's who could be made available to his patients for what he himself could not provide them.

He entered his patient's room. The boy appeared to be asleep. As always now, the top of his bed had been cranked nearly upright, and Mark lay in pillows against it, eyes closed. His face was strained and very pale. There were dark circles under his eyes. Earnshaw observed that his nail beds had a bluish cast, though his lips were pink enough. He was breathing hard. The only other sound in the room was the gurgle of the suction machine drawing air from Mark's chest cavity.

The doctor touched the boy's shoulder. "Mark?"

The eyelids opened. "Oh, hi."

"You had a pretty rough night last night. Do you want to tell me about it?"

The youngster gave the details. Earnshaw was struck by the effort with which he spoke and by the tonelessness of his voice. Even on Monday, reporting on his lung collapse, Mark had been his cheerful self. "I'm all right! Well, I've got this tube in my chest, and it was scary when it happened, but I feel fine!" This morning he obviously felt nothing like fine. Never before had Earnshaw seen Mark in such distress that he could not rally.

Back in the hallway some minutes later, he encountered the boy's mother returning from her shower. When he got close to her, she saw that Daniel Earnshaw had tears in his eyes.

He told her about Perry Smith. He explained why he'd wanted to give Mark the chance he hadn't given Perry. "I knew the treatment would hurt him," he told Ellen, "but I also know that Mark is especially strong. I felt he could bear the pain. That's why I had enough nerve to try the tetracycline with him, whereas I didn't with the other boy."

"Well," she said, gently now, "you could say that's a very nice compliment to Mark."

"I would have done anything to spare him what he went through last night."

For the first time in all the years they had known each other, they embraced.

Finally he said he was going to get in trouble with the hospital board if anyone reported him, and both he and Ellen laughed.

As she left him to return to Mark's room, he watched her go. For some years after coming to Children's, Earnshaw had done his job having no real understanding of what it meant to live with a child with cystic fibrosis. Then the family of one youngster had invited him to go fishing with them. Earnshaw liked to fish, so he had spent a day with the family on their cabin cruiser.

And every ten or fifteen minutes, the child would cough. Every ten or fifteen minutes all day long, Earnshaw had been reminded that the boy had cystic fibrosis, that the disease was active, that the child's life would be short. A few hours on that boat had given Earnshaw some inkling of how it must feel for a family to be given such reminders every day of their lives.

He did not know how parents stood it.

Ø

Candy Rudolph had made such good progress since her surgery on Monday that had there been a bed available on one of the floors, she could have transferred out of Acute on Wednesday afternoon.

Her face remained quite swollen, which was to be expected. But her vital signs were stable. Though still congested as a result of the anesthesia, she was off oxygen and breathing room air. Her pneumothorax had almost completely resolved. She showed no signs of infection. Her urine output was fine. Both her bladder catheter and the arterial line in her left wrist had been removed. While still receiving IV fluids, she was tolerating juices and clear soups without difficulty. She was increasingly active. She'd been out of bed to sit in a chair and in her mother's lap.

However, the child was neither comfortable nor happy. Thanks to morphine she was still sleeping a lot, but awake she was restless, fussy, and irritable. She spoke only to say "No" or "I want to be held." She said no to juice, no to baths, no to a change of pajamas, no to the nurses doing anything for her when her mother was nearby and sometimes when her mother wasn't. Yvonne took consolation in the fact that the child's condition was improving. Irritable as Candy was, she seemed less agitated today than yesterday. In only five more days she'd be going home to her grandparents'.

Thursday, December 6

Early in the morning Rolfe Lorimer and chief plastic surgery resident Dean Whitehill arrived in Acute to remove Candy Rudolph's bandages and take out her chest tube. The latest x-ray showed complete resolution of the pneumothorax.

She was sitting up in bed with turbaned head bowed low. A nurse stood holding her hand, talking to her quietly. When the doctors greeted her, Candy began to fuss apprehensively.

"Here's your dolly," said the nurse. The child accepted Baby Diaper Rash but with her free hand felt for and found a bar on the raised side rail of her bed. She gripped it.

The mass of gauze was crisscrossed with adhesive tape. Whitehill snipped the tape with scissors. The patient protested in soft cries. As the nurse stroked her arm, the resident tried to calm her with chitchat.

"You're doing fine. We let Mommy know that you're going to look like a big pumpkin for a while, but that'll go away. I know you wish I'd quit bugging you, Candy . . ." He unwound some gauze, then lifted off the mound remaining. It came easily.

"You may not be able to see, Candy," the nurse said. "Your eyes are real swollen."

Her eyelids bulged out as if each concealed a whole walnut. Both were purplish-red. The right lid actually drooped slightly onto the child's cheek. The new contours so carefully crafted by Lorimer in the operating room had disappeared in bloatedness. Candy's head might have been a reflection in the distorting mirror in the Children's Hospital lobby. The fringe of hair in back was stiff and spiky from blood now dried—as ropy as the yellow tresses on Baby Diaper Rash.

The doctors examined the incision. The gash had been closed by more than fifty black sutures which together resembled a zipper across the bald scalp. The surgeons were pleased to see that the incision was dry and that the edges of flesh were beginning to knit.

Lorimer tore open a sterile gauze pad from the patient's bedside table. "Honey," he said smoothly, "I'm going to open your eyes."

She replied without petulance. "No."

"I know they're swollen," Lorimer continued, placing the pad against one eyelid. "Honey, put your hands down," he said as the nurse restrained her. "It won't hurt."

As soon as she realized this was true, she stopped whimpering.

When he had lifted both lids, which were far too swollen to stay open on their own, the surgeon gently depressed her skull with his fingertips. "Does this hurt, Miss Candy?"

"Uh-huh."

"Where does it hurt?"

She pointed to her eyes.

"Yes, you have a little fluid in there. It's only water. It's like a sprained ankle. It'll go away soon." In fact the swelling that follows craniofacial surgery is usually at its peak three days postop. Unless a problem developed, Candy's puffiness would begin to decrease dramatically in a day or two.

Arriving in Acute about 9:00 A.M., Yvonne Rudolph saw in her daughter's bed a child so grotesque as to be almost unrecognizable as herself.

Ø

Two floors up, Mark sat in bed holding a small mirror in one hand, combing his bangs with the other. The hair on the right side was sticking out at an angle. He'd been sleeping on that side because of the chest tube. Dipping the comb into a glass of water on the bedside table, he wet the hair and used his fingers to plaster it flat against his forehead.

"Gorgeous!" This from Kate, who had come in to take his temperature. She was wearing a red sweater, a heavy denim skirt, and knee socks with her loafers.

He frowned at the mirror. "You should have seen me when I was younger. I was a really cute baby! I have to admit it!"

"Who says?"

"Everybody says. Ma, wasn't I a cute baby?"

Ellen sat watching a soap serial on the television set suspended from the ceiling in one corner. "Oh, absolutely," she replied, catching Kate's eye. "He was adorable. If Mark says so, it must be true."

"Ma!"

"What?"

"That's not what you're supposed to say!"

He felt much better this morning. His pain from the tetracycline had been so severe that the pain he had from the chest tube seemed mild by comparison. With the help of codeine and Tylenol, he could stand that pain. He had caught up on his rest, too, since yesterday morning.

He was also breathing more easily. He had been in the hospital exactly a week. Seven days on antibiotics had knocked some of the infection from his lungs. He did still have decreased breath sounds on his left side because that lung hadn't fully reexpanded. But as the degree of collapse had decreased from twenty-five percent to five, the CT surgeons had told Mark this morning that they might clamp the tube tomorrow and take it out.

This had greatly encouraged him. He calculated that at most he would only have to be in the hospital another week to finish getting antibiotics. He probably wouldn't have to come back in at least until the middle of January. All through the Christmas holidays he would feel fine.

"Kate, can I get up in a little while and get my hair washed?" He had been out of bed only once since the pneumothorax. Tuesday afternoon, before the tetracycline treatment, he had sat in a wheelchair beside his bed for twenty minutes.

"Sure!"

As usual his day was filled with visitors.

The first was social worker Dick Jacoby, a lanky man of thirty who had been at Children's about a year. In that time his contact with Mark Price had been so routine as to be superficial. This was not unusual. Since children in for tune-ups become well enough within a few days to socialize with other kids, they feel no need for someone like Jacoby. Though the worker felt, as the doctors did, that Mark knew his time was beginning to run out, Jacoby was reluctant to urge the boy to talk about his fears unless Mark raised the subject.

He felt he had a bigger role to play with the patient's mother. Ellen Price was preparing herself for the inevitable. She needed a lot of support, yet wouldn't necessarily acknowledge that she did. So Jacoby sometimes found it difficult to talk to her. But he genuinely sympathized with her and always made a point of seeing her often whenever Mark was in.

Mark's second visitor Thursday morning was his nutritionist, a petite, energetic mother of two teenagers with a master's degree in her field. To Beryl Kaiserman the CF kids were all tough cases, and Mark was especially tough because he was finicky about food. He existed on snacks. Though he'd have a meal now and then, he refused to eat a balanced diet. His disregard for good nutrition puzzled Daniel Earnshaw, who saw it as a blind spot in Mark, because otherwise the boy took very good care of himself.

Earnshaw and Kaiserman had tried all kinds of ways to improve Mark's nutritional status, but either the measures hadn't worked or Mark had tired of them. Now he was in pain from the chest tube and often dopy from the pain medications. Today he felt better and was trying to get food down. But since the pneumothorax, his intake had been mainly cola. If cola wouldn't help him, neither would good nourishment cure him.

So Beryl Kaiserman had few suggestions to offer Mark this morning. She visited him because she was paid to, because she still hoped to find a way to make some small contribution to the life he had left, and because she liked him.

Soon after lunch came Clara Bowman, Mark's favorite respiratory therapist, thirty-four and buxom, mother of two young sons. When Mark's spirits were in the cellar, Clara could make him laugh. As the doctors now thought it best for his breathing treatments and percussion to be stopped again temporarily because of his lung collapse and his pain, her visit today was purely social. She had known Mark most of his life. In the early years they had read comic books together and exchanged jokes and played tic-tac-toe, which Clara had let Mark win. More recently they had played electronic games, which Mark won without Clara's help. They also had religion in common.

She found him now reading a magazine. He seemed so improved over the way he'd felt when she'd seen him yesterday that she commented on the change. "Something good must be happening. You sound better."

"They're maybe going to take my chest tube out tomorrow. And Bob is coming in tonight. He's going to get my mother and take her home."

Clara was always impressed at how Mark's spirits went up anytime his new father was due to come in. She said, without planning to, "He sure must be a beautiful person to do what he did. This man loves you."

"I know. And I love him."

"As I've told you, I myself was a foster child at one time. I still remember how it felt to go back to people who loved me. Promise me you'll be as nice to Bob as he has been to you."

"I am nice to him."

"Yeah, but promise me you'll keep on being as nice to him. Bob loves you. Not many men to have done what he did. Promise me you'll be a son to him."

"I am. I will."

And about 3:30, when he had finished cleaning rooms and buffing floors on the Adolescent Unit, Dennis May came to play a game of chess with Mark.

May was twenty-three and married, the father of a daughter four and a son five. He had met Mark Price the very first day he had worked on Adolescent and continued to enjoy his company whenever Mark was back in the hospital. He found the boy a down-to-earth person whose disease didn't seem to bother him. They had gotten into games right away. On the Adolescent bumper pool table Mark was unbeatable. Unlike the other patients, May could at least give him a little competition. They'd play on his break or at the end of his workday. Mark always won. Finally one day May had said to him, "My game is chess. Do you play chess?"

Mark did. So then they'd started playing chess three or four times a week on May's lunch hour, or even while he was working. He'd play one move, go around the room with the wet mop, and then come back to the bedside and play a couple more moves. Mark had never beaten him in chess. The boy had a nice game, in May's opinion, but he himself had been playing for thirteen years. Once in a while May was tempted to let Mark win—until he reminded himself that Mark had never shown *him* any pity at the pool table!

Ø

At noon Candy Rudolph had been transferred out of the Acute Unit and into a four-bed room on Six Surgical.

She was miserable for the whole afternoon. "Where's my hair? Why can't I open my eyes? Where's Poppa? Where are we? I want to go home! I want some French toast! I don't want any juice! I want Mommy to give me my juice! I want to sit on Mommy's lap! I want to get back in my bed!"

She'd sleep for a while, then wake up and be unhappy. Aspirin suppositories helped. But Yvonne's efforts at comfort were of little avail. At one point she began to read aloud from "The Three Bears," Candy's favorite story. Blind as she was from the swelling, the child yanked the book out of her mother's hands and threw it down on the bed.

Early Thursday evening, on doctors' orders, she was served the first solid foods she had had since the night before her operation. She was unable to manage the steak sandwich that came up on her tray. But with her grandmother's help, Candy ate all the melted cheese that covered the steak and also polished off a whole bowl of peaches and most of the chocolate ice cream brought by her grandfather from McDonald's.

Ø

Mark felt well enough at suppertime to eat his first good dinner in days. All evening he was just short of ebullient. When he wasn't playing cards with his father and mother, he was laughing and socializing with the nurses. He was medicated twice for pain with codeine and Tylenol. If he felt concerned about his mother going home after staying almost literally at his side for five days, he gave no sign.

Ø

Had Mark been born healthy, surviving adolescence would have been for him almost a foregone conclusion. Such a statement could not have been made in this country—or any other—until relatively recently. Until well into the twentieth century, death at an early age was a distinct possibility for virtually every child emerging live from the womb.

In America in the 1600s children died of smallpox, diphtheria, scarlet fever, measles, tuberculosis, whooping cough, malaria, yellow fever, and a fierce dysentery known as bloody flux.

In the 1700s colonial children lost their lives to smallpox, diphtheria, scarlet fever, measles, tuberculosis, whooping cough, malaria, yellow fever, and diarrheal disorders, particularly the "summer complaint," or cholera infantum, that killed thousands of babies under two in the hot months of the year.

In the 1800s young Americans perished from smallpox, diphtheria, scarlet fever, measles, tuberculosis, whooping cough, malaria, diarrhea and enteritis, cholera, cerebrospinal meningitis, congenital syphilis, and poliomyelitis.

During the first three decades of this century American children died of smallpox, diphtheria, scarlet fever, measles, tuberculosis, whooping cough, malaria, summer and other diarrheas, meningitis, congenital syphilis, poliomyelitis, typhoid fever, rheumatic fever, and juvenile diabetes.

In America today more children die from injuries than from the next nine leading causes of death *combined,* including birth defects, cancer, heart disease, pneumonia, and meningitis.

The field of pediatric medicine has·changed more radically in the past half century than in any similar period in recorded history. Gone are the dreadful epidemics of infectious diseases that plagued the race for so many generations and that at their most savage could obliterate whole families of children in a week's time. Thanks to vaccines, those diseases themselves are dying out. Smallpox held sway on this planet as long ago as the sixth century. As of May 1980 it has been eradicated from the earth. Diphtheria reached its peak in America in 1921 and afflicted nearly 207,000 persons that year. In 1983 there were five reported cases of diphtheria in the United States.* Polio, which commonly killed a fifth or more of its victims, struck more than 21,000 Americans in 1952. In 1983 just twelve cases were reported.

*Most recent available statistics from U.S. Centers for Disease Control.

Progress almost as dramatic has occurred in whooping cough and measles. The incidence of pertussis in this country decreased from a high in 1934 of well over a quarter of a million cases to under 2,500 in 1983, while measles dropped from a 1941 high of nearly 900,000 cases to an all-time low in 1983 of fewer than 1,500 cases. The number increased somewhat in 1984, but experts are optimistic that with greater diligence they can eliminate such outbreaks. Rubella, or German measles, has also been reduced to a couple of thousand cases a year. An epidemic in the mid-1960s produced congenital rubella—rubella present at birth—in more than 20,000 newborns. In 1983 the reported cases of congenital rubella in America numbered six. Typhoid, tetanus, and mumps have also been substantially tamed by immunization.

Statistics worldwide are somewhat less impressive. But in this country, except for chicken pox, for which a vaccine is now being perfected, all the formerly most common infectious diseases of childhood have become rarities. Once in a great while when a youngster with measles comes into the Children's Hospital Emergency Room, residents whose parents probably both had the disease are invited in to take a look at a case of a sort they may never see again.

Vaccines are but one explanation for the changed topography in contemporary pediatrics. Childhood deaths from diarrheal disorders have also diminished markedly over the past five or six decades. Prior to the 1920s, for as long as records had been kept in this new land, diarrhea had killed more children under five each year than had anything else. In large part the improvement resulted from the subduing of summer complaint. Always predominant among infants whose mothers could not or, following fashion, would not nurse them, summer diarrhea claimed as many as eighty to ninety percent of all babies fed by bottle in certain periods and localities in the nineteenth century, and as the twentieth began remained, in the words of pediatric historian Thomas E. Cone, Jr., M.D., "a prevalent and serious disease without an effective method of treatment."

By that time, however, a connection had been recognized between illness in young children and dirty cow's milk. With the coming of pasteurization in America also came refrigeration and public health measures that improved sanitation, housing, and food production and distribution standards and assured the population an uncontaminated water supply. Physicians started to understand the body's need for fluid balance, which began to reduce the number of deaths by the most lethal complication of cholera infantum, dehydration. Mothers were urged to breast-feed their babies if they possibly could.

In 1922 diarrhea slipped to third place as a cause of childhood mortality, behind malformations and diseases of early infancy and pneumonia. Today diarrheal disorders rank seventh as a threat to the lives of children under one year and are so far down the list over the age of one as to be hardly worth mentioning. Even among infants the ranking is deceptive. Babies under one who died in 1981 numbered 43,305.* Almost exactly half died of conditions associated with prematurity. Only 489 died of diarrheal diseases. Among the reasons for the vast improvement in these figures over 1930 was the development of sanitary and inexpensive infant formulas.

A growing appreciation of the elements of good nutrition has also contributed to diminishing mortality rates in young Americans. Vitamin and iron deficiencies were widespread in the nineteenth century. Among children, rickets was commonplace. Nutritional disorders intensified during the Depression years. In 1930 they constituted, along with infections, a chief cause of childhood illness and death. Disturbingly high levels of malnutrition continue to be documented in this land of plenty. But rickets, scurvy, beriberi, and goiter have virtually disappeared, thanks in part to improved living standards which enabled more Americans to avail themselves of healthier diets.

Mortality in children has been further reduced by such drugs as cortisones, steroids, broad-spectrum antibiotics, and, more recently, anticancer agents. Though persons who contracted the ailment as youngsters continue to be seen in adult hospitals, rheumatic heart disease in the pediatric population has all but vanished. While still a serious cause of illness and death in certain other parts of the world, tuberculosis has become uncommon in America, and so has death from tuberculosis. Scarlet fever has been reduced by penicillin to two or three cases a year. Congenital syphilis is rather rare, though its increased incidence since the early 1970s is a cause for concern. Meningitis is treated successfully far more often than not. That it is

*Most recent available figures from National Center for Health Statistics.

usually curable while continuing to rank as a leading cause of death in youngsters under five conveys succinctly a profound truth of pediatric medicine in the modern era. As one pediatrician puts it, "Children aren't dying of very much anymore."

They certainly aren't dying of diseases much anymore. They are also dying from injuries at a much lower rate than once was true. In 1960 injuries took less than half as many young lives per hundred thousand children in the population as in 1920. Furthermore, in 1980 fewer American children under fifteen died of injuries than died in this country in 1916 of whooping cough alone. Injuries have become the primary cause of death in young people all over the Western world not because accidents themselves have increased but because all other causes of death have so greatly decreased.

Yet more than ten thousand children under fifteen die from injuries every year in America. Since 1950 the rate has improved rather slowly. In the general population, injuries rank fourth behind heart disease, cancer, and stroke as a cause of death. But injuries account for fully half of all deaths in persons between the ages of one and twenty-five. Moreover, accidents permanently cripple or disfigure one hundred thousand American children every year. Two million more are incapacitated by injuries for two weeks or longer. According to historian Cone, "Accidents and acts of violence have replaced microbes as the major threat to lives of children and adolescents in contemporary American society."

Not all children are equally vulnerable. Injuries are the leading cause of death for children in the aggregate and for all children over the age of one. Babies under one are likeliest to die of problems associated with prematurity. Most such deaths occur within a month of birth. In fact, forty percent of all deaths in children less than a year old occur in the first twenty-four hours of life.

For babies who survive the first seven days, the biggest threat is sudden infant death syndrome. Considered by most experts to be a definite disease entity—though the experts don't know what causes it—SIDS kills between six and seven thousand infants in the United States annually and is the leading cause of death in babies between a week and a year old.

During the first twelve months of childhood, injuries as a cause of death rank fourth. These fatalities are due primarily to falls from unprotected surfaces, suffocation by bedclothes or plastic materials, ingestion of food or objects into the respiratory passages, motor vehicle collisions, and mechanical strangulation often involving either portable cribs with mesh sides or cribs in which slats are spaced more than two and three-eighths inches apart.

A youngster over one year of age is more likely to die in an automobile accident than from any other single cause. Though people are most often injured in various kinds of accidents around the home, auto accidents are more likely to be fatal, especially to children.

Children's bodies are small and light. In a collision, a child is much more susceptible than an adult to being bounced around the inside of the car. Struck on the street, children are likelier than adults to suffer head injuries. Being shorter in stature, they receive the impact higher up than do adults, who tend to incur more injuries to the pelvis and lower extremities. Children may die from car accidents that would produce only minor harm to their parents.

Other causes of fatal injury in childhood vary by age group. A child's chances of dying from injury rise significantly when he or she begins to walk. After auto deaths, children one through four are particularly susceptible to lethal injury from falls, fires, burns, scalds, electric shocks, colliding with heavy objects, choking on such items as coins, toy parts, or soda can "pop tops," and poisoning from common drugs, vitamins being a chief culprit, as well as from a huge variety of household cleaning agents and insecticides.

Relatively speaking, the elementary school years are a safer time for children. While the automobile continues as the primary agent of death by injury, children five to fourteen are a little less likely to die in car accidents than are preschoolers. Head injuries decrease sharply during this period, as do burns, poisonings, and internal injuries. However, drownings, playground and athletic injuries, and firearm fatalities increase. Youngsters in this age group may also be killed by knives, matches, engines and electrical equipment, tools and farm implements, and sports equipment such as bicycles, baseball bats, and skateboards.

By far the period of greatest danger from death by injury is between a person's fifteenth and twenty-fourth birthdays. More than twice as many young adults die from injuries each year in this country than do all children under fifteen combined. Many more young adults die of injuries than do their elders in any age category.

Though fewer die in falls and fires than do younger children, more die in drowning, and many more die in motor vehicle crashes. Two-thirds of all deaths by injury among Americans fifteen to twenty-four involve automobiles or motorcycles. A large proportion involve alcohol as well. The toll is high: 23,582 in 1981.

The second and third major causes of death in this age group are homicide and suicide, respectively. Both have increased alarmingly in the past few decades. Together these two forms of violent injury claimed more than eleven thousand young adults in this country in 1981—nearly three times as many as died from cancer and heart disease combined.

The homicide rate is highest among nonwhites. In fact a young black male in America is more likely to die of homicide than of any other cause and five times as likely to be killed in this manner as a young white. Murder is associated more often than not with poverty and frequently with alcohol abuse as well.

Suicide is increasing among both whites and nonwhites. It is also increasing among the youth of other industrialized nations. Experts attribute the trend here to stress brought on by such factors as the dissolution of the family, economic hard times, pressure to succeed despite inadequate schooling and a pinched job market, changing moral codes, and the feelings of anonymity that accompany over-crowding. Alcohol is often a factor. Most suicides as well as most homicides among the young in America are committed with handguns.

After injuries and conditions associated with prematurity, the third leading killer of American children is congenital anomalies, more commonly known as birth defects. In 1981 these disorders were fatal to eleven thousand youngsters, the vast majority under a year of age. With exceptions, anomalies serious enough to be lethal tend to cause death within months or even days of birth. In infants these disorders are the primary cause of death behind prematurity. In children one through four they are second to injuries, and they are third behind injuries and cancer in children five to fourteen.

They drop to sixth place in young adults between fifteen and twenty-four. In this category fewer than six hundred persons died from birth defects in 1981. The downward curve is somewhat deceptive. Certain conditions present at birth do not manifest themselves until much later. The classic example is Huntington's chorea, the disease that killed musician Woody Guthrie in his prime and that typically remains silent until after its victims have turned forty.

The scope of mortality and morbidity resulting from congenital anomalies in this country is considerably broader than the above statistics suggest. As calculated by the March of Dimes Birth Defects Foundation, established in 1938 as the National Foundation for Infantile Paralysis, congenital defects figure in half a million miscarriages and stillbirths in America annually, account for some sixty thousand deaths and the hospitalization of more than a million Americans of all ages each year, and affect the daily lives of about fifteen million Americans, both victims and families. Of the infants born alive in this country each year, more than a quarter of a million—one in twelve—have birth defects of one kind or another. The incidence of most has changed little over the years. Like injuries, they loom now as a large problem of childhood because larger problems of childhood have been solved.

The term "congenital anomalies" means abnormalities present at birth. Some are primarily genetic in origin—that is, they are inherited. Others originate in external factors of which the well-known examples include the tranquilizer thalidomide, the food fish poisoned inadvertently in Japan by mercury, and maternal rubella, or three-day measles. The specific causes of the majority of birth defects, however, remain elusive.

Experts group the genetic causes into three categories. Chromosomal disorders, which are relatively rare, result either from too many or too few chromosomes, the threadlike bodies in cell nuclei that carry genes, or from displaced chromosomal material. Among liveborn infants the most common chromosomal anomaly is Down's syndrome. About five thousand American children are born with Down's each year.

Gene disorders are those caused by abnormalities in a single gene or by one abnormal gene from each parent in combination. Parents may be affected themselves or may simply be carriers. Gene disorders include cystic fibrosis, hemophilia, sickle cell anemia, Huntington's chorea, colorblindness, and the disease of the "elephant man," neurofibromatosis. While each is rare in itself, together these disorders account for approximately five percent of all hospital admissions.

The third and largest category of gene-related birth defects comprise those considered polygenic or multifactorial. Among them are many of the most common malformations: clubfoot, which appears in about 9,300 newborns each year in America; cleft lip and/or palate, about half as common as clubfoot; and imperfections of the heart, which affect nearly 25,000 new babies annually in this country.

These disorders are poorly understood. A genetic component has not been proved. Yet it seems likely that genes make some contribution, since these defects tend to run in families. Scientists theorize that genes confer susceptibility which is then triggered by something in the environment. The precise role of environmental factors also has yet to be ascertained. Some have yet to be even identified.

But there are known hazards: fetal exposure through the mother to cigarettes, alcohol, drugs, lead, x-rays, viruses, venereal diseases. Poor maternal nutrition puts a fetus at risk. So does inadequate prenatal care. While implications for humans aren't yet known, certain pesticides and chemical wastes can cause birth defects in laboratory animals.

Some birth defects are of little or no consequence. Most urinary tract anomalies can be corrected with surgery that does not require overnight admission to a hospital. An extra finger or toe can likewise be taken care of in one brief trip to the operating room. A baby born with undetected galactosemia can become retarded and die within weeks, but if the child is diagnosed, taken off milk, and kept on a special diet for the first six years of life, he or she will be fine. A child born with cystinuria will be fine so long as he or she drinks a prescribed amount of water. Much more serious defects may also be successfully treated or even cured by surgery. A child born with internal organs outside an open abdominal wall, a life-threatening defect horrifying to behold, can live normally and fully after surgical repair.

Far too many children are at the opposite end of this spectrum, unfortunately. Far too many born with congenital anomalies are destined for a lifetime of disability or an early death or both. Like cystic fibrosis, Tay-Sachs disease, sickle cell anemia, hemophilia, thalassemia, and muscular dystrophy are all incurable. Thanks to medical advances, many youngsters with these diseases now live longer than once was possible and also better: more comfortably and with greater mobility, less pain, less isolation. Sicklers who get past their first five years usually live at least into their thirties. The life expectancy of most hemophiliacs now approximates that of the general population, and living with this disorder is enormously more tolerable today than in the past. Yet after bleeding, the second most common cause of death among persons affected by hemophilia is suicide. (The impact of AIDS on mortality among hemophiliacs is not yet known.) Few children who inherit any of the rest of these diseases will survive their twenties. That many will take pleasure in their lives even so—will enjoy, aspire, accomplish, and bring pleasure to others—does not alter the fact that every one of their stories is ultimately tragic.

Some of these tragedies may be averted by abortion of an affected fetus or by a decision on the part of known carriers to adopt rather than conceive a child. The most dependable and least risky form of prenatal testing is amniocentesis. Done primarily in women over thirty-five to identify Down's syndrome and other chromosomal abnormalities associated with advancing maternal age, this procedure can reveal the presence or absence of a growing number of major and minor congenital anomalies including Tay-Sachs disease, sickle cell anemia, and myelomeningocele, or spina bifida.

However, amniocentesis does carry a small but decided risk to the fetus. Widespread use of this procedure is also limited by practical considerations of cost and timing. Thus it is offered only to rule out those abnormalities for which a given baby is known to be at risk. Many abnormalities are undetectable by any form of prenatal diagnosis.

Scientists have recently announced that a test may be in the offing that could ascertain through gene analysis a family's degree of risk for having a Down's child. Other means of preventing birth defects seem far off. About genetic susceptibility the experts can do nothing. With persistence and luck they may one day pin down the environmental culprits. Since many hereditary disorders are relatively rare and attract neither researchers nor research dollars in significant numbers, they may be among us for a long time to come.

The fourth leading cause of death among young persons in this country is cancer, which is actually a rare disease in childhood. Ma-

lignancies killed some 4,500 Americans under twenty-five in 1981—
less than half as many as died from birth defects, one-seventh the
number who died from injuries. Most were five years of age or
older. Cancer is especially rare in infants and preschoolers. While
nearly 9,000 infants twelve months old or less succumbed in 1981 as
a result of congenital anomalies, fewer than one hundred died of
malignant disorders.

Told through survival statistics, the cancer story is one of the
happiest in modern medicine. Before 1940 children diagnosed with
the disease in any form were sent home to die. Rarely did they live
longer than a few months. However, with improved surgical techniques, the discovery in the 1960s that chemical agents used in combination were more effective against some cancers than any drug
used individually, and the concurrent discovery that irradiating
"sanctuary areas" unreachable by drugs could prevent localized relapse, survival rates improved in all age groups but—for reasons
having to do with the physiology of growth—especially in the
young. In the 1970s some pediatric oncologists dared to claim that,
if caught in time, certain pediatric malignancies could be and actually were being cured.

Today experts say they are curing or achieving long-term remis-
sions that may equate with cure in nearly sixty percent of all children diagnosed with cancer of any kind. In particular forms the
odds are even better. Those with the best prognosis are Hodgkin's
disease, Wilms' tumor, which starts in kidney tissues, and acute lymphocytic leukemia. Progress against the latter has been hailed as one
of the medical milestones of the twentieth century. ALL is the most
common cancer in childhood. In the late 1940s a youngster with
that disease would die within weeks of being diagnosed. Between
1964 and 1979 survival rates improved from fifteen or twenty percent to seventy percent at some major research centers, Children's
Hospital among them. In the treatment of no other form of malignancy have the strides been more dramatic.

The battle, however, has yet to be won. While mortality rates are
decreasing among children with cancer, the reduction of childhood
mortality from other causes means that more children are living
long enough to develop malignant disorders, so that reported incidence of these disorders in Americans twenty-four and under is actually increasing. Certain forms of pediatric cancer have proved

stubbornly resistant to the new therapies. In the words of the Oncology chief at Children's, "There are still too many children who
for different reasons can't be cured." Though a child growing up in
America is more likely to die of homicide or suicide, cancer still kills
more young persons than does any other disease.

The two other illnesses that rank as leading causes of mortality
in children are heart disease and pneumonia. Together they accounted for about the same number of deaths among the young in
1981 as did cancer alone. Cardiac disorders in adults are usually
acquired and degenerative. In children they tend to derive from
congenital malformations, a fact that statistics don't always reflect.
Thirty-three hundred persons under age twenty-five were reported
to have died of heart disease in 1981. Most were between the ages
of fifteen and twenty-four, while the majority of some 1,500 deaths
from pneumonia occurred in babies twelve months old or younger.
Many of these deaths, too, were probably associated with congenital
anomalies or with chronic diseases.

Scientific advances have made pediatrics a much happier field
today than at any other time in history but also, in some ways, far
more complex.

Progress has virtually redefined pediatric illness. As acute diseases have gradually lost their power over children, the attention of
pediatricians has focused increasingly on youngsters with chronic
illnesses. Some are disabled by incurable inherited diseases with
which one may now live two or more decades. Others are disabled
as a result of extreme prematurity, significant birth defects, severe
trauma, and acquired diseases of extraordinary virulence which
only yesterday would have killed them outright.

Many more children are somewhat disabled from less serious injuries or by illnesses that flare up from time to time and are usually
treated successfully, among them asthma, which affects a million
and a half children in this country and represents a major public
health problem. Experts disagree as to whether the incidence of
chronic disease and disability has actually increased or whether reporting has simply improved. Either way, chronicity among the
young has become a major concern in pediatrics.

Specialists are also concerned about more subtle disorders in children arising out of social factors: divorce, child abuse, drug and alcohol abuse, venereal diseases, adolescent pregnancy, depression, alienation, homicide, and the impulse to commit suicide. "Increasingly," writes historian Thomas Cone, "pediatricians are asked to support parents and children in facing up to the psychological and environmental challenges of modern society." Thus the practice of pediatrics has now begun to concentrate on handicaps in the very broadest sense. As a group these disorders have come to be known as "the new morbidity." The term was coined in the 1970s. The problems to which it refers defy solution by pills, injections, or anything else in the doctor's black bag.

Progress has also raised exceedingly difficult ethical questions about the treatment of severely damaged newborns, questions which also apply to the treatment of infants born weeks too early. Not so long ago medicine had little to offer these babies. In due course they died. Today such infants can be saved by therapies routinely employed in the intensive care settings of referral centers such as Children's. Whether these babies *should* be saved is a matter of controversy in and out of pediatrics. Two critical questions lie at the heart of the issue: what should be done, and who should decide?

The dilemma is dramatically illustrated by children born with significant open spine disease. Doctors know this disorder as myelomeningocele, a form of spina bifida. Mild cases are rather common, cause few if any problems, and may go entirely undetected. In severe spina bifida some portion of the spinal cord fails to close as the fetus develops, and the child is born with a visible lesion on the spine: an opening small or massive or a skin-covered cyst. Surgeons can remove the cyst or cover the opening. In fact if they don't close the back, and even if they do, the baby may die from meningitis.

But the most successful surgery cannot cure a child whose central nervous system has developed abnormally. In the severest cases, so many problems await such a child that doctors and parents may agree not to operate. In his office one afternoon, Children's neurosurgeon Guillermo Perez described to a visitor the anguish involved in making these decisions:

"This morning a couple had their first child. The baby had open spine disease. A few hours ago the parents had never heard of it. Everybody's heard of muscular dystrophy because of Jerry Lewis.

This is less common, but it's more common in children than cancer. The baby was put in an ambulance to come here, and the doctor said to the father, 'Go over and talk to Guillermo Perez. He'll close the spine, and it'll be okay,' or words to that effect.

"This child will probably be paralyzed. She will probably be retarded. There's a good possibility that she will have poor bladder and bowel control, that she will need surgery for a shunt to divert fluid from her head to her abdomen, that she'll need orthopedic surgery as time goes on, and that she'll require pediatric care for years. I tell the father that our options are two. We can do nothing and wait until the child dies, or we can go all out and get the best possible child, and we don't know how good. At the time of birth you can't predict.

"The father collapsed and cried. He called a priest. He called the baby's grandfather. They'll make a decision, and whichever it is, they'll be sorry. If they let the baby live, I could talk for a day and they wouldn't have any idea what they're getting into, the number of operations, the pain. . . ."

Perez sighed. "In Great Britain, they've come to the conclusion that it's not worth it. They tilt it in a way that parents will reject the idea of supporting the child. I don't have to tell you that any doctor can tilt so parents will say anything he wants them to. There all these kids are dead within six weeks. It's said that they're fed on demand, but if you give a baby morphine and he slips into a coma, there is no demand.

"In our experience, if you do nothing—put the child in an Isolette and give antibiotics—a good fifteen or twenty percent will survive. Eventually we'll find a nursing home. . . ." Perez mentioned a nearby institution where, he said, "there are full wards of these kids. One has a head bigger than its body. It doesn't move, but it talks. If you see it, you never forget it.

"Within ourselves we don't know what to do," Perez continued. "My colleague Dr. Kendall will tend to tell parents not to do anything. I tend now to be a little more optimistic. The former chief surgeon would get a judge [a court order] to operate. The longer I live, the less I know about how to handle this. In the whole U.S. there are only twenty or so pediatric neurosurgeons. At meetings when we are sitting around the bar in the evening and someone says, 'What will you do with a newborn myelo?' we have three-hour discussions. Nobody agrees with anybody else."

Thirty years ago most children born with open spine died in their first few years of life. Those who did not succumb to meningitis died from complications of hydrocephalus, which occurs in the great majority of cases. Antibiotics and improved technology have reversed these odds. With aggressive early treatment, most children born today with spina bifida will grow up to be productive adults with a number of health problems who will conduct their lives from wheelchairs. At least in theory they can expect long lives. Thanks to the development of the shunt in the 1950s, more than in the past will grow up with normal brains.

Citing these advances, the Spina Bifida Association of America has declared itself strongly opposed to a policy of nontreatment and is working to educate doctors out of their "negative" attitudes toward infants born with myelomeningocele.

But the physician overseeing the outpatient rehabilitation clinics at Children's until her death recently had a less sanguine perspective on youngsters growing up with this disease. Asked to comment on the myelo patients in her care, this doctor readily cited those who were doing well, then went on to observe that most in clinic were retarded and badly involved, that some would never live on their own or support themselves, that for those who might the transition from extraordinary dependence to self-sufficiency was made with great difficulty, that one patient old enough and well enough to hold a job and drive a car talked rarely of friends, that the quality of this young woman's life was "not so good." Sometimes the doctor wondered privately whether the shunt truly represented advancement for these patients. For her their tribulations were "matters of the soul."

In the past few years the dilemma posed by the birth of a child with serious defects has become a public matter. On at least four occasions since 1980 the courts have ruled on such cases. Two of those rulings were handed down in 1981. One involved Siamese twins born in Danville, Illinois. Reportedly, within moments after the delivery, the obstetrician and the father of the infants, himself a physician, had agreed not to support the twins. An order reading "Do not feed in accordance with parents' wishes" was written into the medical chart.

A week later the Illinois Department of Children and Family Services was notified by an anonymous caller that the twins were being neglected. The Department investigated, then filed for and was granted temporary custody. The parents and the obstetrician were charged with conspiracy to commit murder and with endangering the life and health of children—the first time criminal charges had ever been brought against parents and physicians for denying food or medical treatment to a newborn with significant anomalies.

Charges were dropped when no one came forth to testify against either the parents or the doctor. Eventually the twins went home with their parents and were separated by surgery at the age of one year.

Also in 1981 the parents of Elin Daniels, a child born with spina bifida, asked a Miami court for permission to let nature take its course. Permission was denied; the baby was treated. Early in 1982 the Indiana Supreme Court upheld the right of the parents of "Infant Doe," a little boy born with Down's syndrome and a deformed esophagus, to withhold treatment and nourishment. The child died as lawyers were preparing an appeal to the Supreme Court of the United States.

In October of 1983 a child was born on Long Island with spina bifida, hydrocephaly, and an abnormally small head. The parents refused surgery for "Baby Jane Doe." Though a lower court ordered the surgery, the parents' decision was endorsed first by the Appellate Division of the New York Supreme Court and then by the state's highest court, the New York Court of Appeals.

By this time, largely in response to the Infant Doe case in Indiana, the federal government under President Ronald Reagan had assumed a watchdog stance over anomalous infants. In March of 1983, having warned hospitals receiving federal funds that denying care to infants on the basis of handicaps was discriminatory and unlawful, the U.S. Department of Health and Human Services issued regulations requiring hospitals to post notices to this effect. Toll-free hot lines to HHS were installed to encourage the reporting of infractions. Hospitals were informed that government investigators were to have ready access to medical records.

Angered by what they saw as Big Brother intrusiveness, concerned that government review could cause delays that would themselves be harmful to infants, the American Academy of Pediatrics and twelve other organizations representing physicians and hospitals filed a suit against the Department. Among other things, the plaintiffs protested that the new rules had not been subject to the sixty-day comment period required in such circumstances.

The judge agreed. Weeks later, in July of 1983, HHS issued a revised set of regulations, this time inviting comments. Some sixteen thousand were received in the two months allotted. According to HHS officials, the overwhelming majority expressed support for the government's stand. Nevertheless, in an effort to neutralize the continuing opposition of the American Medical Association, among other groups, the Department retreated from its original stance, proposing that cases in question be reviewed first by voluntary hospital committees set up for the purpose and by the federal government only as a last resort. The regulations took effect in February 1984.

Meanwhile, since the government's right to accept complaints from citizens had never been at issue, the hot lines had remained hooked up. By the time of Baby Jane Doe's birth on Long Island in the fall of 1983, some forty cases had been or were being investigated. In none of the cases that had been closed had discrimination been substantiated. Though certain doctors and hospital administrators had expressed public dismay over the tactics of the so-called Baby Doe squads, the government had encountered no unsurmountable obstacles until, alerted to the New York case by a citizen having nothing whatever to do with it, HHS investigators requested the medical records of Baby Jane Doe.

Citing confidentiality, hospital officials said no.

HHS put the question to a judge, marking the first time the federal government had taken a case of this kind to court.

Federal Judge Leonard D. Wexler rejected the government's request. He saw no evidence of discrimination, he said. In view of medical forecasts that surgery would afford the child a very compromised, painful, and foreshortened life, it seemed to that judge that the parents were acting out of genuine concern for their daughter's welfare.

The government appealed. While the appeal was pending, the lesion on Baby Jane's back healed over, and fluid built up in her head to dangerous levels. To spare her needless discomfort, her parents agreed to shunt surgery. In April 1984 they took her home. In June the courts issued an order which in essence nullified the HHS regulations and imposed a permanent nationwide injunction against any further government actions of this nature. Again the Department appealed; again it lost.

In the fall of 1984 Congress passed and President Reagan signed legislation that both broadens the definition of child neglect and abuse to include "the withholding of medically indicated treatment" from disabled infants with life-threatening conditions and so strictly delimits the circumstances under which nontreatment may be justified as to in essence obligate physicians to treat any infant who is not indisputably dying or irreversibly comatose. Under this law, an amendment to the Child Abuse Prevention and Treatment Act of 1974, hospitals must designate a staff member responsible for reporting cases of suspected medical neglect; and states are asked to set up machinery in state child protective agencies through which such reports may be received and acted upon.

States are not required to comply. Those that do not, however, may lose federal support for their child abuse prevention programs. In addition to the above-mentioned provisions, the bill encourages hospitals to establish committees charged with, among other duties, "offering counsel and review in cases involving disabled infants with life-threatening conditions."

The new law is the product of intensive negotiations between liberal and conservative members of Congress and representatives of twenty-one medical, pro-life, and disabled rights organizations including the American Academy of Pediatrics and the National Association of Children's Hospitals and Related Institutions. By many or even most of those party to it, the bill is considered a compromise. The AAP and NACHRI among others see state oversight as vastly preferable to the federal intrusiveness which so rankled these groups in 1983. Militant right-to-life groups would have vastly preferred a bill endorsing an aggressive federal role.

The impact of this legislation on babies, their doctors, and their families will not be known for some time. Much will depend on the implementing regulations to be issued by HHS in the spring of 1985. In order for agreement to be reached among the various organizations involved, the bill was drafted in language general enough, observers feel, to permit a whole spectrum of interpretations.

Conceivably the regulations will be written in a way that effectively alters current practice very little in America's birth rooms and neonatal units, leaving the decisions about infants in crisis to family members and professionals directly involved in those cases. This is what pediatricians most hope will happen. Ethicists such as John Arras, philosopher in residence at Montefiore Medical Center in New York, further hope that the hospital committees proposed and encouraged by the legislation will be permitted the latitude to make "prudent moral judgments," including judgments that "go beyond the very stringent standards set by the federal government," as Arras puts it.

But there is no question that HHS could construe the law very narrowly indeed, or that stern regulations rigorously monitored—whether by the state or by pro-life groups—could result in a Big Brother intrusiveness considerably worse than the federal interventions of 1983. Fear of precisely this outcome caused the American Medical Association to withdraw from the negotiations that yielded the new law.

"Our basic position," says AMA Associate General Counsel B. J. Anderson, "is that these are the kinds of decisions that should be made by the family, with the physician providing whatever information and consultation the family wants or needs." For the most part, Anderson continues, AMA officials believe that these decisions as currently made are made appropriately.

As passed, the law makes no provision for parental discretion in the cases at issue. Treatment deemed medically beneficial must be given unless the baby's condition is clearly hopeless. "If there is to be any parental discretion," says John Arras, "it'll have to be carved out in practice by doctors and parents and hospitals."

Should HHS interpret the so-called Baby Doe legislation with restraint, the controversy engendered by the unprecedented court rulings and federal intercession of the early 1980s may ultimately be viewed as having performed a valuable service. By focusing attention on the issue, they have engaged the general public in a debate that has broad public ramifications.

At the very least a full airing of facts and opinions and feelings in this realm could afford parents confronted with a badly damaged baby a sounder basis for making a decision about that baby than has customarily been possible. Untold numbers of parents have faced these excruciating decisions virtually alone. Some have had the compassionate guidance of physicians who were nonetheless strangers.

Others have had little professional guidance, have encountered strongly opposing views in their own families, and have been nearly overwhelmed, in some cases, by a sense of isolation.

"I find it really comforting to know that this is somehow coming out of the closet and into the open," says a former head nurse at Children's. "Everybody suffered from being in the closet. The public attention is letting air into a deep, dark place, providing other viewpoints on matters which parents incompletely understand and which are thus decided on the basis of superstition. I'm happy about the debate."

More generally the discussion could help society as a whole reassess its priorities. Many staff members at Children's Hospital find it ironic that the same administration which has taken extraordinary measures to preserve the lives of handicapped infants has also cut back sharply on programs benefiting disabled children and adults. Some of those programs were inadequate to begin with. For the kind of child being saved in this decade, community supports are all but nonexistent. Where resources do exist or can be made to appear, they may be absorbed by children with severe disabilities at the expense of other children.

Should the government assume responsibility for extending life without making a commitment to nourish it? Do citizens wish to pledge tax dollars to that effort? Do parents have a right to say "Do everything" for a child who will not only be unable to contribute to society but may actually deny resources to a youngster who might better utilize them? These are questions deserving of the most careful public scrutiny.

Other large issues relating to the health and well-being of children are likewise matters of public policy. Infant mortality rates remain higher in America than in sixteen other nations. Among blacks infant mortality is twice as high as among whites. The overall death rate for black youngsters is considerably higher than for whites, one indication, according to the author of a standard pediatrics text, of "palpable differences in access to health care and other aspects of health maintenance between the haves and have-nots in our society."

Though injuries are far and away the leading cause of death and disability among the young in this country—in fact among all citizens under the age of forty-four—America has been remarkably slow to commit to injury prevention resources that are commensurate with the magnitude of the problem. Federal dollars are much more likely to go to disease prevention. One recent comprehensive study showed that although motor vehicle injuries cost the American economy nearly two-thirds of what cancer cost in 1975 in terms of medical and legal expenses and forgone earnings, tax moneys spent in cancer research and prevention totaled more than twenty-one times those spent on injury research and prevention.

Further insight into skewed federal priorities is offered by the organization chart of the National Institutes of Health. The U.S. government's principal medical research arm, NIH comprises eleven separate institutes, each dedicated to a major category of human ailment: cancer, heart disease, neurological disorders, infectious diseases, aging, and so on. There is no Institute of Injury at NIH. There is a program devoted to burns and trauma in the Institute of General Medical Sciences, but it is by no means the focal point of GMS, which also oversees programs in genetics, pharmacological sciences, physiology and biomedical engineering, and the cellular basis of disease.

Similarly, the federally funded Centers for Disease Control have yet to make a major effort to control injury. Asked to name the best federal programs in the field as a whole, William Haddon, Jr., M.D., a pioneer in injury research and currently president of the Insurance Institute of Highway Safety in Washington, D.C., replied, "As far as I am aware, there are *no* federal programs in injury research and prevention worthy of being called 'the best federal programs.'"

Until quite recently the medical profession itself has shown surprising indifference to injury prevention. Haddon believes that this is beginning to change among pediatricians in particular. But the newest editions of classic pediatrics textbooks, which run three or four inches thick, typically dispose of the major cause of childhood mortality and morbidity in one or two chapters or subchapters and some scattered references.

The reason appears to lie in the traditional belief that the accidents which lead to injuries result from chance, fate, or bad luck. Viewed as random events owing to errant human behavior, they are considered to be unpreventable except by modifications of behavior and are thus not seen as the business of the sciences, or at least of the physical sciences.

But experts now believe that "injury is no accident," as one researcher titled a 1978 article on the subject. The experts actually avoid using the term "accident" because it implies a randomness in patterns of injury that in fact does not exist. For example, boys are more likely to be hurt than girls, injury rates are higher in nonwhites than in whites, aggressive children have more accidents than timid children, hungry children are more at risk than those who have just eaten.

While behavior is a factor in accidents, many injuries can be prevented by means that don't depend on the individual. Deaths among young Americans have been reduced by the fifty-five-mile-per-hour speed limit, seat belts, and infant car seats; by smoke detectors and school crossing guards; by protective surfaces in playgrounds; by lifeguards and physical barriers in swimming areas; by campaigns against lead paint and the development of the "Mr. Yuk" warning label for toxic substances; and by childproof caps on medicine bottles—a partial list. Many more deaths could be prevented, experts believe, by such measures as raising the legal drinking age nationwide, restricting the sale and use of handguns, and abandoning driver education programs, which, because they have increased the absolute number of teenaged drivers on the nation's highways, have actually contributed to adolescent mortality from motor vehicle accidents.

Efforts to control accidents by changing behavior have often met with little success. Seat belt campaigns are a prime example. Furthermore, holding individuals responsible for getting hurt reflects an "obsession with blame," according to one expert, which disregards, according to another, the role played in injuries by the "social, political, economic, and physical environments that largely determine behavior." The new researchers are attempting to redirect society's thinking and its policies on environmental contributions to injury. They are also trying to convince physicians that prevention of injuries, the leading cause of death from birth till middle age, is no less the province of medicine than is the prevention of disease.

Staff members at Children's Hospital are sometimes asked why they or anyone would choose to work with sick children. Hearing the answers, one almost wonders why anyone elects to work with sick adults.

A pediatrician: "It's too depressing to take care of eighty-nine-year-olds dying of uremia. Though much of what I do is also depressing, I can always go see a kid with pneumonia who'll go home in a few days."

The chief of radiology: "Most adult medicine is not curative but allows the patient to maintain some sort of life-style despite a deteriorating body. Children are usually healthy before they get whatever brings them in here. After being one hundred percent sick, they're likelier than adults to bounce back to one hundred percent well. With kids we're dealing not with a few years but with fifty or sixty years of useful life."

A nurse: "I couldn't stand the complaints and whining in adults. A lot try to manipulate you. Kids may try to manipulate you too, but when kids complain, it's different."

Another nurse: "It's much easier to lift or turn a child than an adult who weighs two hundred pounds!"

A resident in general surgery: "Adults don't like having their bellies tickled!"

A pediatrician: "It's a lot of fun getting down on the floor and examining these kids while you play with them! Also, to overcome a child's fear, you have to be quite skilled. I felt that was a challenge."

Another pediatrician: "Kids forget quickly. After a shot, when the kids cry, I say, 'Give me a kiss,' and they do! It's great. Kids don't have the knowledge we have. They accept their handicaps. They accept pain. Adults *know* surgery is supposed to hurt, but we rarely use pain medications postoperatively for kids."

A resident in cardiac surgery: "Kids are innocent. You always feel you're making a contribution if you help one. You help a rapist who's been shot as you would anyone else, but you certainly have reservations. You don't have reservations with a child."

Sooner or later almost everyone mentions physiology. Though adults have more reserve, children have more resilience and more reparative powers. Infants have the ability to regenerate certain organs. Children's skulls are more flexible than those of adults and tolerate certain kinds of trauma much better. Children's brains can recover from insults that would leave adults vegetative. Children's systems are, in general, more elastic.

Illustrations are happily cited. "When a kid has a hernia, we operate on the child in the morning, he goes home in the afternoon, and he's riding his bike the next day," says the granddaddy of pediatricians at Children's. "Granted, it's different from hernia repair in an adult, but adults are out of work for three or four weeks, and they're holding their sides for a week.

"Yesterday a patient of mine had her nose bobbed. She's sixteen or seventeen and has colitis. A couple of hours after surgery I found her eating a McDonald's hamburger!

"We had one kid of thirteen who got Reye's syndrome. She went into a coma for about ten days. When we got her over the acute phase, she was still comatose. Just nothing. On Friday I went on vacation. On Wednesday I got a call telling me she woke up. That was in August. She went back to school normal in October. If that had happened to you or me, it would have been Karen Ann Quinlan."

The chief radiologist at Children's says the children's resilience keeps him humble. Whenever he begins to cherish the notion that professional intervention has contributed significantly to a diagnosis or cure, the doctor reminds himself that the child actually does most of the work in recovering and often just needs "a little push" to get better.

In acknowledgment of this bounce-back ability, the granddaddy pediatrician offers a piece of advice: "If you have to get sick, get sick as a kid."

Friday, December 7

The fifth-floor clinic waiting room was noisy with the happy sounds of children playing and of small birds chirping. The birds, brightly feathered, inhabit two cages rising to the ceiling from a low, carpeted island which also holds a free-form playhouse. Nearby are two huge tanks of tropical fish. Expanses of city are visible through windows along two walls of the waiting room, but this afternoon as usual, the view was getting no attention from clinic visitors.

A child with a ponytail watched the fish, her nose pressed flat against the glass. Behind her an older boy clambered headfirst into the playhouse through a porthole. Elsewhere in the room a mother shot marbles with her toddler son, a little boy drew a face with a marker on a white balloon, several children chased each other in a game of tag, several mothers exchanged news, and a bald, buxom teenager sat reading. Toys and books cluttered the floor in a cheerful mess reminiscent of a kindergarten. The young parents pushing their tot through the room in a wheelchair had to clear a route for themselves and for the boy's IV pole.

The child's face was pale and thin. What remained of his hair was an aura of gold filaments, a gossamer record of what had been, like the faded print of the old moon. The faces of his mother and father were drawn and solemn. Nowhere else in the building had more effort been devoted to neutralizing fear than within these particular four walls. But reality could not be dispelled. It hangs in the air of this room. Sooner or later and usually repeatedly, advances in treatment notwithstanding, reality lays a cold grip on the shoulder of anyone with business here. The sign in the hall reads ONCOLOGY CLINIC. This is the hospital's outpatient treatment center for children with cancer.

It is approached through the hallway by a path of red and yellow linoleum tiles. Gina DeRose and her parents came down that path and entered the waiting room at 3:30. They were carrying their coats. Despite the usual Clinic chaos, their arrival was noted immediately by one of two secretaries at adjoining reception desks to the left of the entrance. Charmaine's greeting was full of warmth. "Hi, Gina!"

Handing her coat to her father, the child veered left. She was chunky and a little too heavy, thanks in part to treatment, with alabaster skin and the dark brown eyes that ran in her tribe. Medicine had puffed her cheeks. Her brown wig had the wave and spring of natural curl. She was dressed in her school uniform: navy jumper and knee socks, light blue blouse, navy and white saddle shoes, the gold pin she had received upon making her first holy communion.

She'd been six then. Today she was eight-going-on-nine, an honor student in the third grade. Before being dropped for missing practice, she'd also been a cheerleader. She felt better now. She'd been in remission for six weeks. Despite her illness, she was a child in bloom. When feeling well—not full, not tired, not frightened— Gina Marie DeRose was irrepressible.

At Charmaine's desk, turning suddenly self-conscious, she

dropped her eyes. They happened to light on a full bowl of jelly beans.

Charmaine grinned. She was young and slim, with a short Afro and a model's features. "Help yourself! I see you brought your dad for a change." Gina's parents were settling themselves nearby on some molded blue chairs.

"Yeah, it's sleeting out, so he can't do construction today."

"Where's that cute little brother of yours?"

"*Cute?*" Her attempt to make a face fell apart in a giggle. "He's over at my grandmom's!"

"You feeling okay?" This from the other secretary, Ellie, who was older than Charmaine, white, and had short frosted hair. She had just hung up her phone.

"Yeah, know why? 'Cause I'm eating Charmaine's jelly beans!" When Gina was relaxed, her words nearly tripped over themselves in their haste to leave her mouth. She felt a tap on her shoulder. Whirling to face two more of the people she liked in Clinic, the child opened her mouth wide and pointed a finger at her back teeth.

"Cindy, see, the dentist just put fluoride on my teeth! Angie, see the vitamin on my teeth? It tastes orange!"

Cindy Strickland was head nurse in the Oncology Clinic, a tall, slender, composed woman in her late twenties. She was clad simply, in a beige dress and jacket. The woman with her was senior nurse's aide Angie Thomas, a flamboyant grandmother in her early forties, black, who favored sweaters in hot colors with her jeans and had a laugh that broke up her whole frame. She looked at Gina's parents and rolled her eyes. "Where'd you plug her in?"

Marie DeRose feigned exasperation. From her knitting bag she drew a crochet hook, a handful of precut lengths of thick acrylic yarn, and a rectangle of heavy white mesh, the backing for a rug with a *Star Wars* motif. "You want her? You can have her!"

Gina's mother was a very large woman, a hearty cook and an enthusiastic consumer of the delicious Italian fare she served her family day in and day out. Her husband, while stocky, was trim and compact. In personality he was also quite different from his wife. Marie was open and easygoing; she loved to talk and loved to tease. Her feelings were usually visible unless she was working to hide them.

Tony contained his feelings. Though genuinely warm in his way, he spoke only when he had thought out what he wanted to say and exhibited pleasure through slow smiles. Despite these dissimilarities, however, no one who had seen the DeRoses in the hours and days after Gina's diagnosis had had any doubts about the soundness of their union.

Gina went with Angie into the only office that opened directly onto the waiting room. By now she knew the whole routine very well: first Angie, then the lab, then the treatment room, then Dr. Sam, or sometimes Dr. Sam before the treatment room. At first the child hadn't wanted to go anywhere in Clinic without her mother and her father too, if he was there. Now she preferred to go to Angie and the lab by herself.

"Okay, Miss DeRose, up on the scale."

Gina took her shoes off and stepped onto the platform.

Angie tapped the weights. "All right, that's . . . forty-one point four kilos."

"What does that mean again?"

The senior nurse's aide pointed to a metric chart on her wall. "Remember I said a kilo is two point two pounds? So here's forty-one kilos. That's a little over ninety pounds. Then you add a little more for the four-tenths. It's about ninety-one."

"Did I lose?" She had decided on her own to diet.

"Maybe a few ounces. You still hitting the potato chips?"

"Not so much!"

"Gotta work on those salads!" Angie wrote Gina's weight in a notebook.

"I love vegetables!"

"Those too! Height!"

Still in her stocking feet, Gina backed up against a paper measure taped to the wall near the scale. She looked up into the face of the woman reading the numbers behind her. Angie was one of Gina's favorites. Angie had held Gina when she'd gotten the first needle in her back. Now she held her every time. Angie liked to talk too, so they matched. Angie made Gina laugh and made her forget about the needle while they were doing it to her.

"Has anybody else come in with leukemia?"

"Yeah, a lot." She entered Gina's height in the notebook. "In the beginning they don't feel so well. Then they get to feeling terrific. You know that yourself."

Gina nodded vigorously. "Yeah, and know what? We were visiting my aunt, and me and my cousin were playing and running all over the place, and when we got done, my cousin said to me, 'I thought you were sick!'"

"There you go! See what I mean? Now open your mouth, and let's get your temperature . . . that's good, just slow your motor and sit quietly for a minute, and then . . ." She opened a drawer. "And then we'll see what kind of sticker you want today."

The patient spoke around the thermometer. "Oh, goody!"

Deep down Gina did not like coming to Clinic. It was hard, because she did get to see Cindy and Angie and her social worker, and she liked seeing Charmaine and Ellie too. They were nice. Sometimes they gave her a job. Because she was there anyway and was always looking for something to do while she waited, she'd told them she wouldn't charge. Even so, Charmaine had given her fifty cents once for stamping papers. Sometimes they let her use a typewriter, and she typed poems from a book.

But Clinic ruined Gina's day. Sometimes she got home so late that she couldn't play outside very much. Also she missed a lot of work in school. Usually there were spelling bees on Fridays. She missed the spelling bees. And gym. On the days of Clinic she never felt like going. The worst was if she was going to get a needle in her back. Though it never hurt as much as she thought it was going to, she always felt scared.

From Angie's office Gina went back to the lab. She carried a piece of paper Cindy had given her to give to Bonnie. The lab is a narrow room with walls of white, cabinets of gray, countertops of black, and machines and microscopes in gray and silver. On one wall is a color poster of Raggedy Ann framed in orange. On another wall is a color picture of two bulldog puppies cut from a calendar. When nobody is talking in the lab, the sounds there are hums, whirs, buzzes, and an occasional beep.

"Hi, Gina! You're back!" Bonnie's thick black hair was swept back into a knot. With her gold hoop earrings, the young woman seemed dressed up even in slacks and low shoes.

"Hi." Gina was beginning to worry about the finger stick. She always had to tell herself that it didn't really hurt that much. It was like a pinch, and then drops would start coming out, and Bonnie would get like a regular drinking straw except regular straws don't bend, and press it over, and the blood would come out into the straw.

She sat down. She watched in silence as the technician made preparations. When Bonnie got ready to put the alcohol on, Gina held out her forefinger. In the beginning she had pulled her hand away.

Bonnie picked up the blade. It was a pediatric lancet, the only piece of equipment in the lab tailored especially for children. A standard lancet might go right through a child's finger. The blade was so small that Gina could hardly see it.

"Ready?"

"Real fast, okay?"

"Okay. One, two, three . . ."

"Ouch!"

Sticking a child's finger as Bonnie stuck Gina's yields about four drops of blood. Some tests involved in cancer treatment require larger amounts. For those a nurse draws blood through a needle in a vein. But finger sticks are used for routine studies in the Oncology Clinic at Children's. This is partly because a child's veins are small and hard to find and partly because the oncologists try to save the blood vessels in a youngster who might one day need every available sound vein for transfusions of blood, medicines, and the other fluids typically summoned for a life in crisis.

With the mouthpiece end of a narrow white tube between her lips, Bonnie touched the other end to the quivering red sphere on Gina's finger and sucked the blood into the tube.

Gina watched the drop disappear. "What do you call that thing again?"

"Micropipette."

"Do you ever get blood in your mouth?"

Bonnie smiled. A familiar question. "That's happened a couple of times."

Placing the free end of the white tube into a clear plastic cup, the technician blew the blood into a small amount of buffer solution. She covered the cup with a plastic cap. From there the blood would go into six tiny vials and onto two slides. It would then be analyzed under a microscope and by machine. That would take about half an hour. When the testing was finished, Dr. Sam Silver would know whether Gina was still in remission and whether she was in more danger from her medications than she absolutely had to be.

For no known reason, her bone marrow had suddenly begun producing too many white blood cells—so many that they had hoarded all the nutrients necessary for the production of red cells and platelets, the clotting factor in the blood.

Leukemia takes two forms, depending on which white cells are involved. Gina had acute lymphocytic leukemia, the commonest malignancy in childhood. "The good kind," it is called by doctors and nurses at Children's, because a child with ALL is more likely to come through it alive than are patients with any other form of cancer. So her prognosis was excellent.

But she could relapse at any time.

If she continued in remission three years without a relapse, her doctors would be able to conclude that her leukemia was probably not going to come back. Only when the child had been disease-free and off medication for five years, however, would the doctors begin to speak of cure.

That day was a long way off. She had just been diagnosed in late September.

The first day she could remember feeling sick was a Tuesday. She'd come home from school too tired to play. At suppertime she'd felt too full to eat. On Wednesday after school she had felt too sick to go to cheerleading.

Thursday morning had been better. But on Thursday afternoon she had felt tired enough to lie down on the couch. Her throat had been sore. She'd felt full again. That night she had vomited and run a fever of 101 degrees. Her mom had given her Tylenol. On Friday her fever had been 103 degrees.

Gina had been worried about the fever. She'd been afraid that her mother would take her to Dr. Potts to get a needle from Simone. Simone gave hard needles. Knowing she was just getting a cold, Gina hadn't thought she needed a shot.

But Dr. Potts had come to the house that Friday night and had given her a needle himself. He'd told her to stay in bed and take Tylenol. On Sunday her fever had gone up to nearly 105 degrees.

On Monday her mom had taken her to Dr. Potts's office. He had checked her and said it was probably a virus. He'd told her to keep up the Tylenol.

But she hadn't gotten better. She'd missed school all five days. The next Monday, in his office, Dr. Potts had given Gina a blood test and told her mom that he would call tomorrow with the results. That day Gina had known she had something bad.

And tomorrow had never come. Dr. Potts had called that same night and said she would have to go to Children's Hospital the next morning. He had already made reservations for her.

She had been so scared. Knowing she'd have to stay, thinking she was going to get an operation, Gina had been more scared than she'd ever been in her life. She had already had one operation. When she was five, she'd had to get her tonsils out at another hospital. She'd had to stay then too. They'd given her a needle to make her fall asleep, and they'd put bars up like a crib and taken her upstairs to where the operating room was, and Gina had started jumping up and down because she had not wanted whatever they were going to do to her. She'd wanted her mother.

"Is my mom coming?" she had asked the nurse on the way.

"Yes," the nurse had told her. "She has to get your bed ready for you and do a few things, and then she'll come straight upstairs and you'll see her."

Thinking this would really happen, Gina had calmed down a little. They had taken her into a room with black balloons all over the place. The doctor had said she had to blow up a big black balloon. A nurse had held the balloon around her nose and mouth, and Gina had breathed through it and fallen asleep, and they had put a needle down there and taken her tonsils out. She hadn't felt a thing.

Even so, she hated hospitals.

She'd only known two other kids who'd gone to the hospital. One was her cousin who'd gotten hit by a car. He'd broken one leg and had a concussion, but he'd been all right.

The other boy had been in the first grade when Gina had been in second. Running after his ball one night, he'd gotten all shmushed by a bus. Bones all over the street. Her girlfriend's brother had known the boy. Real small. Red hair. He'd gone to a hospital and died there.

That first day in the Clinic she had cried when they'd taken her blood and screamed bloody murder when they'd given her a needle in her back to take some marrow out to get the results, but whenever she wasn't feeling scared about the needles, she'd felt scared about having to stay.

The doctors had taken her mom and dad away to talk to them alone. A social worker had stayed with Gina. When her parents came back, Gina had noticed that her mom's eyes were all red and tears were coming down.

"She'll have to know," Dr. Silver had said gently toward the end of that initial conversation, and at first the child's father had resisted.

But listening to the doctor's explanations, Tony DeRose had become convinced that Silver was right. Gina was to be admitted to the Oncology Unit that afternoon. She would hear the term. The doctors and nurses would be doing a lot of things to her. A child her age would need to know why, especially a child as smart as Gina, who was already asking many questions. Treatment would be long and drawn out. If she knew what she had, she wouldn't always be wondering.

Chances were she would find out anyway, by accident, Silver had suggested. If they told her the truth now, she wouldn't have any fear that her parents would lie to her in the future. She would trust them. If she knew, the doctors wouldn't have to duck her questions. They could teach her as much as she wanted to learn. Understanding the disease would help her cope with it.

It wouldn't be necessary to tell her immediately, Dr. Silver had said. They could wait a day. If Marie and Tony wanted to tell her themselves, fine. If they'd prefer that the doctors tell her, fine.

At this point the DeRoses had been at Children's a little more than four hours. Tony had been impressed with the Clinic doctors. They had shown a lot of concern. They had treated Gina very well. They'd sat with her, talked with her, explained everything to her, which had taken time because the child had been so frightened.

Her father had been especially impressed at how the doctors had gone about taking a sample of bone marrow from Gina's pelvis. She'd been absolutely terrified. They had treated her with gentleness and kindness and had not made a move without telling her what they were doing. "Now Dr. Silver is washing his hands. Now he's moving his chair. Now he's opening his pack. Now he's taking out the needle. Now Angie is going to rub a spot on your back with alcohol on a gauze pad, and it will feel cold. Now Dr. Silver is getting the medicine ready." Like having a mirror there, Tony had thought. Every single thing they had done they had told her first, and everything they had told her had been the truth.

If he had had any experience with them before that day, perhaps Tony DeRose would have let the Clinic doctors tell his oldest child and only daughter that she had cancer. As it was, he'd thought Gina would accept that news better from him.

She had sat before him white and scared on a hard table in a place she'd never been before surrounded by people she had just met.

Everything her father knew about her disease at that moment he had learned in the past half hour.

In his whole life Tony DeRose had known of only one person with leukemia: the son of comedian Red Skelton. Tony had been a kid himself when he'd heard about it. The boy had died.

After talking on the phone with Dr. Potts Monday night, Gina's father had hung up thinking in terms of weeks. Now, the next afternoon, the doctors at Children's were saying they could probably cure Gina. That news, too, had been totally unexpected.

Tony had looked over at his wife. She'd been staring past him, eyes full.

Taking Gina's hand, he had told her as much as he could find it within himself to say. When he'd choked on the word, the doctors had provided it for him.

Her dad had told her that she had a bad disease of her blood. Leukemia. She had never heard the word. The doctors had said they didn't know how it started. It was like it just came from air. Though the doctors hadn't explained it this way, Gina had understood them to say that her bad cells were taking the place of her good cells, like one country taking over another country. The doctors had to try and get that country to be the good cells again so all the cells could do their duty, instead of just one doing it and the others couldn't.

The doctors had said her kind of disease was the easiest because they had medicines that could help her. But she would have to stay in the hospital for a few days. After that she would need treatments for a long time.

They had asked her if she had any questions.

She had asked them how long she would have to stay.

They had said she could maybe go home in five days or a week. They had told her that her mom could stay with her in the hospital all night.

She had asked if she was going to get an operation.

They had said no.

She had not been able to understand why this was happening to her. Why her? Her dad had said "disease." Diseases were serious. She must have done something wrong. God was punishing her. But what had she done?

Crying, throwing her arms around their necks, she had begged her parents to take her home.

Gina had never wished for anything that her father wanted more to give her.

Moments later, while her parents were talking to the doctors, Gina had asked her social worker in a very small voice if she was going to die.

The social worker, a graduate student specializing in work with sick children, had looked down into the eight-year-old face beside her and taken a calculated risk.

The child had been admitted that same afternoon to the twelve-bed Oncology Unit around the corner from Adolescent on the sixth floor. There, within hours, she had begun treatment. Discharged after six days, though still tired, Gina had felt better and looked better. Unless she relapsed, she would probably never again need to be hospitalized for leukemia.

Treatment for her disease takes place in three phases. Gina had completed two of them by Thanksgiving. The first, begun that week in the hospital and known as Induction, had killed off leukemia cells in vast numbers and flushed them from her system, putting her into remission within twenty-eight days.

The second phase had begun exactly one month from the date of diagnosis. Known as Intensification, this part of treatment is aimed at preventing the disease from spreading to the central nervous system. Five days a week for two weeks running, Gina had received cranial irradiation at the university hospital next door to Children's. Before, during, and after that period she had, at Clinic, received six injections into her spinal fluid of Methotrexate, the first anticancer drug successfully used against leukemia. Four days after the last of ten visits to the radiotherapist, Gina had returned to school.

In principle she was now in the third phase of therapy, Maintenance. She was supposed to be taking orally, at home, a precise combination of four drugs which, along with periodic injections in Clinic, were intended to maintain her remission with a minimum of side effects. Gina was supposed to be coming to Clinic only once a month.

However, she was experiencing minor problems from one of the drugs. The oral Methotrexate was causing her liver to produce a surplus of enzymes. In itself this posed no immediate danger. Sometimes the liver merely needs time to adjust to the unfamiliar chemicals. Left unchecked, however, the malfunction could in time result in severe damage to the organ.

Gina's doctor had taken her off Methotrexate temporarily. He wanted to give her liver a chance to regenerate. Yet the child could relapse if she received lower doses of the drug than were considered optimal. So Dr. Silver was working to ascertain the maximum dosage of Methotrexate that the patient's body could tolerate within prescribed limits and to get her on that dosage as soon as possible. Even a minimized dose of Methotrexate would be better than the next-best anticancer agent of its type.

As long as the enzyme problem remained unsolved, then, Gina would be coming to Clinic every week or two.

On a Sunday evening two weeks after her discharge from Children's, Tony DeRose had sat reading in the living room across from his daughter, who had also been reading, and she had suddenly burst into tears. When he'd gone to her, she had sobbed against him. "I don't want to die!"

He had taken her into his lap. "You're not going to, Gina. You're not going to."

"But I'm real sick."

"You *were* real sick. But you're mostly better now. You're still not all better. You've still got to take your medicine and go for your treatments. But you're mostly better."

"How long do I have to take it for?"

"It might be for a month, it might be for a year, it might be ten years."

"*Ten years?*"

"What's ten years? Other people take medicine every day just like you do, Gina. Your grandfather takes medicine every day for his ulcers. It's no big thing. The important thing is that you're okay again."

Which was what the child's father had chosen to believe himself.

Now she felt like she always had, except when she had to take the medicines. Gina hated taking them. Some she had to take in the morning, some when she got home from school, some before she went to bed. Her dad had put a chart up on the refrigerator. Bactrim, the long green pills, one in the morning, one and a half at night, on Monday, Wednesday, and Friday. 6MP, the white pills like aspirin, one and a half every day. Methotrexate, the little yellow pills, eight on Fridays. Prednisone, the white pills shaped like aspirin but smaller, only some days, nine a day.

At first she had not known how to take a pill. In the hospital she had practiced with TicTac candies and gagged on every one. Now she squished the pills in a spoon, stuck them in a glass of water or soda, and drank them down. Some of them didn't taste so good. But Dr. Sam had told Gina that the medicines she was getting weren't as bitter as what some other people took, because her disease was the easiest kind, and they had it under control.

Before the medicines, before the hospital, Gina had felt too sick to do anything. Now she could do anything she wanted.

She could do anything she'd done before, and she looked better, and she was back in school, but she was still not the old Gina, in her mother's opinion.

Before getting sick, Gina would go upstairs by herself at bedtime and read before going to sleep. Now she waited for her dad to go up with her. Before getting sick, she'd turn on the stereo in the living room every afternoon after school and do disco and sing.

Now she might do that once a week. She didn't talk and laugh at the dinner table as much as she once had. She still played outside after school, but while before getting sick she was constantly wanting to go out, now some days she preferred to lie down. Her family saw the old Gina at times. But she just wasn't as bouncy or happy-go-lucky now as she had been before she got cancer.

Her mother kept reminding herself that things were better. Things *were*. Sitting awake that first night at the hospital, seeing Gina's fear, her whiteness, her helplessness, thinking her daughter as good as dead, Marie had thought her heart could not bear the hurt she knew must lie ahead for all of them.

The first week home had been no easier. Gina had scarcely let her mother out of her sight. She had watched Marie's reactions constantly. For the first time in her life, Marie had envied her husband. A man at work could cry. She could not cry while Gina was watching her. So she had forced herself to postpone her tears, concentrating instead on trying to learn the names of medicines she could not pronounce, checking Gina's temperature, taking care of her, making time for Little Tony, who was two, and going back and forth to Clinic three times a week. But as soon as Gina had gone to bed, her mother's head would fill with unendurable pictures. Night after night Marie had cried herself to sleep in Tony's arms.

Then when she had finally begun to feel some hope, to believe that Gina might actually make it, to get back into a routine that resembled normalcy, the problem had developed with the liver enzymes.

When Dr. Silver had first told her they were elevated, Marie hadn't understood what he was talking about. But she had understood that something was wrong, because he had taken Gina off the Methotrexate. It had been obvious to Marie that Dr. Silver would rather not have done this. So now she was holding her breath again. She was always holding her breath. It changed everything, Gina having cancer. Marie DeRose was never free of the fear that one day the doctors were going to say, "Well, it doesn't look good."

They had gotten her into remission, but she could still die.

Before the enzyme problem developed, Gina's mother had found herself able to push such thoughts from the front of her mind to the back of her mind. She could do that once in a while.

At Children's, never. Coming back was always hard. Marie always arrived in Clinic with lumps in her stomach and fighting tears. She had been relieved this morning to see that none of the children in the waiting room had looked too sick. Even the boy in the wheelchair didn't look as bad as some Marie had seen.

She'd seen children looking really bad, especially in the mornings, when Clinic was busiest. Marie kept remembering a little black girl, thin as a toothpick, with no hair and one very swollen foot like a ball at the end of her leg. The child had been too weak to walk or even sit up. Sometimes there were kids with visible tumors. Every time she saw a child who didn't look good, Marie would think, *That could be Gina next week.*

She did not like coming to Clinic in the mornings. One saw sights in the afternoons too. But somehow the afternoons were better.

Cindy had directed them to wait for Dr. Silver in Examining Room 5, a boxlike space furnished with a desk, two straight chairs, and a standard examining table covered by a white paper runner. Gina sat on the table fully dressed. Sam Silver's appearance was without formality, in part an accident of nature. The doctor's body had the lank and looseness of a basketball player's. His presence as a threat was further diminished by worn spots in the knees of his fading pale blue corduroy trousers. Silver was twenty-nine and tall, with black-rimmed glasses, a mustache, and tousled brown hair cut like a monk's.

"Hi, everybody." He took a moment to greet the adults. Marie appreciated this. Whenever Dr. Sam called her with test results, he always asked first how everybody was.

He stood in front of Gina. "And how are *you?*"

"I'm fine, know why? Because I don't have to get a needle in my back today!"

He nodded. "That's right, you're not due again till . . . when is it, end of next month, I think?"

"And I'm never going to have a bone marrow unless you give it to me!"

Behind the doctor's back Marie looked at Tony and rolled her eyes. Gina had insisted on this arrangement from the first day—insisted on Dr. Sam to give the needles in her back, insisted on Angie to hold her, insisted on Cindy to draw blood from her vein when staff needed more blood than could be yielded by a finger stick, insisted on Cindy for chemotherapy injections. When Angie or Cindy wasn't available, Gina would accept a substitute. For the bone marrow she would have nobody but Dr. Sam. If he was busy, she'd wait for him.

"What have you been doing in school?" He glanced at the numbers Angie had written in the chart.

"Well, my girlfriend was over last night because we were doing a project for Catholic Schools Week."

"What's the project?" He laid the chart aside.

"We had to get a big poster and glue on some pictures of our family and bring it in."

From the desk drawer he removed a tongue depressor. "Sounds like fun," he said cheerfully.

"Yeah, it was! Hey, Sam, wait a second—see that cup on the desk that says DOCTOR?"

"Yeeeess?"

"We got one like that for my dad for his birthday that says SLAVE!"

Silver laughed but moved closer to her. "Okay, Gina, open your mouth."

"Don't put that on the back of my throat, okay? Just stick it on my tongue. . . . Aaaaagggghhh!"

She had been one of his first patients here. On the morning her parents had brought Gina in for diagnosis, Silver had happened to be the doctor in Clinic with the fewest ongoing cases and thus the most time available. He'd been at Children's a matter of months. Born in Rhode Island, he had gone to medical school in Illinois, done a four-year residency at a pediatric hospital in Pennsylvania, and come to Children's to specialize in the treatment of pediatric cancer. His title was oncology fellow. The fellowship was to last two years.

"Okay, Gina, will you slip your jumper top down and lift up your blouse so I can listen to you breathe through the stethoscope?"

When he laid the metal on her skin, she jumped.

"Oooh! Your hands are cold!" Giggle.

"Oh, sorry." He hung the stethoscope over his wrist and rubbed his palms together to warm them. When he touched her again, she shivered.

"Still cold! What did you do, put your hands in the refrigerator all day?"

He laughed. He had liked Gina from the start. Once feeling better, she had turned into a real character—bubbly, vivacious, delightful, incredibly sophisticated. Some eight-year-olds in Clinic were almost sullen. Silver always felt he knew what Gina had on her mind. He could talk to her.

This hadn't happened overnight. After being hospitalized, she had come to Clinic terrified, especially about getting a needle in her back. The first time he had had to give her one, she had threatened before he'd even touched her to scream bloody murder, and she had. The second time she had screamed less. The third time she'd said it was "fun."

About then she had begun to exhibit a very good eight-year-old's understanding of both the disease and the treatments. Hair loss is devastating for any child, but Gina had handled hers well. This was not atypical, in Silver's experience. Most kids he'd known had displayed an amazing ability to rebound and were more sophisticated than people gave them credit for. Still, Gina was a special personality. She had coped with her disease remarkably well.

He removed the stethoscope prongs from his ears. Letting them rest on the back of his neck, he checked the child's eyes and ears, felt the glands in her neck and under her arms, asked her to lie down so he could feel her abdomen, told her she could sit up again and put her jumper top back up, and then he remembered to ask about her hair.

Her response was offhand. "It's growing in! But it itches."

"Do you want to show it to me?"

A shrug. "Okay."

A shrug. Her hair had been medium brown, naturally frizzy and unusually thick—"bushy like a witch's hair!" she'd say, laughing— and had hung halfway down her back. It had been cut only once in Gina's lifetime: the day before she had received her first communion. One afternoon six weeks after the first chemo treatment, her hair had begun to come out in her brush. The next few mornings she had picked it up in handfuls from her pillow. What remained of her witch's bush had then disappeared almost overnight. She had grieved in bouts of weeping that had broken her parents' hearts.

They had tried to get her to look on the bright side. "At least you're healthy and you're here," they had told her. "Isn't this better than being sick?"

Marie had even ventured a little affectionate teasing. "If anybody says anything about you being bald," she had advised the first day her eldest had worn the wig to school, "just pull your wig off and show them! Shock the hell out of them!" The child had reacted by laughing. "Mom, you're crazy!" When feeling well, Gina could take such teasing from her mother. She accepted it from no one else and now refused to discuss her feelings on the subject of her hair with anyone including her mother.

Snatching off her wig for Dr. Silver, Gina became instantaneously a creature from science fiction in a Catholic school uniform. "It's coming in black!" the child informed her doctor.

He could see that it was. Often this first growth was frosted and curly, which made boys furious. Gina's was a field of fine, dark stubble.

"Oooh, my head's hot! Feel my head!"

He rested his palm on her scalp. "Are you wearing your wig all the time?"

"Yeah, except I can take it off when I'm home with my family."

After making a few notes, the physician gave his patient and her parents some news that brought the adults a considerable measure of relief. The blood tests from last week had shown enough improvement in Gina's enzyme levels, Silver said, that he had decided to put her back on the full dose of Methotrexate.

A moment later he excused himself to check the finger stick results, and he returned with more good news. The blood counts were fine. This told the DeRoses without his having to spell it out that Gina was still in remission.

Her parents felt no need to question the doctor further. He had stressed from the beginning that he would keep no secrets from them. When things were going well, Silver had promised, he would tell them so. If things began to go less well, he would tell them that. In Tony's mind, this had been one of the best things the doctors at Children's had done for him: they had let him know that he could trust what they said. They pulled no punches. They answered any question straight from the shoulder, good or bad.

They had also offered him a shoulder to lean on. They tried to help him and his family in any way they could. Tony had observed this to be true of all the people in Clinic. He could see it wasn't just a job for them. They really cared.

"Okay, Gina, that's all, except the nurses will need to draw some blood again for the enzyme studies. You won't have to come back next week . . ."

"Yay!"

". . . so I'll see you the week after. I'll call Wednesday or Thursday with those results," he added to Marie.

Goodbyes were said. The doctor turned to go and was stopped by the voice of his patient.

"Hey, Sam, do you say nine and five *is* thirteen or nine and five *are* thirteen?"

He appeared to think this over. "Gee, I don't know."

"They're both wrong! Nine and five are fourteen! Do you know why Uncle Sam wears red, white, and blue suspenders?"

Hand on the doorknob, he exchanged glances with Marie and Tony. "Nope. I guess you'll have to tell me."

"To hold his pants up!" She giggled. "Do you know how much dirt there is in a hole two feet by two feet by two feet?"

"Gina . . ."

Once again he claimed ignorance.

Delight and triumph gathered in her face. "None!"

Sunday, December 9

Mark's lung had started to collapse again.

As planned, Dr. Cipriani had discontinued suction and clamped the chest tube on Friday afternoon. All Friday night and the next morning Mark had been fine except for pain. But yesterday's x-ray had shown a small increase in the size of the air cap in his pleural cavity, meaning that the lung was still leaking, that the hole hadn't sealed over, that the lung wasn't staying up without suction. Dr. Cipriani had had to unclamp the chest tube and restart the suction.

Mark had been very upset. He had not expected a setback.

Worse news had come this morning. He had awakened having

unusual trouble breathing. As time passed, he had grown more and more air-hungry. Finally they'd done a chest x-ray which had shown a twenty-five percent pneumothorax—the same amount of collapse that had occurred that first night. After eight days, he was right back where he'd started—except he'd had a chest tube in him for eight days that hadn't worked.

Disappointment had hit him like a punch.

Dr. Cipriani had come back to Adolescent and had turned up the dial on the wall suction to make it as strong as possible. Another x-ray had been done. Mark was waiting now to hear the results. If there was no improvement, he might have to have another chest tube.

He feared it. He feared the pain of the insertion. He feared the pain of having two tubes in him when one already hurt. The pain was constant. He needed codeine and Tylenol several times during the day and chloral hydrate at night so he could sleep. Once on Friday he had refused the codeine and Tylenol, but he hadn't been able to tolerate the pain.

He was afraid that he was going to have to stay in the hospital longer than another week. Not least he feared the effects of a second chest tube on his appetite. The pain medications made him feel too spaced out and sleepy to eat. He wanted to get off them. He had already lost several pounds since coming into the hospital. He could not afford to lose any more.

He tried to control these fears by not thinking about them. He reminded himself that Christmas was still more than two weeks away.

Ø

Two floors down, oblivious of the coming of Christmas, Jody Robinson played by himself in his stainless-steel crib in the Intermediate Intensive Care Unit. Though connected to a respirator by two fat accordion-pleated plastic tubes that dropped down his PRE-CIOUS CARGO T-shirt from a brass swivel under his chin, though endowed with "Charlie Brown cheeks," as the nurses called them, from a lifetime of artificial ventilation, a full-moon face that concealed his tracheostomy and all but concealed his neck, the child looked neither sick nor miserable. He was a chunky baby of eighteen months with a crisp Afro, an oversized belly, and a lump for a belly button, and his attention had just been captured by a 50 cc. syringe—plastic, no needle—in a white paper sheath.

He found a way to open the sheath. Pulling out the syringe, he studied it, turning it this way and that in his pudgy brown hands, then made several attempts to put it back. He got interested in the wrapper. Dropping the syringe, he began to wave the paper furiously in the air over his head, brushing it against the wooden pole tied to his crib from end to end which held his rings and trapeze. The paper crackled. Jody beamed. He set the wrapper down on his bare toes. He moved a toe and watched, fascinated, as the paper drifted toward him about a third of an inch. He looked around the unit to see if anyone might be available to share in this fun.

The view from Jody's mattress was actually only half of Intermediate. Five cribs lay on the other side of a partition. He could see only the two patients in the cribs on either side of him and the two in cribs opposite. Of course he could also see any adults who happened to be in the vicinity. At the moment there were several: a couple of parents, a couple of nurses. One was Jody's primary nurse, Marla Meyerle, who was busy bathing another baby. Neither she nor anyone else was looking Jody's way.

He watched her for some seconds. Then he began to survey his own belongings. Toys surrounded him on his mattress: a calico bunny, a teddy bear, a stuffed dog, a stuffed owl, a fuzzy monkey in a red jacket who clapped tiny cymbals together when wound up, a block on wheels, a yellow plastic cowboy, a big yellow plastic top, a red plastic telephone, a red plush heart decorated with white ribbons and red letters spelling I LOVE YOU. At the foot of the bed was a small white laundry bag crammed full of Jody's clean clothes.

He moved down the bed and reached for his cowboy. He examined it, then flipped his arm sharply and let the cowboy go. It startled him by landing between his legs.

He regarded it there. After a moment he picked it up and threw it again. This time it clattered to the floor.

Scooting forward on his diapered bottom, he pressed his forehead against two side rails and peered down.

"Jody, what did you do?" Marla had turned to look at him.

He gazed at her and waited for clues.

"Poor Jody! Did you drop your cowboy?"

Grinning, he slapped his hand against the full laundry bag.

The hand bounced high. This surprised him. He went back for more, slapping the bag again and again, delighted, until Marla, pretending to scold the child for beating up on his poor laundry bag, came to Jody's bedside and reached over the rails.

He grabbed her hands. Standing him up, she kissed the top of his head. Marla was large-busted, built like an English teacher, she had always thought—a creamy-skinned woman of thirty, older than many of her colleagues in Intermediate, and divorced. Her hair was blond and frizzy, swept back on either side with silver barrettes. She had been at Children's a year and a half, almost exactly as long as Jody.

"You're a silly!"

He gave her his fabulous laugh. Any other description would demean the truth. Jody's laugh was one of a kind. First his whole face became transfigured by a toothy smile of joy so pure, so unreservedly trustful of the moment that to see it was to feel joy reaffirmed in oneself and the world; and then, throwing his head back, the baby let himself be overcome, opening his mouth wide in extravagant, soundless rapture, drawing his top lip down over his two top teeth, a personal signature, hunching up his shoulders, and squeezing his eyes so nearly shut over his chubby brown cheeks that Marla kept warning him he was going to crack his face in two. Jody's laugh was soundless because the hole in his throat through which the ventilator gave him breath made him mute. But his laughter shed light and warmth in such measure that people who saw it stood waiting for it to happen to them again.

Laughing with him, Marla picked up his cowboy for him and gave her patient a careful hug.

He had been born a month early to a nineteen-year-old unmarried drug addict who had had no prenatal care. To what extent her addiction accounted for her son's condition at birth may never be known. In his first moments outside the womb, the baby had appeared to be normal. Every finger, every toe was perfectly formed. But when a nurse had tried to suction him, she had been unable to get the tube down his throat.

He had been transferred to Children's Hospital at the age of three hours. There he had been discovered to have significant internal defects. Bluntly put, his insides were a mess. His trachea or windpipe was completely blocked by a thick web, an extremely rare anomaly that allowed no air to pass to or from his lungs. His esophagus ended in a blind pouch, which meant he could not take nourishment by mouth. He could not have digested food in any case because his lower intestine also ended in a blind pouch. He had no anus. He had a small heart defect, a hole between two chambers.

He had other malformations, which, by an astonishing quirk of fate, had actually kept him alive long enough to even get to Children's. In a normal baby the esophagus and the trachea are wholly separate ducts. In Jody the two were connected by passageways of tissue. At one site a split or cleft in the trachea adjoined a cleft in the esophagus where nature had simply failed to finish a task. These anomalies permitted the flow of oxygen to and from the baby's lungs despite his blocked airway. Without such defects Jody Robinson would have died, probably within hours.

A decade earlier he would have died anyway. The technology of medicine would not yet have been sophisticated enough to keep him alive. Born when he was, he would have died had he not been turned over to experts.

Doctors at Children's had never seen a tracheal blockage such as Jody had, and his combination of anomalies was peculiar to him. But individually, except for the web in his windpipe, the baby's defects were all familiar to the Children's physicians. All had been treated successfully in other infants. While treating the combination successfully was a much greater challenge, the alternative to trying was to lose the patient. The child could not survive with minimal respiratory function and no digestive function. His anomalies were incompatible with life. At Children's, however, they were deemed to be correctable, at least in principle. As complicated a case as Jody Robinson presented, he was not the most complicated newborn the Children's experts had ever seen.

In the first eight days of his life the baby went to the operating room four times. He went back fourteen times over the next twelve months. Several of the operations were small ones that amounted to checkups. Most of the surgery was major repair work: the opening into his throat through which the child could be ventilated, an opening into his stomach through which he could be fed, a colostomy through which he could eliminate fecal waste, closures of the abnormal connections between his trachea and esophagus, revisions of repairs that had broken down.

In one of the earliest operations surgeons also cut off the closed end of Jody's esophagus, leaving a short but healthy segment which they rerouted sideways to a small incision in the side of his neck. This gave the baby's saliva a point of exit. The diversion was also a way to keep the esophagus in working order against the day when the surgeons hoped to provide the patient with a functioning digestive tract.

Months later they were able to make some progress toward this goal. On Jody's first birthday they made him an anus, fashioning a sphincter out of the patient's own muscle. To this new orifice they sewed the lower end of his colon, from which they had cut the tip off the pouch. Combined with the closing of the colostomy a month later, this surgery gave Jody one half of a working digestive system.

He had had his most recent surgery at the age of fifteen months. At that time the ear-nose-and-throat specialist had improved the architecture of the child's larynx with pieces of a rib harvested from Jody's chest. A normal larynx, the structure which houses the vocal cords, is rather stiff with muscle and cartilage. Lacking some of this firm framework, the patient's larynx had tended to collapse in upon itself. The surgeon's solution had been to sew two strips of rib along the outer wall of the passageway, one on either side, anchoring the ends of each strip to the skeleton of good cartilage above and below the underdeveloped section at the entrance to the trachea.

Insofar as planned surgery was concerned, two major operations remained on the docket for Jody Robinson. One was a bigger and riskier procedure than almost any the child had had to date. When the time was right, surgeons would open the baby's abdomen, free a short piece of colon from the rest of the intestine, leaving it attached to the wide strip of tissue and vessels that runs along the bowel and serves as its blood supply, and swing the segment up into Jody's chest to become the link between his esophagus and his stomach. In a second operation, surgeons would close the patient's gastrostomy, the abdominal opening through which he now received nourishment in the form of blenderized formulas. Ideally these two procedures would enable the child to eat and digest ordinary food.

Exactly when the colon interposition would be done was under debate. So far the doctors involved had agreed only that they would postpone the operation until the patient had become considerably bigger and stronger than he was presently and until his respiratory competency had improved. The child was and had always been totally ventilator-dependent.

The ventilator performed three functions for Jody. It actually took breaths for him, filling his lungs with oxygen and then withdrawing it, letting the lungs deflate. It made oxygen available to him for the breaths he was able to take on his own. The machine also encouraged his initiative by exerting continuous positive air pressure on Jody's lungs, thus keeping the millions of tiny air sacs perpetually inflated and giving the child a head start on every breath he took himself.

If and when Jody ever became free of the respirator, it would be a great day in his life and in the lives of those closest to him. He had been undergoing a wean for some months. Very gradually and cautiously, his primary physician had been attempting to decrease the amount of support Jody was getting from the machine in the hope that as the child grew and developed, his own system would begin to take over. There had been some progress. Jody now needed the machine to breathe for him only three times a minute. The rest of the breaths he needed he took unassisted. He needed less oxygen than he once had, less positive pressure than he once had.

But the machine remained essential to the child's survival. Every so often the staff got dramatic and frightening reminders of this fact. Once in a while Jody would become disconnected from the ventilator. The brass swivel would pop, or a defective string would snap, or a thin piece of metal would break under stress, or the child's own movements would sever the connection. Whenever such a thing occurred, alarms would go off, nurses would come running from every direction, and Jody would begin to turn blue almost immediately.

Weaning is almost invariably a long and frustrating process involving minute advances and frequent setbacks, and Jody Robinson was hardly an ideal candidate. He lost ground every time he had surgery. There were setbacks between operations as well. While he was apparently nearing the point of being able to draw all his breaths by himself, conceivably within a month, it could be many months or even years before he came off the machine entirely— assuming he lived that long.

His prognosis was questionable. Medically speaking he was a time bomb. On the good side, he was growing, well-nourished, and able to defend himself against infection. His gut from his stomach down was intact and functioning. There had been no further break-downs of previous repairs. Doctors were optimistic that Jody's heart defect would resolve itself with growth. His ventilatory status was as good as could be expected.

Neurologically he was fine. Though ventilator-dependent, he was like Karen Ann Quinlan in no other sense. Jody's brain was sound. At one time he had carried a diagnosis of developmental delay because he was not doing the things a child his age should be able to do. He had never learned to crawl. Though he could sit for long periods without support, he still couldn't get from his back to his bottom unless he used his trapeze. He couldn't stand without support. Standing with support, holding onto the trapeze bar or the crib rail, he couldn't make the transition into a sitting position with-out help. His knees would lock. However, doctors attributed his slow pace to the fact that he'd been so sick. Once he'd gotten rela-tively stable and the nurses and therapists had begun working with him, he had made so much progress developmentally that he had almost caught up with himself.

He was tough. A survivor. He had a lot of potential. In the right environment he could become a productive human being, make a tangible contribution to society, accept love and offer it. If nothing disastrous happened to Jody, it was possible that he would continue to improve, learn to walk and talk, and live to a ripe old age with not much more handicap than a voice that sounded slightly odd.

Yet his future was by no means assured. He had had half a dozen surgical procedures in his airway. He had had nearly that many in his abdomen and several more on or in the vicinity of his esophagus. In all those areas he was at risk of scarring that could cause him a variety of problems, including permanent muteness. Somewhere along the way he had contracted hepatitis—secondary, perhaps, to a long course of intravenous nutrition, which tends to stress the liver. Though he was no longer on IV feedings and had recovered from the inflammation, the organ had been scarred. It was possible that he had developed cirrhosis. Five years down the line he could have the lungs and liver of an alcoholic. He could run into serious trouble when the doctors did his colon surgery. He could get a big infection and die at any time.

He had been reasonably stable for some months. But he had never been well enough to leave the building for even five minutes. Except for the first few hours after his birth, Jody Robinson had spent his entire life at Children's Hospital. The east bay of the Intermediate ICU and the rectangle of sky he could see through the Intermediate windows were his whole universe. He left the unit only to go down the hall to the operating room.

One would expect such adversity as Jody had known to dampen a person's spirits very considerably. This person behaved as if his life had been charmed. He entered into it with remarkable zest. There was a lot of activity in Intermediate, and Jody was entertained by all of it. He loved to sit in a walker or a playpen and watch. If someone happened to be standing in his line of vision when people were walking in the door of the unit, he'd crane his neck around the obstructing presence to get a look. At social interaction Jody was a prodigy. He loved people, loved attention, loved to put on a show. He'd do anything if somebody did it with him. Unless feeling very poorly, he engaged so readily and so wholeheartedly in play of all kinds that hospital staff members having a bad day sometimes visited Jody Robinson to cheer themselves up.

This is not to say he bestowed his affections indiscriminately. He didn't. He could look someone up and down without betraying the slightest interest in carrying the relationship one step further. Jody chose his friends.

But he could be won with sincere courting, and what he gave in return made the impulse to court him virtually irresistible. Small wonder that he had friends in Housekeeping, in Central Supply, in Public Relations, in Respiratory Therapy—indeed, all over the hospital. So many people greeted him in the hallway whenever he was wheeled to the OR that on one occasion a resident accompanying him finally demanded of the patient whether there was anybody in the place who didn't know him.

There were those at Children's who believed that Jody's extraordinary personality was an amalgam of coping skills devised by a child who sensed himself to be without natural allies. Jody's mother had been in jail off and on nearly all of his life. Most of her offenses had been drug-related. Recently, however, she had tried to kill a boyfriend with a knife. She had visited her son at Children's fewer than half a dozen times. On one occasion the nurses had had to point out to her which little boy was hers. Sabra Robinson telephoned even less often than she visited.

When she appeared, she was Jekyll and Hyde. During several visits she had been very loving with Jody, showering him with affection, begging the nurses to show her how to take care of him, asking questions and listening to the answers, promising everyone that she was going to become a better mother. "I'm getting myself together," Sabra would say. "I'll be in next week and take his dirty clothes home to wash."

On other visits she had ranted and raved. "He doesn't need any clothes! He's just a baby! All he needs is a diaper! I ought to know; I'm his mother! He doesn't need to see me!" She had spoken abusively and belligerently to the nurses and had actually threatened them with physical harm. Some of the nurses were afraid of her. They were not comforted by seeing fresh track marks on her arms, though Sabra vehemently denied ever using drugs.

Once she had come in with a buggy saying she had a taxi waiting and was going to take her baby home. Once or twice she had sent heartbreaking letters of contrition to Intermediate head nurse Jan Haver. She was going to straighten out her life, Sabra had written, so that when Jody was well enough to leave the hospital, he'd have a home. Once in a great while she mailed money to Jody and asked the nurses to tell him she loved him. Once she had asked Marla Meyerle whether Jody's lungs were so bad because she herself had smoked four packs of cigarettes a day while pregnant.

This past June Sabra had given birth in jail to a normal baby girl she had named for herself. That child was now living with cousins of Sabra's: a woman and her grown daughter, both with young children of their own. The cousins had visited Jody perhaps three times. Once they had brought his little sister, who looked exactly like him. The two babies had taken to each other instantaneously.

The cousins had made very tentative inquiries about the kind of care Jody might require when and if he could be discharged from Children's, wondering aloud if they might be able to take him themselves. At first the nurses had jumped at this idea. The cousins seemed to be warm, goodhearted people who could give Jody the familial affection and attention of which he had so long been deprived. Intermediate staff had urged the cousins to become more involved. But there was no denying that the women already had their hands full with their own children and Sabra II, as the nurses called her. Invariably after their visits to Jody the cousins would not be seen again for weeks on end.

The whereabouts of Jody's father were unknown.

In essence the child had been raised by his caretakers. Most of his clothes had been bought or made by nurses. Most of his toys had been gifts from nurses and other hospital staff members. The nurses took turns doing his laundry at home in their free time. They did this not out of obligation or pity but out of love. The nurses cherished the child as if he were their own, which in a sense he was. Jody's doctors loved him too, as did many of his other friends at Children's Hospital. One could even argue that he had gotten a better start in life than had he been born healthy to a nineteen-year-old drug addict. But he was tucked in at night by one nurse, dressed in the morning by another, awakened from his afternoon nap by a third. Never once had Jody Robinson experienced the feeling of being prized by someone who belonged to him.

Staff concern about his social status had begun to intensify in recent months. Most of the child's scheduled surgery was now behind him. If he got strong enough and arrived at a certain point on his ventilator settings, there would be no medical reason to keep him in the hospital. While the colon surgery still lay ahead of him, he would certainly not need to sit in Intermediate and wait for it. From a psychosocial point of view, the sooner he got into a more normal environment the better. One other child had gone home from Intermediate with complicated care problems very similar to Jody's. More than a dozen had gone home on ventilators. All had done well.

But all had gone into the bosoms of their own families. Would someone who had not borne Jody be willing to make the huge commitment that would be required to give him proper care outside the hospital? Would someone who had not borne him be willing to love a child who faced surgery he might not survive? If the cousins wouldn't take him, who would?

Underlying this question was a fear on the part of some staff members that Sabra Robinson might one day claim her son and somehow succeed in getting him, that a first-rate medical system which had made an enormous investment of time and money in the boy—to say nothing of the personal investment made by those closest to Jody—would finally get him in good enough condition to leave the hospital and would be forced to turn him over to a sociopath incapable of giving him any real chance in the world. Staff felt sorry for Sabra but saw no indication that she could provide for Jody the care and affection he needed and deserved.

For these reasons Children's social worker Lynn Story had undertaken to convince local officials of the state Welfare Department to evaluate Jody's case and to consider filing for formal custody of him. This would make the child a candidate for adoption or foster care so that if and when he did leave the hospital, he could go into a home with a person or persons chosen for their willingness to give him at least part of what he needed.

Meanwhile Jody was biding his time at Children's. He was waiting: waiting to be weaned off the ventilator, waiting for a decision to be made about surgery, waiting for a decision to be made about custody, waiting to grow enough that his body could tolerate what remained to be done to it, waiting, ultimately, for a home to be found.

He had his bad moments. Sometimes, for reasons not yet apparent, he gagged so violently that every vein on his head stood out. He hated to be suctioned. He fought it, crying, kicking, rolling around on the bed, sometimes actually striking out at the nurse who was doing the job, punching her arms, which only made the procedure more difficult for him, and worst of all he'd clamp down on the tube somehow so the nurse could not pull it out of his throat. This would make him turn blue from lack of oxygen, and his heart rate would drop. Sometimes he turned blue when he wasn't being suctioned. He often turned blue from gagging.

Otherwise, except when he had a cold or became disconnected from the respirator, his days passed uneventfully, which was precisely how staff wanted them to pass: without setbacks.

Scientific advances over centuries accounted for the child's presence in Intermediate. He was the product of the most sophisticated technology civilization had ever known. He owed his very existence to it. Technology had saved Jody, had worked incredible miracles on him. In this sense he was a glass half full.

But he was also a glass half empty. So far the technology had failed to either cure him or make him normal. So far it had given him life on a mattress, life on a machine, life in a universe big enough to accommodate five cribs. Technology had saved the child, but it had made him no promises.

Even the doctors said this: Jody Robinson represented the best and worst of space-age medicine.

They all did, the children of Intermediate. "The losers of Children's Hospital," a former head nurse had called them, a term not of judgment but of anguish over the gap between what nature or God had made wrong and what medicine could make right; anguish, too, over what the children would lose out on by accidents of nature. Few could anticipate normal lives.

There were eight of them now. For months all ten beds had been occupied by patients with major problems requiring long-term intensive care. Staff morale had become a serious problem. The nurses had found it increasingly difficult to come in day after day to ten children who weren't going anywhere very fast and might never go anywhere at all. Fearful that her staff would grow careless or begin quitting, head nurse Jan Haver had persuaded the anesthesiologists in charge of Intermediate to keep two beds open for short-term patients. Seeing kids get well and go home recharged the nurses thought by some people at Children's to have the least enviable jobs in the entire hospital.

Some of the eight long-termers had been born prematurely and developed chronic lung disease as a result of the ventilator therapy that had saved their lives. The others, like Jody Robinson, had been born with significant anomalies alone or in combination—spina bifida, abdominal or heart defects, urinary tract deformities, ambiguous genitalia—and suffered among other things from hydrocephalus, paraplegia, and retardation. Whatever their diagnoses, the eight long-term patients in Intermediate had one thing in common that defined the unit and set it apart: they all were, or until recently had been, ventilator-dependent.

Thus amidst the routine sounds of Intermediate one rarely heard the voice of a child. Every long-termer in the room had a tracheostomy. Until a patient came off the ventilator and the tracheostomy could be closed, air would exit the patient's trach tube without ever passing the vocal cords. Babies burst into tears or laughter without making a sound. Nurses talked to their patients all the time but almost never had the satisfaction of an oral response.

In the old hospital, Intermediate had not existed. It had opened with the new building as a stepdown unit for children over three months of age who were too sick for a regular floor but not sick enough to be in Acute.

By the late 1970s, however, advances throughout medicine but especially in respirator therapy and other aspects of critical care had begun to save children who in the early 1970s would have died: tiny premies, children suffering crises relating to fatal neuromuscular diseases; surgical patients such as Jody Robinson who had survived big, complex operations so unusual as to blaze trails in the field. These children were on the frontiers of medical progress. While in one sense all who survived were success stories, a small number of them became ventilator-dependent.

At Children's they ended up in Intermediate. In less than half a decade the unit had become a repository for patients whose hospital stays would be measured not in days or weeks but in months or even years. At the beginning the outlook for most of these children had seemed very bleak indeed. Those with fatal diseases would eventually die no matter what was done for them, and the others were exceedingly vulnerable. There was no body of evidence to suggest that they could last even a year, let alone a normal lifetime, or that they would ever come off the breathing machines.

As these youngsters had begun stacking up in Intermediate, the unit had become the subject of controversy at Children's. Some staff members believed that in treating such patients, the hospital was doing them no favor, and that limited health dollars should not be spent on children who seemed likely to be dependent on their parents and on society for the rest of their lives. To some staff members the unit was an embarrassment, a burden, even a travesty. Residents working there bestowed upon Intermediate some ugly nicknames during this period. The Back Room. The Eternal Care Unit. The Garden, as in vegetable garden. The Indeterminate Unit. Ventilator Villa. Trach City.

The criticism had not died out altogether. But by Jody Robinson's first birthday it had diminished considerably. A number of factors were involved in the turnaround, but it was due primarily to two people who happened to be on the scene at the same time:

anesthesiologist Peter Crossin, now medical director of Intermediate, and Sara March, Jan Haver's predecessor as head nurse.

Youngest son of a nurse and a surgeon, Crossin had by his own admission grown up "a rather irresponsible sort" who had applied to college to please his parents and had signed up for premed thinking, *Why not? I'm never going to last here anyway.* But he had become interested in medicine. In his senior year he had made the dean's list and discovered the rewards of accomplishment.

He'd begun his internship thinking neurology. That year he had met a nurse he wanted to marry and switched to anesthesiology thinking it would guarantee him a temporary military deferment. Instead Crossin had been drafted to run a huge anesthesia program in an American military hospital not far from Children's. After paying his debt to Uncle Sam, he had completed his anesthesia training at Children's and at the university hospital next door. Wanting the good life, he'd applied to a hospital in a wealthy suburb. That same week he'd been offered a job at Children's. Flattered, Crossin had taken it thinking that if he didn't like it, he could always leave.

He had had no special responsibilities in Intermediate when it first opened. Like his colleagues, he had rotated in and out. But as the character of the unit had begun to change, the rotation system had become a source of frustration and anger to parents. Some couldn't figure out who their child's doctor was. To help ameliorate the situation, Crossin had begun spending more and more time in Intermediate.

He would bristle at the suggestion that his reasons might have roots in his own family. Crossin's eldest sister had cerebral palsy. She had had numerous operations to straighten her spine, had been confined to a wheelchair for many years, had been imprisoned off and on for years in body casts. Crossin thought of her as an intelligent, courageous person who, though dependent, had never been morose. He felt it had been a valuable experience for him to grow up with her. But he denied a relationship between his sister and his job.

As he put it, "I don't want people thinking I'm doing what I'm doing because of my parents or my sister. The only relationship I can see is that I'm like my mother: if there's something to be done, I get it done." Whatever the reason, it was obvious to all concerned that Peter Crossin exhibited unusual sensitivity toward the children of Intermediate and toward their families. He became their advocate long before he agreed to serve as unit medical director.

If asked, he would claim to have learned about advocacy from then head nurse Sara March. The only nurse in the unit who was herself a mother, March had specialized in growth and development with youngsters having mental deficits. She was eager for the patients in Intermediate—virtually all of whom were developmentally delayed because of illness—to reap the benefits offered by her field. She was also eager to teach parents skills that would make them partners in the effort. Her plans had meshed perfectly with a desire of Crossin's to have children lose as little ground as possible while they were his patients.

With the anesthesiologist's enthusiastic support, March had begun with her staff. The nurses had almost all been young, and inexperienced in growth and development. Nonetheless, they had seen right away the value in what March wanted to accomplish. Moreover, her goals had provided them with an opportunity to be creative. As the nurses had learned, they had taught the families, and then nurses and parents had worked together with the children. Help had been systematically enlisted from the hospital's speech, physical, occupational, and recreation therapists. Progress had been slow, but almost every child had made some.

Concurrent with this effort, Crossin and March had begun sending children home on ventilators. This had been done with two patients in the earliest days of Intermediate, not with any idea that the children were pioneers in a pilot program—there was no program—but because they were thought to be dying. Both had fatal diseases. One eight, one twelve, they had been sent home to die at home. Instead they had gotten better. Recovering from astonishment, the staff of Intermediate had credited the improvements to the very attentive one-to-one nursing care the children had received from their mothers, to the tonic for the child of being at home in a normal setting, and to the decreased risk of infection away from the hospital environment. Both youngsters were still alive. One had weaned herself off the respirator. The other used the machine only at night. Both had gone camping and been to Disneyland.

Meanwhile a number of children had come into Intermediate who would not have required hospital care had they not been dependent on respirators. They were stable. Their beds were needed by patients who weren't. Administrators began to pressure the anesthesiologists to resolve the situation. Crossin's solution had been to discharge the kids into the care of their parents.

At the time, this had been a revolutionary notion. Children had once gone home in iron lungs, but the ventilator is one of the most sophisticated pieces of equipment known to modern medicine. Life was at stake. Could laypersons be trusted to operate and troubleshoot such machines?

It was Crossin's opinion that they could. He'd already seen it happen in two instances. Even a ventilator is a closed system, and Crossin thought parents were much smarter than sometimes is recognized. Further, he and Sara March both strongly believed that living at home was in the patients' best interests.

So he and the nursing staff had taught the parents what they'd needed to know, and ten children had been discharged. While the community had been very slow to embrace them, medically the children had done surprisingly well. None had died. Most had gotten better. Several had become less dependent on respirator support. Several had parted company with the machines entirely.

Their progress had not convinced all critics of Intermediate that patients who seemed destined for very limited lives should be supported either by the nation's health care system or by Children's Hospital. However, the strides achieved by both the children who had gone home on ventilators and those who remained in the unit had made it difficult for critics to maintain that Intermediate was nurturing vegetables incapable of meaningful response. Crossin and March had shown that while the children's physical powers had been severely compromised, their mental faculties had not necessarily. Most had good brains. Some had good potential.

During the grimmest period in the brief history of Intermediate, the intensity of the criticism had pushed the anesthesiologists to hold an open meeting in the hospital auditorium to defuse the controversy and explain their goals in the unit. Peter Crossin had run the meeting, assisted by Sara March and a general surgeon. The three had been bombarded, especially about one child who was both paralyzed and profoundly retarded. How could Crossin justify giving a bed to that patient and turning away a child with a better prognosis?

Ironically, this was a case in which the doctors involved at Children's had been reluctant to support the child. They had gone ahead only at the parents' insistence that everything possible be done. Even Crossin had reservations about continuing to treat this patient.

But he had long since answered the critics' question in his own mind to his own satisfaction. Since medicine had given these children life, medicine could not responsibly abandon them. Not in Intermediate had the die been cast for those patients. In every case the original decision to sustain life had been made elsewhere. Crossin had not been with those children at the fork in the road. His job, as he saw it, was to pick up the pieces. He did that job in the only way he could have that allowed him to live with himself: by making sure the children got what he felt they were owed.

Marla sat Jody back on his mattress and lowered his side rail. Leaning on it, she began a game with him, calling him by the Yiddish nickname her mother still called her.

"Shane punim. Pretty face. Where's my button?"

He pointed immediately to the top button on her open-necked blouse.

"And where's my nose?"

He pointed to his own.

"Not your nose! *My* nose!"

He rectified his error.

"How big is Jody?"

Grinning, he raised one arm.

"Right!" She raised the other. "Soooo big!"

But he was looking beyond her. He suddenly began to blink. Marla turned to see a respiratory therapist winking at Jody. Every time the therapist winked, Jody blinked. After a moment the patient put a hand over his left eye, thus giving himself the impression when he blinked again that only one eye was closing.

Marla laughed and rubbed his head until he laughed back.

Ø

The results of Mark's second x-ray, which reached Darryl Barth in the Adolescent nurses' station about 1:45, gave Barth no reason even to smile. The film showed that despite the increased suction, the pneumothorax was a little worse.

Barth put in a call for Drew Cipriani. Arriving back on Adolescent about 2:00, the CT resident ordered an Emerson for Mark, a machine ordinarily used with adults that provides more powerful suction than is available through a wall hookup. Cipriani warned Mark that if the Emerson did not work, he would probably need another chest tube.

The Emerson arrived at about 2:30. Shortly after it was attached to Mark's chest tube, an x-ray technician took the third chest film the boy had had in fewer than five hours. The x-ray showed that the Emerson was having no effect on Mark's pneumothorax.

At this point Neil Martinson himself came up to Adolescent to examine the patient. The cardiothoracic surgeon beheld a sickly kid in misery from a bad respiratory tract infection and the chest tube he already had. Martinson did not think the boy's pneumothorax was life-threatening at present. A cystic's lungs are stiff and full of mucus, like a sponge full of glue. If stiffness had kept Mark's lung from reexpanding in a hurry, the surgeon reasoned, it was also likely to impede swift collapse. The pneumothorax was potentially correctable with one or more additional chest tubes. A strong reason for going ahead with another chest tube was to give the tetracycline every chance to work. Unless Mark's lung and pleural surfaces were in direct contact with each other, scarring could not take place.

But Martinson had reservations. Would a second tube help this child live through a crisis only to die soon afterward?

Back in his office, the CT surgeon called Daniel Earnshaw. Told by Earnshaw that if Mark could get past his acute difficulties he would probably be able to finish high school, Martinson decided to go ahead with a second chest tube as the next logical step in the direction of discharge.

He gave some thought to placement. Normally it doesn't matter where a chest tube goes in a pneumothorax patient. Air rises. Ordinarily it settles in the apex, the top of the space. For that reason, surgeons usually try to place initial chest tubes rather high when treating pneumothorax, and had done so in Mark's case. Yet the tube had not worked, perhaps because Mark's chest had been deformed by his efforts to pull air into his lungs. So Martinson and the CT residents decided to place the second tube a little above the first.

This was accomplished just after supper. As Mark did not feel up to going into the treatment room, the second tube was put in him in his bed. At Dr. Earnshaw's request, he was premedicated with three milligrams of morphine. Even so, he was very upset and anxious throughout the procedure, which took about thirty minutes. Darryl Barth and a nurse did what they could to calm him. The surgeon explained what was happening at each step and asked Mark at each step how he felt. Barth was impressed with the surgeon's honesty and with his concern for Mark's emotional well-being. Drew Cipriani was over six feet tall, but he had a baby face which, combined with a sweet disposition, made him appear to Barth as a person who had somehow stumbled into surgery.

When the metal burst through the sensitive pleura into his chest cavity, Mark shed tears into his hands. Some minutes later, he calmed down and said this insertion had hurt him less than the first one. The tube was attached to a Pleur-evac and hooked up to wall suction. A chest x-ray taken soon thereafter showed considerable improvement. The pneumothorax had been reduced to around five percent.

When the morphine began to wear off, Mark's pain became acute. A dose of codeine and Tylenol failed to relieve it. Dr. Barth ordered a little more morphine, which helped.

About 9:00, when Mark's mother had started for home after spending the weekend at Children's, a fifth and final x-ray was done; and it was Darryl Barth's great pleasure to report to the patient that this film showed no change from the prior study. The lung was apparently staying up.

Monday, December 10

Winter sun came in the big windows of the Intermediate Unit and lingered on Jody Robinson's tight black curls, making them glisten. Wearing only a diaper, he sat in his crib with his feet dangling out through the bars of the lowered side rail. Next to him Marla chatted with a surgical resident about the child's upcoming bronchoscopy.

Three months had passed since the ear-nose-and-throat specialist had braced Jody's trachea with rib grafts. The surgeon
wanted to inspect the organ under anesthesia to see how the stint
job had healed. As Jody was still his mother's son, her permission
was required for all scheduled surgery. The resident was wondering
whether anyone had been able to contact Sabra at the prison.

"She's not there," Marla told him, pouring some water into
Jody's green cup. "I thought you'd heard. The social worker
phoned out there at the end of last week and was told she's out on
probation. But she does keep in touch with the cousins, so maybe
she'll find out from them that we're looking for her."

The nurse snapped the lid on the cup. The lid had a small spout
which looked like the mouthpiece of a whistle. As the resident
moved away from the bedside, she called after him, "Don't worry,
she'll turn up! She always has in the past."

With the patient watching, Marla folded a white towel and
tucked it around his right hip over his diaper.

"Time for your sham feeding, Punkin. Are you ready to have a
little drink of water?"

He nodded, looking pleased. He had finally learned that the signals for yes and no were different. For weeks he had answered
every question by shaking his head from side to side like a puppy
with a bone.

She handed him the cup. That he could use it she considered a
kind of miracle. Since he had never been able to take nourishment
by mouth, he had never experienced the oral stimulation involved.
He'd never even had a bottle. The nurses had tried him on bottles,
but every time a nipple had entered his mouth, he had thrust it out
with his tongue.

This had been cause for concern. Nutrition is often a problem
for babies fed intravenously or by tube over long periods. When it
finally becomes possible for them to eat normally, they can't do it
very well because they've never learned how. The nurses wanted to
accustom Jody to the sensation of something in his mouth and to
the mechanics of swallowing a foreign substance. To their great relief he adored his green cup. Marla always gave him a sham feeding
just before she gave him his regular tube feeding in the hope that
he'd make the connection.

He reached for his cup with both hands. Closing his lips over the spout, tilting his head back, the baby drank deeply. The water flowed through Jody's esophagus, streamed out the hole or esophagostomy in the right side of his neck, washed over his shoulder down his tummy, down his back, down his arm, and drenched the towel put there for the purpose. The feel of the water made the child stop drinking to laugh.

"You like that, don't you! You just love getting yourself and the bed all soaked!" Marla gathered the towel and blotted the wet skin. "In case you don't know it, that's why I don't change your bed till last!"

He got his real feedings every four hours: a blend of yogurt, junior fruits and meats, baby rice cereal, and pasteurized egg yolk mixed up by the nurses according to a formula worked out by Marla and a dietitian. The thick beige brew was poured into a 50 cc. syringe attached at one end to the foot-long gastrostomy tube anchored in Jody's abdomen and at the other to the bar across the top of his crib and was pushed slowly through the tube into his stomach by a nurse wielding the plunger.

Usually the process took half an hour. The nurse could leave the bedside, but not for long. For one thing, Jody often tried to play with the gastrostomy tube, an activity as natural for him as playing with his toes; for another, he had been known to yank the syringe free of the heavy-duty rubber band that held it to the overhead bar and to splatter formula all over himself and the bed. Marla stayed busy trying to distract him.

"Here, Jody, put the lid back on the formula bottle."

Concentrating, he tried to put it on upside down. He made several attempts. Marla watched without directing him. In a moment he turned the cap over in his hands and placed it on top of the bottle.

"Good boy! You did it!"

Scarcely a day went by now when she didn't see him accomplish something he hadn't done before. Recently he had begun the imitative phase normal to toddlers his age or a little younger. He was picking up a lot of new things very quickly. It seemed to Marla and her colleagues that his whole personality was suddenly emerging.

He had not always been so responsive. In common with many other babies transferring in from Acute, Jody had been very sick and scrawny when he'd arrived in Intermediate. At nine months of age he had weighed only six and a half pounds. He had needed a lot of ventilator support. He would turn blue in the split seconds it would take two nurses to change his trach tube. He'd had frequent unexplained episodes of lowered heart rate. He had kept to himself in those days, and small wonder. He'd had strength to do nothing more than sleep or lie quietly in his crib. Learning to accept affection had taken him a long time. Almost the only way the nurses had found to please him at the beginning was to wind up a fuzzy giraffe from the Play Therapy Department. The giraffe had played a lullaby and moved its head, and Jody had liked to have it lying next to him.

He had been no great favorite of the nurses during that period. Jan Haver had been his primary nurse then, but almost nobody else had sought him out. He'd been a mass of tubes: a huge nursing responsibility from a physical point of view and, for a variety of reasons, not a particularly pleasant one. In addition, he had made progress extremely slowly. Moved along too quickly, he'd regress, which was unrewarding to his caregivers. Some nurses had shied away from Jody because of his family situation, wanting, understandably, to avoid the emotional hazards inherent in commitment to a child who to all intents and purposes had been abandoned.

It was precisely the family situation that had prompted Marla to become involved with Jody. The full implications of that situation had hit her in an instant one day when she had gone to check the baby's IV and discovered that the tip of the needle had pulled out of his vein and was lying just beneath the fragile skin. The tiny hand had been inflamed and swollen. As Marla had removed the needle, Jody's blood had come out on her fingers.

Such accidents happen in any unit. But almost any other youngster might have a mother at the bedside, someone who had learned enough about the child's care to notice when something went wrong and would alert the staff.

Jody had no such person. He had Jan Haver, who at most was with him five days a week for eight hours a day. It had become suddenly obvious to Marla Meyerle that somebody as vulnerable as this baby needed people to look out for him at other times too. Then and there, wiping Jody's blood from her fingers, Marla had decided to become one of them. Though once in a while she had backed away from him, protecting herself from pain he had to endure, she had never been sorry.

Off and on Marla had talked about adopting Jody. Convinced that the best placement for him would be in a black home with a father as well as a mother, she also felt that if he were ready to leave the hospital and had no place to go, then perhaps she would take him, though not without serious reservations if the child's mother were still in the picture. Marla herself had never had any problems with Sabra. But she felt a healthy fear of the woman's potential for doing harm. The nurse had no wish to live in a state of apprehension. Nor did she wish to set herself up as a target. Much as she loved Jody, Marla did not believe she would be willing to go that far for him.

She had grown up in Poughkeepsie, New York, and followed a brother to the University of Iowa intending to study dental hygiene. Soon after arriving in Iowa, she had switched to a nursing program. As she would later tell friends, "They dropped me off in pediatrics." Hired in Intermediate soon after graduation, she had worked there happily for well over a year. Recently, though, wanting a change, she had applied for a job as assistant head nurse in the Operating Room. She was waiting to hear.

Her leaving would solve a problem for her supervisors. Jan Haver considered Marla Meyerle to be a good nurse and a nice person who gave Jody Robinson excellent care. However, in Haver's view and in Peter Crossin's, Jody's nurse had grown too involved with her patient, as in the past she had grown overly attached, they thought, to other patients.

She had become less than objective where Jody was concerned. In assessing his condition day to day, instead of stating facts verifiable by any observer—"Jody has a fever this morning" or "His skin is very dusky"—Marla would make such comments as "Jody's not himself today. He doesn't look good," speaking less like a professional than a parent, which, in Crossin's view, compromised her professional effectiveness. He sometimes saw her as the kind of grandmother who worried over every bowel movement. More often Crossin felt Marla had appointed herself surrogate mother to Jody.

A delicate matter. To some extent all the Intermediate nurses become surrogate mothers. However hard a nurse may fight the impulse, it is difficult not to fall in love with kids who stay so long. But these attachments exacted an emotional price, in Crossin's opinion. He had seen it happen many times despite his own and Haver's efforts to guide the nurses around such pitfalls.

Jan Haver had initiated a number of conversations about objectivity with Marla Meyerle. During one of them, Marla had broken down and cried. She hadn't realized that her assessments had become so subjective, she'd told Haver. She did know that she tended to get overly involved with her patients. Yet even if she could change, she wasn't necessarily willing to in Jody's case. If her assessments weren't objective, where was the harm? If she didn't say motherly things on Jody's behalf, who would?

The head nurse had found it difficult at the time to contest Marla's point and difficult since then to press for change of which the other woman might truly be incapable under present circumstances. Perhaps the problem could be resolved only by Marla taking a new job in another unit.

Marla set Jody's yellow plastic tub on the floor beside his crib and filled it with warm water. "Bath time! Otherwise you get sleepy after breakfast and take your nap too early, right?" As she took his diaper off, he kicked and squirmed and played the ham, beside himself with anticipation.

"You look like a dirty little kid!" Lifting him, she bore him naked through the air, ventilator tubes and all, and sat him down in the water. He laughed, smacking the water with his hand, splashing her legs.

"You turkey!"

"Marla?"

The voice, another nurse's, sounded odd. Marla turned to see her colleague standing at the counter along the wall with the phone receiver in her hand, her palm over the mouthpiece and a look of astonishment on her face.

"For you. It's Sabra."

Marla recovered in a hurry. "Get ENT on the phone so they can get permission for surgery," she whispered, clapping her own hand over the mouthpiece, "and get the social worker in here fast. And the resident. I'll stall her as long as I can."

She put the receiver to her ear. "Hello, Sabra! How have you been? What can I tell you about Jody? Oh, your cousins told you he needs surgery? Well, the resident will be here in just a minute, and I'll put him on so he can tell you exactly what's happening. . . . Where are you?"

The social worker had likened keeping Sabra on the phone to doing suicide intervention. One never knew when she would hang up. It was impossible to call her back because she would never give a clue to her whereabouts except to say she was "on the streets." Always her calls precipitated a mad scramble to line up the people who wanted to talk to her before she disappeared again.

Today, as once or twice before when she'd called, her voice was slurred and her conversation confused. She wanted to know why her baby had "that thing" in his neck. She wondered whether he was talking. She wanted to know if they were taking him away. Not knowing whether Sabra had received the social worker's certified letter informing her that the Welfare Department was being asked to file for custody, and not wanting to incite Sabra's anger in case she would then refuse permission for the bronchoscopy, Marla replied, truthfully, "No, he'll be here at least a few more months and probably longer."

Jody's mother stayed on the line. She talked to the first-year resident about Jody's medical status; she gave oral consent for surgery to an ear-nose-and-throat resident with a nurse listening in as a witness; and she assured social worker Lynn Story that she had indeed received the certified letter about the Welfare Department. Then she asked to talk again to her child's nurse.

Sabra told Marla that she wanted nothing further to do with her son. In the next breath she promised that she would be up to see him tomorrow. Just as the nurse was about to ask what time, the line went dead.

Ø

Upstairs on Six Surgical this morning, Candy Rudolph was not being prepared for discharge. Ordinarily a child having craniofacial surgery leaves Children's seven days later. But one full week after Candy's operation, her face remained extremely swollen, and she still could not open her eyes. She would have to stay on Six Surgical until the swelling decreased.

At least from a medical standpoint, she was otherwise fine. Her vital signs had continued stable. Her body had resumed normal functions without difficulty. The long incision line in her scalp was healing dry and clean. In fact the doctors had come around early this morning and removed two-thirds of the stitches in Candy's head.

But she looked frightful. Her eyelids still appeared to have walnuts behind them, and they had turned from purplish to brownish-red. The right lid still drooped onto the pale cheek. The child's forehead was bruised yellow. Puffiness had given an almost sinister quality to Candy's face. Her bare scalp was now shadowy with sprouting hair. Seeing her on Saturday for the first time since the surgery, Bill Rudolph had thought his daughter looked gruesome. In the afternoon, making excuses, he had left the hospital and taken a long walk by himself.

She had seemed to feel as bad as she looked. Apparently her misery over the weekend had stemmed less from physical discomfort than from the confinement of being unable to see. Ordinarily by now a patient who'd had this kind of surgery would be able to look at books, watch television, participate in quiet games, and go to the playroom by herself. Candy couldn't even go to the bathroom by herself. Unless someone walked with her, or took her for rides in a wheelchair, a child accustomed all her life to normal activity had to stay put in darkness. She walked fearfully even when someone held her hand.

Small wonder that she'd been cranky all weekend. Instead of asking for her doll or a glass of milk, she had reverted to babyhood and cried or whined her requests. A number of times she had simply pleaded, "I want, I want," without ever finishing the sentence. After begging to be held, she'd then beg the person holding her to put her back to bed. She'd refused both food and fluids.

On Saturday morning when her mother had suggested a bath, wanting to wash the dried blood out of what was left of the child's hair, Candy had screamed at the word, though ordinarily she loved baths. She had cried a good part of Sunday—"I can't see! I want to go home!"—and had rejected comfort from everyone but her father. She had even cried when being held by her grandfather.

Nonetheless, she'd felt well enough to converse on Sunday. She had also felt well enough to play her sister Amy's piano for a while and to eat a cheeseburger and drink a milkshake. She had loved being taken for wheelchair rides. "Keep going, keep going!" she had urged when the person pushing her had stopped for any reason. That Candy could take pleasure in anything at this point had convinced her mother that despite the child's misery, her condition was definitely improving.

This morning the patient's spirits had risen considerably. She had lost one of her front teeth. The tooth had been loose when she'd been admitted to the hospital, and Candy had been wiggling it so hard over the past couple of days that finally after breakfast this morning, as Tammy Torrence was washing her back, she had worked it free. Thrilled, she had immediately told Tammy all about her pink Tooth Fairy pillow with the green pocket.

Now Candy was telling Tammy what she intended to do with the Tooth Fairy's quarter for this tooth. She would take that quarter and buy her sister Amy three presents because Amy was three years old. Candy announced this plan while sitting on the toilet trying to go. She announced it in the direction of the bathtub, where Tammy, perched on the edge, sat waiting for her to go.

The nurse was dressed in khaki and plaid. She had long, straight brown hair held back at the sides with barrettes. At twenty-two, Tammy Torrence had a face so young that she sometimes had trouble convincing parents to rely on her and a professional dedication so intense that it sometimes interfered with her relationship with her boyfriend. She had always been crazy about kids. On a peds rotation at Children's during nursing school at the university hospital next door, she had loved taking care of anyone old enough to talk, especially patients who'd had surgery. Asked on the Children's job application to list in order three units she'd like to work on, she had listed Six Surgical in all three spaces.

Tammy loved the little stories Candy would tell her and was charmed by Candy's plans for her tooth money. Most six-year-olds Tammy had met preferred to spend their money on themselves. The nurse suspected Candy's proposal as a ploy by which the child hoped to impress the person taking care of her. Given the trauma involved in craniofacial reconstructive surgery, for Candy to solicit support through ingenious methods was perfectly fine with Tammy Torrence. She was also glad for anything that distracted the patient temporarily from her misery and frustration.

That Candy felt miserable was clear to Tammy from the child's unwillingness to cooperate. The nurse had been trying to get the little girl to help wash herself. Candy wouldn't. Tammy had been wanting Candy to drink her medicine herself. While willing to take the medicine, antibiotics with a taste she liked, Candy refused to hold the cup. On those occasions when she agreed to eat something, she had refused to feed herself. Whenever Tammy tried to clean her eyes with a Q-tip, Candy put up a fight. She had been very unwilling to do anything except lie in bed. Having met Candy during the youngster's tour of the hospital, having found her a very friendly little girl with a delightful personality, having cared for many patients too young to understand why they felt so punk, the nurse understood that Candy had turned ornery as a way of exercising some control over her situation.

Tammy's heart went out to her. Though she would continue to encourage the patient to do as much as she could for herself, the nurse felt it would be unreasonable to expect independence from Candy until the child could see at least a little.

At suppertime Candy made her first trip to the cafeteria since the day before her surgery. There, in the company of her parents and grandparents, she had a jelly doughnut, three-quarters of a cup of yogurt, and some grape drink. Though she tired quickly and wanted to return to her room, she enjoyed the outing.

Monday had been a better day for her than Sunday or Saturday. In the morning she had listened appreciatively to a tape of "Snow White." Though she'd refused lunch, Tammy had put in a special order of peaches for her, and the patient had eaten them all. During her nap the Tooth Fairy had come.

Perhaps best of all, Candy figured out toward the end of the afternoon that if she pushed up her left eyelid with a finger, she could see.

But as her family was leaving to go home for the night, she begged them tearfully to take her with them.

Tuesday, December 11

Bright and early, Jody Robinson was taken to the operating room for the bronchoscopy to which his mother had consented on Monday. It was performed by ear-nose-and-throat specialist Jim Palardy, who had done all the reconstructive surgery on Jody's trachea. The checkup took no longer than twenty minutes. Palardy simply inserted a long metal tube into Jody's throat that illuminated and magnified the tracheal tissue for the surgeon's scrutiny.

Both the surgeon and the attending anesthesiologist were pleased by what they saw. Their reactions were enthusiastically relayed to the Intermediate nurses by the anesthesiology resident who accompanied Jody back to the unit when surgery was over.

"They found an itsy-bitsy little hole, like a pinhole, where his secretions might be leaking just a tiny bit," the resident reported, "and they said some of the tissue was rattier than a rag bag, but they were in raptures! Their eyes positively lit up! Palardy thought he looked great—for him!"

Along with the bronchoscopy, Jim Palardy had performed a small procedure that he and Peter Crossin hoped would cut down on the child's gagging. They had theorized that the hole in the side of Jody's neck to which his esophagus had been diverted had failed to grow with the patient; thus secretions were backing up and causing the child to gag. So Palardy had dilated the hole, inserting a long three-sided metal tube and twirling the tube to widen the corridor, hoping thereby to eliminate some moments of discomfort for Jody.

While the child was still in the operating room, a decision was made about him in rounds. They were held in a small conference room next to the Isolation Unit across the hall from Intermediate. Peter Crossin presided; nurses, residents, fellows, and the social worker attended. It was the opinion of one fellow, a doctor who had recently completed training as an anesthesiologist and was now at Children's learning to be a specialist in critical care, that Jody Robinson was doing very well—so well, the fellow said, that she would like to wean him down in the next day or two from three breaths a minute on the ventilator to just one.

An anesthesiology resident questioned a two-step decrease. Several months ago, he pointed out, Jody had been lowered from five breaths a minute to three. Though he had done well at first, he had started to sleep a lot. Tests had been done, and the appropriate setting on the machine had been moved from three to four. On four breaths a minute Jody had been fine. Just that minor change had made an important difference for him.

Crossin considered, pulling at his short beard. He wore wire-rimmed glasses and a scrub suit. The Intermediate medical director was thirty-eight and balding, but his beard, salted with gray, was thick and curly. "A bear of a man," a newspaper reporter had called him once in print, though Crossin was husky, not heavy; a hard tennis player when he could find the time. The teasing had gone on for weeks. Crossin had accepted it with enough good humor to suggest that the description had not displeased him. He was the father of two young daughters. Before finally adopting a child and then conceiving one who'd lived, Crossin and his wife had lost five pregnancies—three stillbirths, two early miscarriages.

On the subject of Jody Robinson he appreciated the resident's cautiousness. Big jumps rarely work for the children of Intermediate. However, Crossin himself believed on the basis of the evidence—the numbers in the chart, his own observations of the patient over the last few days—that the child could tolerate a two-step decrease in ventilator support. The doctor okayed it on condition that the fellow herself be present in the unit while the setting was changed and for several hours thereafter, and that she remain readily available for the rest of the day should the nurses need to call on her.

Talk turned from medical to social matters. For those few present who hadn't heard about it, Jan Haver recounted Sabra's phone call on Monday. She said she seriously doubted that Jody's mother would make good on her promise to visit; nonetheless, Haver wanted to alert everybody to the possibility.

When the head nurse had finished, social worker Lynn Story added a twist to the story of the telephone call. She spoke with the helpless humor of exasperation. Yesterday morning Jody's mother had told Story on the phone that she had received, read, and understood Story's certified letter sent to her at the prison informing her that the Welfare Department was being asked to take custody of Jody. Yesterday afternoon the letter had shown up on Story's desk. It had been returned from the prison unopened. The social worker was sending it out again this morning in care of the cousins.

Crossin shook his head in silence. In a way, he thought, it was Jody's good fortune that his mother had resorted to violence in her own life. A charge of attempted murder would make a strong case for getting the child away from his mother and into an environment where he'd have some prayer of thriving.

Ø

Candy Rudolph had eaten a good breakfast of pancakes assisted by Tammy Torrence, who had helped the patient guide her fork. Now Candy was asking Tammy to take her to the playroom so she could paint.

The nurse was startled and thrilled at this request. She hadn't thought Candy felt well enough to want such activity.

"Will you help me?"

"Of course."

When the patient's mother and grandfather arrived on Six Surgical at 9:30, they were directed to the playroom. There they saw Candy in her robe and slippers sitting in a tiny red chair at a long table, applying colors to paper with a small sponge as Tammy Torrence, having been instructed by the patient to do so, leaned forward from a chair directly behind her, left hand curving lightly over the bristly bald expanse of Candy's swollen scalp, and held the child's left eyelid open.

Wednesday, December 12

Mark sat on the examining table of the Adolescent treatment room, breathing hard and sweating, yet joking with Kate and with Darryl Barth, who was about to premedicate him. "Hey, Darryl, am I going to get fifteen of meperidine?"

Bending to inject Demerol and Phenergan into Mark's IV line, Barth shook his head. "Meperidine, the kid says. Did you hear that, Kate? I'm going to kill this smart-alecky kid."

"Yeah," Kate said, "he knows too much."

"I wouldn't know it if you didn't bring me the drug index anytime I ask for it." He was watching every move Barth made.

"Blame it on me. I'm tough enough to take it."

"Yeah, you're a pretty tough lady."

Just about as tough as you are or Darryl is right now, Kate thought. *We're all faking.*

He now had three chest tubes in him, as of yesterday. The third had gone in above his left nipple and was attached to yet another Pleur-evac. His chest x-ray this morning showed a pneumothorax of between fifteen and twenty percent. Neil Martinson was on his way up now to replace the third tube with a new tube through the same incision. The surgeon hoped to advance that tube into the apex of the patient's chest cavity.

Kate wondered how much more Mark could take. On Sunday he'd gotten a second chest tube. On Monday that tube had been replaced because the surgeons had thought it might have become clogged with mucus. Yesterday a third tube; today another manip- ulation. He had refused breakfast this morning because of pain. He had refused lunch out of anxiety over what Dr. Martinson was going to do to him. Though the Adolescent treatment room was directly across from his room, he'd felt too weak to walk. Barth had had to bring him over in a wheelchair, Kate pushing the Emerson behind them. Again this morning, for the fourth day running, Mark had wanted Kate to bathe him. This amazed her and made her sad. Always before he had insisted on doing his own A.M. care. Now he couldn't move without pain, and because he was eating poorly, he was growing weaker.

She wondered how much more she herself could take. Mark's discomfort was wearing her down. His whole situation was wearing her down. Once or twice recently when talking about him with her roommates, Kate had cried. The more involved she got with him, the more she felt she was running out of the energy she needed to support him.

Darryl Barth was in a similar state, and for similar reasons. His relationship with Mark had become almost a voodoo attachment, in Barth's mind. Like Kate, he felt Mark's pain almost as if it were his own. In three days Barth would be finishing his rotation on Adoles- cent. Thanks largely to Mark Price, he had become more depressed during those six weeks than at any other time in his brief medical career and perhaps in his life.

From Neil Martinson's point of view, the case was becoming a major nuisance. Day after day he and the residents were doing big heart and chest operations, and they had acutely ill patients all over the hospital, yet whenever they made rounds, they spent more time discussing Mark Price than almost anybody else. His care was also demanding emotionally. Mark was miserable. No one wanted to make him any more miserable than he already was. So Martinson was eager for several reasons to get Mark's pneumothorax resolved, which was why he had decided to bypass his residents this time and tackle the problem himself.

Arriving in the Adolescent treatment room about 1:00, the surgeon soon found out what the residents had been up against. In normal anatomy, the ribs are three-quarters of an inch apart. Because of his deformity, Mark's ribs were almost touching. It was impossible to push a tube between them except at certain points, and Martinson, working blind, could not find a space beyond which there was free access to the apex, which had never happened to him before. The procedure outlasted the effects of the Demerol and Phenergan and was extremely painful for the patient, who also needed oxygen while the surgeon was working.

"It's over," Kate said when Martinson had finally given up and accepted a compromise, but Mark replied, crying against her, "It's never over."

An x-ray showed no improvement in the pneumothorax.

Martinson ordered a second Emerson. Because this piece of equipment was not immediately available, he requested a Y connection and attached both the second and the third chest tubes to the Emerson Mark already had.

Martinson's plan once the second Emerson had arrived was to wait a day and see if two adult machines pulling air out of Mark's lungs through three chest tubes would resolve the pneumothorax or reduce it. If neither happened, there was a possibility that Mark would need a fourth chest tube.

At 2:00 Kate McDevitt and a dozen other Adolescent nurses gathered in the playroom for a meeting with psychiatrist Charles Tanish. A slight man in his mid-thirties with a particular interest in adolescent psychiatry, Tanish met monthly with the nursing staff on the Adolescent Unit to offer support and suggestions.

December was turning into a bad time on the ward. With the holidays just around the corner, there were some very sick kids in the unit. Mark was one. His roommate was another. Down the hall was another child who was also in coma but from a brain tumor.

Next door was a boy with an unusual and very painful inflammation of his capillaries and small arteries.

And Janet was back in, a seventeen-year-old cystic whose older sister had died of CF and whose younger sister also had the disease. Admitted in November in heart failure, she had come in this time, too, with heart problems. Dr. Earnshaw had let it be known some time ago that Janet was probably dying. While the Adolescent nurses did not for one minute think of Janet and Mark as being at the same point in their illness, Mark's current trouble along with Janet's readmission just three weeks after her most recent discharge had given the nurses a sense, suddenly, that all the cystics they knew were turning around. So the meeting with Dr. Tanish this after-noon focused almost entirely on the two CF patients currently on the floor.

In Janet's case the nurses were most concerned about the young woman's readiness for death. Janet had always handled her disease by denying its power over her. The sicker she became, the more she pushed herself. Right now she had her heart set on making the senior class trip to Florida over Easter. Because she rarely commu-nicated beyond small talk with the staff at Children's, the nurses didn't even know whether Janet had acknowledged to herself that she was dying, let alone how they could help her. The psychiatrist made several suggestions. He also emphasized the importance for the patient of letting in reality at her own pace, even if she did not reach acceptance before her last admission.

The nurses' worries about Mark related mainly to his frustration and their own over his recurrent lung collapse. Pain and fear had made him very demanding. As with Janet but for different reasons, the nurses did not know how best to help him. Several nurses found it difficult even to know how to speak to him in his present distress.

The staff was also concerned about his mother. Whereas over the past year Ellen Price had expressed to several nurses an under-standable wish that Mark would die and get some rest, she was scared now. She was telling certain people on staff that this admis-sion was different, that this might be the end for her son. Before this admission the nurses had never seen her scared.

They had also observed that more than is usually the case, this patient's mother was often alone in her vigil at Children's. Though her husband came in whenever he could, the distance between the

Prices' home and the hospital was long. The kids at home also needed a parent. Occasionally Ellen was spelled by Mark's natural father or joined by her good friend Sandy. But for a variety of reasons there wasn't the steady stream of aunts and uncles and grandparents some families can count on when a child is hospitalized. Ellen did talk to other mothers and occasionally had dinner with one of them. Because Mark would not allow her to be gone long, however, her life had essentially been confined to his room for more than a week.

Discussing these matters with Dr. Tanish proved fruitful for the Adolescent nurses. They concluded that since Mark was very close to his parents and drew a lot of support from them, the nurses might be of most use to him indirectly by giving all the support they could to his parents, thus making the Prices the strongest possible resource for the boy.

The nurses thought it likely that Ellen would be receptive to such efforts. In past admissions she had apparently needed nothing from the staff beyond a little pleasant conversation over a cigarette in the hall. Now she seemed to welcome longer talks, particularly with Kate and Carol. Since almost all the nurses found Ellen easy to get along with, they resolved to make themselves available to her as much as time allowed.

As the meeting drew to a close, Kate described to Dr. Tanish and the other nurses her feeling that she was too involved with Mark. Dr. Tanish was sympathetic. He asked Kate how she wanted to solve this problem. She replied that perhaps she should take a day off from Mark and work with another patient. Dr. Tanish agreed that this was a good idea.

The head nurse suggested that perhaps one of the recent graduates should have Mark for a day. When several of these nurses confessed that they didn't know how to behave with a boy and his mother who knew more than they did themselves about CF and its treatment, Dr. Tanish encouraged them to look at Mark's knowledge as something other than a threat.

"This boy is an example of a system that has worked," Tanish told them. "He *should* know more than you. He's been living with this disease a long time. His confidence and mastery are a product partly of his own hard work, yes. But that he has come to see himself as an expert, and be seen as one by you, is also proof that doctors and nurses at this institution and on this floor have spent a lot of time explaining things to him. You can look at it as a threat if you choose to. I choose to see it as something you can all be proud of."

As the Adolescent nurses discussed with Dr. Tanish how they could best help Mark and his mother, Ellen Price sat alone at one end of the long wooden bench in the sixth-floor hallway. Smoking, staring into space, she was remembering May, the end of May, a few weeks after Mark had been discharged from the hospital for the third time in half a year, when what lay ahead was becoming all too plain. Had there been one moment, one incident that had made his future suddenly seem so pointless to her?

She could not recall. She knew only that on an afternoon in late May, she had gone down on her knees beside her bed and had asked God to please either cure Mark or take him, thinking at the time that a mother could do nothing harder in the world than ask God to take her child.

In the last week she had discovered that there *was* something harder. It was harder for a mother to watch her child suffer as Mark was suffering, and to be able to do nothing about it, and to know that no one else could do anything about it.

Ellen saw Clara Bowman coming toward her through the hall. Inwardly she blessed Clara. Though Mark wasn't getting any breathing treatments now, his friend the respiratory therapist visited him every day.

"How's Mark?"

"Oh, Clara. They're talking about a fourth chest tube. They say they'll take him down to Radiology for this one and do it under fluoroscopy so they can see what they're doing, but they want to try to push it up really high into the chest, and they say it will be very painful. . . ."

Her voice broke. When Clara gripped her shoulder, she added vehemently, "I don't want him to have it."

"I don't blame you."

"It's not as if we're going for a cure."

"If he were mine, I'd feel the same way. But if they haven't done it this way before, maybe it will work."

"I don't think he's going to make it through Christmas."

"It's funny, isn't it," Clara said, "how we say, 'Lord, do your will,' but sometimes His will is death. It's hard to understand."

Ellen nodded, unable to reply.

Clara bent over her. "Pray. Leave it in God's hands. Whatever happens, it's His decision."

"Yes, I know."

"Whatever happens," Clara said, "stick together."

Thursday, December 13

Standing at the Adolescent nurses' station at 7:30 A.M., Dr. Daniel Earnshaw paged through Mark's chart reviewing the events of the patient's week thus far. Four painful procedures in four days. Three tubes now in place, each contributing to the misery that had come to characterize Mark's days and nights.

The record was full of references to his pain. "It hurts so much," a nurse had quoted Mark as saying. "Please give me something for pain." "Boy, that codeine and Tylenol didn't help at all," he had told another nurse. To another: "I'm not hungry. Can I have some more pain medication?" To still another: "The pain got much worse when I was coughing so much."

The effects on his nutrition were also obvious from the chart. No breakfast or lunch at all yesterday. Then at dinnertime he had eaten everything on his tray and sent his mother down to McDonald's for more food. At about 10:00 he'd been given chloral hydrate for sleep. Twenty minutes later he'd thrown up the chloral hydrate along with 100 cc. of hamburger and Coke. This morning he had thrown up another 100 cc. of undigested food. He was running a slight temperature.

And the CT surgeons were talking about putting in a fourth chest tube.

Earnshaw was prepared to believe that the boy needed it. But he also wanted Mark to have a day off if possible to collect himself. One day of relative peace.

The doctor wrote his wishes firmly into the chart, underlining certain words: "I would like to *give Mark a rest* from further chest tube procedures today." At the patient's bedside a few minutes later, he promised Mark and his mother that he would make every effort to postpone another invasive procedure until Friday or even Monday if he possibly could. Shortly thereafter Mark's nurse noted that both his spirits and his mother's had improved considerably.

Ø

Mark's view across the court was the unit where Candy Rudolph was recovering. She lay now in her bathrobe on the examining table in the Six Surg treatment room. Rolfe Lorimer stood beside her removing his suit jacket. He asked the nurse for a 20 cc. syringe. The swelling in Candy Rudolph's head had persisted. There was so much fluid under the skin that by pushing at it gingerly, Lorimer could cause displacement that was actually visible on the surface as rippling. The patient's eyelids were still swollen shut. The surgeon wanted to draw off some of the fluid.

"Now, Miss Candy, honey, I don't think this is going to hurt at all," Lorimer said easily, drawing up a stool at the head of the examining table. The child whimpered in fear and was consoled by a nurse she barely knew. The doctor pressed her forehead. "Do you feel this?"

With the nurse's help, she touched her fingers to the spot.

"It's kind of squishy up there, isn't it."

Her "yes" was barely audible.

"Well, we're going to get some of that squishiness out of there so your eyes will open up. You'll just feel a little stick."

All told Rolfe Lorimer removed 90 cc. of fluid from Candy's scalp—approximately three ounces. Though samples would go to the lab for testing, Lorimer had no doubt that the stuff was cerebrospinal fluid, the lubricant that bathes the brain and spinal cord. Somewhere in the patient's dura was a leak. At some point during the surgery, a tear had occurred in that tough membrane covering the brain which may or may not have been repaired at the time but which obviously, in the ten days since, had failed to seal itself off.

In themselves such leaks are more annoying than worrisome. Though they prolong the patient's hospitalization, most often they resolve themselves within forty-eight hours. If the accumulation persists, however, it can exert tension on the scalp incision that can hamper healing and lead to further complications. The danger lies in the possibility of infection. If fluid can get out of the dura, bacteria can get in. A patient could end up with a fatal meningitis.

This danger can actually be heightened by the insertion of needles to remove the leaking substance. In Candy's case Lorimer felt the risk to be outweighed by the need to maintain good circulation in the patient's scalp. Though he took out the excess fluid somewhat reluctantly, he knew from experience that one such procedure is ordinarily sufficient to resolve the problem.

While Candy was still on the examining table, her doctor proceeded to remove the remaining sutures from the incision in her skull and all the stitches from the rib graft site in her chest. In those few minutes the patient grew increasingly restless and unhappy. But when she returned to her room, the outlines of her upper face were visible as they had not been since Lorimer had finally laid flesh back over bone in the OR. Lightened by the absence of fluid, Candy's left eyelid opened up partway by itself for the first time in ten days.

Her mother assumed this meant that tomorrow, Friday, the child would be discharged.

Ø

Because she could now see, Candy was able this morning for the first time to join other children in the Six Surg playroom for play therapy. The therapist arrived with a large basin full of stuffed cloth dolls in pink, tan, and brown without features, clothes, or hair. The children were invited to choose a "patient," to decide who it was and color it accordingly with crayons, and to practice taping a real but needleless IV into the patient's arm.

"You can be doctors or nurses or whatever you want," the play therapist told them, "and the patients are yours to keep." In part the purpose of this exercise was to give youngsters restricted by hospitalization a chance to make some decisions, feel some control, and engage in a bit of fantasy.

The broader aim of play therapy at Children's is to alleviate trauma and anxiety. This is a subtler task than might be supposed. Kids who are afraid for the obvious reasons may also be afraid for reasons that aren't so obvious, based on their own misconceptions. Asked why he was in the hospital, one child replied, "Because I stole candy from my teacher's desk." The notion of hospitalization as punishment is not uncommon in children, perhaps because parents unwittingly invoke the hospital as a threat: "If you don't get down from that tree, you'll fall and hurt yourself and have to go to the hospital, and *then* you'll be sorry!"

Other misconceptions can develop on the scene. Told that a doctor or nurse is going to take their blood, some youngsters become terrified that *all* their blood will be taken. Yet they don't necessarily say so. Thus the job of the nine play therapists on staff at Children's is to design activities that will flush out such fears as well as mitigate them.

In the mornings the therapists are usually busy conducting group programs in the playrooms. Often in the afternoons they work individually with children unable to participate in group play. Occasionally they encounter a child whose illness makes exceptional demands on their ingenuity. One such child was a thirteen-year-old boy who within the course of eight hours had fallen ill with an extremely rare and catastrophic illness and become permanently paralyzed from the neck down. The play therapist assigned to long-term patients at Children's had arranged among other things for the boy to be visited weekly by representatives of the local science museum. During their most recent visit they had put on a light show for him.

This arrangement was unusual in that it involved only one patient. But youngsters at Children's are treated routinely to special entertainments set up by the Play Therapy Department, often in conjunction with Public Relations—everything from monthly visits by zoo personnel bringing snakes and raccoons to occasional appearances by such superstars as Donny and Marie Osmond. Superstars can be unpredictable. One well-known comedian came to Children's and addressed the board but refused to visit the paralyzed thirteen-year-old. The Osmonds, on the other hand, had planned to spend half an hour at Children's, actually spent three times that long, and visited every child in the Oncology Unit. Nationally known sports figures headquartered locally have been generous with their time as well as their money.

The chief play therapist receives a number of calls each month from local groups wishing to entertain the patients at Children's. These groups are carefully screened. Youngsters under fourteen are ordinarily not permitted to come, though an exception was made for the cast of *Annie*. High school musical ensembles are welcome when the participants are fifteen or older. One call came from a home for the elderly offering a production of *The Emperor's New*

Clothes. Wondering briefly if a senior citizen planned to walk in naked, the chief play therapist graciously refused the offer on the grounds that the playrooms would be too small for a cast of seventeen, given that some members of the audience would be in wheelchairs. The caller agreed, saying, "Half the singers are in wheelchairs too."

Besides screening calls and running the department, the chief play therapist is responsible for choosing and ordering all the toys to be found at Children's Hospital. Toys fall into two categories, diversional and therapeutic. Diversional toys are playthings given to patients to allow them to explore, enjoy, and be creative. Staples are paper, paint, crayons, puppets, rattles, and mobiles; but this category also includes VCRs, video games, and such board games as Monopoly, Dungeons & Dragons, and Trivial Pursuit.

Therapeutic playthings include Fisher-Price medical kits, special infant toys made by Johnson & Johnson which are useful in growth and development activities, tape recorders, medical puppets, anatomically correct dolls, and Mylar mirrors for babies.

The annual budget for toys of all kinds at Children's is roughly ten thousand dollars. In addition, the hospital receives donations of toys or money for toys amounting to a value of approximately five thousand dollars a year. The chief play therapist has a wish list ready when donors call. On it presently are free access to videotapes, an ongoing supply of rattles for every baby in the hospital, and plane or car models for every older child in the hospital, with a tube of glue affixed to each.

Used toys are accepted if they are in good condition and can be scrubbed clean. Stuffed toys are never accepted unless they are brand-new and still wrapped. As a matter of policy, toy guns are not used in the Children's play therapy program. An occasional tricycle is donated, but most of the patients at Children's are too sick to ride a trike.

So far the chief play therapist has not attempted to purchase Cabbage Patch dolls. She has not wished to become involved in the hassle that has attended the sale of these hot items, and she avoids buying toys that can benefit only one or two children. The public has been generous in its contributions of the one-of-a-kind human look-alikes. But if the contributions slow, the chief play therapist may have to break down and add Cabbage Patch kids to her budget.

Those dolls with no hair now go through chemotherapy with the Children's oncology patients.

Ø

Candy was napping with her play therapy doll and Baby Diaper Rash when Bob Price arrived at Children's about 3:00. He had taken the afternoon off, ostensibly to bring his wife some clean clothes. But at 3:55, telling Mark that they were going downstairs for coffee, his parents walked over to another wing of the sixth floor to keep the first appointment they had ever made for a conversation with Daniel Earnshaw.

His office was a simple white room small enough to seem cluttered by a few chairs, a few file cabinets, a stack or two of medical journals, and an overflowing in box. On one wall was taped a collection of drawings and paintings done for Dr. Earnshaw by his patients. Inviting the Prices to sit down, he asked how he could help them.

"Dr. Earnshaw," said Mark's adoptive father with difficulty, "I don't want to sound like I have a stone heart, but I . . . Ellen and I are beginning to feel that it would be better for Markie to die than to go on as he is."

Bob's customary optimism was gone from his voice. His wife looked from his face to the doctor's. "Both Bob and I have changed our prayers. We used to ask God to give Mark as long and good a life as possible. Now we're praying for Him to please end this suffering."

Bob nodded. "And we would like to ask you . . ." He began again. "We don't want him to go through anything he doesn't have to, and we would like to ask you to . . . not to take any extreme measures."

The doctor was quite relieved to see that Mark's father had apparently begun to confront the inevitable loss of his son. Bob's resistance to doing so had been a source of concern to Earnshaw.

But also he felt that the Prices were drawing conclusions prematurely about Mark's condition. Yes, the child was deteriorating, and conceivably the lung collapse had somewhat hastened the deterioration. Having to forgo percussion so long as the lung remained unstable was not helping Mark, nor was being confined to bed with no exercise. But the pneumothorax in and of itself did not mean the youngster's death was imminent. Earnshaw fully expected Mark to get past this incident.

"Your feelings are not unique," he told the Prices. "Other parents of CF children have come to feel as you do at a certain point, even when the child has not had a pneumothorax. But I want you to understand that while a pneumothorax is definitely not a favorable sign, it is something other CF patients have recovered from. Another example of a complication that is not necessarily fatal is hemoptysis. Hemorrhaging."

Seeing that Ellen remembered the conference she and Mark had attended on the subject, the doctor went on to tell the Prices that there was nothing about the baseline condition of Mark's lungs to indicate that he could not get better and go home and have a fairly decent life for at least another couple of years.

They looked at him for a moment in silence. Finally Ellen said, "Why is this going on so long? Why is Mark having such a difficult time of it?"

Earnshaw smiled sadly. "This happens to a very few children. We have one hundred patients with cystic fibrosis on our rolls. Mark is one percent of them. He's the only one whose lung has collapsed."

Another silence. This time Bob broke it. "My understanding was that these kids just sort of drift off to a peaceful death from lack of oxygen."

"Yes," Earnshaw said, "that is the way most of the children die."

"Then why," Ellen demanded fervently, "is Mark going through every inch of hell?"

The doctor shook his head. "I'm afraid I can't tell you why."

He addressed the point upon which they had opened the conversation. "You spoke earlier about heroic measures. I'm not quite sure what you meant by that, but when we talk about using unusual methods to prolong life, we're talking about, among other things, respirators. A respirator is usually used in a situation that's reversible to get the patient over a difficult period. I have used a respirator with a few patients. But the opportunity to use that therapy constructively in CF is rare. It is certainly not a good answer to our problem. When children get to the point where we can feel that even if they survive, the quality of their lives would be very low, we will not resort to heroics of that kind."

Because the Prices seemed to be listening very attentively to this, Daniel Earnshaw added specifically that he would not put Mark on a respirator.

They left his office some minutes later. On their way back to Mark's room, his parents commented on how Dr. Earnshaw had spoken to them not just as a doctor but as a friend, and they agreed that he had said everything they wanted or needed to hear.

Clara Bowman, meanwhile, was in visiting their son. She had found him crying.

"All right with you," she had asked, "if I pull up a chair?"

"Sure."

She had barely sat down when he said, "I'd just like to pull out all these chest tubes."

"Don't. Fight a little bit longer."

"I know, but I get so tired." He bent his blond head. "I'm going to die anyway."

"Who told you that?"

"I just know."

She made him look at her. "Mark, sometimes things are not like they seem to be. Once when I was in training for respiratory therapy, I walked in on a dead person. That was my first experience with the dead. It shook me. I went home and told my husband I was scared to death to deal with dead people and wanted out of this work. My husband said, 'No, you have to go back.'"

He listened with interest.

"Then back in '70 I had a pulmonary embolism. Blood clot in the lung. I was in the hospital seven and a half weeks, and for some of that time I was unconscious. When I woke up, I felt as if a door had opened up to death, and I'd gone through it. I'd been there. After that I wasn't frightened anymore. Death may not be as bad as you think it is. People say they don't want to go, but somehow when it's close, people welcome it."

"If anything happens to me, I wonder what's going to happen to my mother."

"Mark, sometimes the weakest person is the strongest. Or the other way around. I may seem strong, but if something happened to one of my kids . . ." She did not finish the sentence. "Strength comes from nowhere if you let it. She's probably going to do well. But you're not going anywhere. You're going to leave here this time. I know you wonder why things happen the way they happen, but sometimes it's better to just be still. God is good. Read the Twenty-third Psalm and the Lord's Prayer. It helps me. It will help you."

He was reading his Bible when his parents returned.

Friday, December 14

Daniel Earnshaw got up an hour and a quarter earlier than usual and arrived in the Cardiothoracic Surgery office at 6:00 A.M. to meet with Drs. Martinson and Cipriani about Mark Price. He had requested the meeting to review Mark's case generally with the CT surgeons and to ascertain for himself the necessity for a fourth chest tube. Though willing to be convinced that a fourth tube was the logical next step, Earnshaw also felt there was a limit to the amount of mechanical intervention Mark could take. He thought the boy ought not be pushed beyond that limit. He wanted to avoid a situation in which the therapy took precedence over the patient receiving it.

The meeting went as smoothly as Earnshaw could have hoped. Basic goals were not at issue. All three doctors wanted to get Mark over his pneumothorax and out of the hospital as soon as possible. Nor did the means prove a stumbling block. The only possible treatment that hadn't yet been tried in the case was to send Mark to the Operating Room for a pleural abrasion. The doctors reviewed this alternative and rejected it. In fact Neil Martinson simply refused to do such surgery on Mark, saying flatly that the boy would be unlikely to survive the operation. Frustrating as chest tube therapy could be, it was the only safe way to proceed.

Martinson assured Earnshaw that sooner or later multiple chest tubes almost always took care of the problem. Martinson's belief that the first three tubes hadn't done the whole job because they weren't in the right place made sense to Earnshaw. So did Martinson's proposal that he take Mark down to Radiology and put the fourth tube in under fluoroscopy, thus enabling the surgeon to see what he was doing.

The sole hitch, a small one, had to do with timing. Earnshaw asked the surgeons whether they could wait until after the weekend to put the fourth tube in. Cipriani resisted. "If we agree that he needs it, why not get it in now?"

"Because he's had a lot of pain, and he's at his wit's end, and he doesn't want another tube right now."

Dr. Cipriani commented to the effect that maybe Mark had too much control over his own therapy.

Daniel Earnshaw replied with a question. "Do we have a choice as to when?"

The surgeons acknowledged that the chest tube could wait till after the weekend, and they agreed to wait, a fact that Earnshaw reported to Mark and his mother soon thereafter on rounds. They could not have been more grateful.

The agreement was to hold for half a day.

Ø

Some three hours after the meeting in Martinson's office, Yvonne Rudolph arrived on Six Surgical to discover that a decision had been made about *her* child for which Yvonne could not feel in the least grateful. Some of the fluid had reaccumulated in Candy's scalp. The doctors wanted to keep her in the hospital another day or so.

This meant that Candy was now beginning her thirteenth day at Children's. Already she had been in nearly twice as long as her parents had understood was customary in such cases.

The thought of one more delay sent the child's mother out to a hall bench in tears. God had His reasons, she knew that. But Yvonne felt that she and Candy both were nearing the limits of their tolerance.

The child had periods now when she seemed able to do nothing but cry. Her intense frustration was extremely depressing to her mother, who was also becoming increasingly annoyed with Candy. Though obviously she didn't feel well, she was turning into a spoiled brat. She was very demanding, rarely said please or thank you now without being reminded to do so, expected presents each morning, got upset if a get-well card contained no money, and insisted on cheating so she could win at Candy Land.

Even if the child had been on her best behavior, the long days at the hospital were wearing her mother out. In the mornings, circling down into the big underground parking lot, Yvonne would feel she was driving into never-never land, or even drowning. *This is going to be my entire universe today,* she'd think in the elevator. Being in a place full of windows that didn't open made Yvonne feel claustrophobic, as if she were in prison. When she drove out of the parking lot at the end of each long visit, the world was dark. She had no time to tend to her personal needs.

Furthermore, the swelling in Candy's head made it difficult for her mother to see what Dr. Lorimer had accomplished. In her worst moments, Yvonne would think to herself, *She'll never look any other way.* It scared her to see the faces of other patients and parents when they caught sight of Candy.

Beyond her concerns about the child who was hospitalized, Yvonne was worried about the one who wasn't. Bill had seen Amy at his parents' home over the weekend. Yvonne had not, nor had she talked to Amy on the phone. She had deliberately avoided calling her youngest out of a desire not to upset the child. But Yvonne now felt torn between her daughters. She found it very hard to keep from calling Amy just to say, "Mommy's here, and she loves you."

Increasingly she felt resentful of her husband. Back on Long Island, Bill was working every day and going home at night to an empty house, which his wife knew was no fun for him. But Yvonne felt that to some extent he was handling the situation by standing back from it. His attitude at times seemed to be "You get this taken care of, and then let's get on with our lives together."

Her parents had been wonderful. But both had other responsibilities and they, too, were getting worn out. Yvonne needed the kind of buttressing that only a spouse could provide. Besides, she loved Bill and missed him.

She could barely stand to think of going through all this again when Candy had the surgery on her jaw.

She had been on the bench only a few minutes when Tammy Torrence came into the hall on an errand. Seeing Candy's mother with her face in her hands, Tammy went to Yvonne, who poured her heart out to the young nurse.

Ø

The second Emerson ordered by Dr. Martinson on Wednesday was finally delivered to Mark's room Friday at 10:00 A.M. When his third chest tube had been attached to it, a portable x-ray was done which showed no improvement in the pneumothorax.

A second x-ray, done at 11:00, was little different from the first. The lung was still down between fifteen and twenty percent.

About 1:00, after consulting with Dr. Martinson, Dr. Cipriani told Mark as gently as possible that he would have to have another chest tube. Today.

The patient put his head in his hands and cried.

But when his mother challenged the CT surgeon, saying she would not let Mark have this procedure unless Dr. Earnshaw were contacted and agreed to it, Mark broke in and said he wanted the tube. "Mom, if the surgeons think I need it to make my lung get better, then I don't see any point in putting it off. Let's just do it." Reached eventually by phone, Daniel Earnshaw, though surprised by his patient's reaction, would see no reason to postpone treatment Mark needed and was willing to have.

The brief, rather heated discussion that followed Cipriani's announcement left the CT resident believing that the decision had been made, the patient's mother that it had not yet, and Darryl Barth that an event had been set in motion which sooner or later was bound to take place. With only the weekend left of his rotation on Adolescent, Barth knew that his opportunities to do something for Mark were running out. Maybe he couldn't spare him the pain of a fourth chest tube, but he could at least help him through the procedure.

"If you do put the tube in," he said to Cipriani as the CT resident was leaving to go back to the OR, "I want to be there."

Ellen Price had a cigarette by herself on the hall bench. In a clinic waiting room across the court she could see a toddler riding a fat plastic tricycle in wide, wobbly circles. She thought of the day Mark had taught himself to ride his two-wheeler. He had been six or seven then. For some reason he had been unable to get the hang of riding even after a lot of practice and help.

One morning he had come to the breakfast table saying he was going to learn to ride his bike that day. He had refused assistance. Instead he had gone out by himself, and he had spent the entire day getting on the bike, falling off it, and getting right back on again. By the end of the day, he had known how to ride.

So why should she have been surprised at his attitude about a fourth chest tube?

He was not six or seven anymore, Ellen reminded herself. He was fifteen, a responsible individual. No matter how his parents felt, it was no longer up to them to say "Do this" or "Don't do that." Mark wanted to live. That was obvious. He would do anything to live. It was his right and his prerogative to make that choice.

"May I join you?"

She looked up into the sad face of Darryl Barth. "Of course."

He had told her that he didn't want Mark to go through the pain of another chest tube. He had told her, too, that he didn't oppose the tube per se. She knew he was hurting badly for Mark and was very discouraged about Mark's situation. In recent days she had also come to realize that he was very discouraged about his whole residency. Earlier in the week she had mentioned his depression to Dr. Cipriani, saying it distressed her to see Darryl so upset because he was such a good doctor. "I hope you'll tell him that," Cipriani had replied, "because he's thinking of leaving medicine."

When the young physician was seated beside her, she took his hand. "Darryl," she said, "let's put that fourth tube in and go for broke."

Dr. Martinson sent for the patient at 2:00. Carol Buchanan, a rosy-cheeked nurse who was a favorite of Mark's, premedicated him according to Martinson's orders and got him into a wheelchair, then with Ellen Price and another nurse took Mark and his two Emersons down to Radiology. No one remembered to page Darryl Barth.

On their return to Adolescent, Carol and the other nurse met him in the hallway. He was very agitated.

"Where's Mark?"

"I just took him down to x-ray."

"I wanted to be called!"

"I'm sorry. I just forgot."

"Did you premedicate him?"

"Yes, Dr. Martinson ordered Demerol and Phenergan."

"How much?"

She told him.

"Jesus," he cried, "that won't be enough!"

He ran back into the unit. In the medications room, he drew up an additional dose of Mark's meds into a syringe, then, brushing past people in the halls, dodging people in the stairwells, he covered the distance to Radiology as fast as he could. Barth felt he had a role here that was not being recognized. Maybe it wasn't much of a role, and maybe it was more important to him than to the patient. He couldn't digest Mark's food for him, he couldn't cough up his secretions for him, he couldn't cure Mark or even make him comfortable most of the time. All he could do was put a hand on Mark's shoulder and prepare the boy emotionally for whatever torment he had to endure. Barth could sleep at night knowing that though Mark was suffering, he himself was doing everything he could to alleviate the suffering. This afternoon that contribution had been usurped.

Ellen sat in the small Radiology waiting area among several parents with their children. Moving toward her to ask where Mark was, Barth was stopped in his tracks by the sound of Mark screaming.

Wheeling, he strode in the direction of the screams and pushed through the door to the room where Martinson, scalpel in hand, had just cut into the base of Mark's left armpit. Next to him, holding the chest tube, stood Drew Cipriani, like Barth a resident, low man on the totem pole; like Barth Mark's friend. Believing that with any other patient under any other circumstances, the surgeons would have been absolutely justified in proceeding with so little warning, believing, too, that these particular surgeons were not mechanics but gentle humanists with a job to do, Darryl Barth lost what cool he had left and told his good buddy Cipriani what he thought of him and his whole profession.

The concept of what he wanted to get across was simple and limited: This kid is not a collapsed lung. He's Mark.

But reflecting as it did the full range of Barth's frustration and emotional strain over Mark's case in particular and first-year residency in general, the outburst was far out of proportion to the

crime committed. Barth let Cipriani have it for Mark's pneumothorax, and then he let him have it for Mark's cystic fibrosis,
knowing with every word that he should have been screaming at
God.

Cipriani felt terrible and apologized.

Barth felt terrible and apologized.

The CT resident asked the pediatrics resident to inject the extra
pain medication. When Barth had done so, both men watched as
Neil Martinson, referring every few seconds to the image of the
inside of Mark's chest projected on an overhead screen, inserted the
first chest tube he had ever found it necessary to put in under fluoroscopy. The procedure was more painful for Mark than anything
he had experienced since the tetracycline treatment.

But Martinson was able to achieve perfect apical placement of
the fourth tube. The chest x-ray done right afterward showed one
hundred percent expansion of Mark's lung for the first time since
his lung had collapsed on the first night in December.

Back in bed, the pain plagued him.

Ever since the pneumothorax, he had received codeine and
Tylenol for the pain he lived with and Demerol and Phenergan only
for procedures. Today the doctors decided to continue him on Demerol and Phenergan at least overnight.

"I hope I don't get addicted," he joked to Carol.

They started him on twenty-five milligrams of Demerol and half
that of Phenergan. When this dose failed to reduce his discomfort,
the Demerol was increased to thirty-five milligrams.

Soon after he got that dose, Mark felt the pain grow dim. Everything grew dim. The noise of the two Emersons pulling air from his
chest, a sound Darryl Barth had said made him think of a distillery,
seemed far away. Mark's own body felt far away. He cared about
nothing. He didn't even care if he died.

He realized in his stupor that the not caring was caused by the
drugs. Sometimes when he felt very sick he didn't care if he died,
but this was different. This didn't scare him.

He made himself a promise, lying there. He promised himself
that when he got so sick that he knew he couldn't get any better, he
would ask for some drugs to make it as easy as possible for himself
to die.

Ø

Mark lay in Adolescent planning how to get medicine when he needed it, and over on Six Surgical, Tammy Torrence was about to talk with Candy about the child's new habit of refusing her medicine except when the person giving it to her was Tammy.

The nurse was pleased that the child was so fond of her. But Candy's shenanigans at meds time had become a problem for the nurses taking care of her when Tammy wasn't on duty. Assuming all went well, the child would be in the hospital only until tomorrow morning. The nurse thought it important for Candy to go home without the bad habits she had learned as a patient.

So while the child's mother was down in the cafeteria getting coffee, Tammy sat at Candy's bedside and told Candy that the nurses did not intend to bargain with her every time they came in to give her medicine. The medicine was to help her get better. If she wouldn't take it, she wouldn't get better as fast, and she wouldn't go home as fast. Tammy emphasized the part about going home. She wanted to make sure Candy knew that her illness wasn't permanent.

"I've never had a child get sicker, and I don't want you to get sicker," the nurse told the child. "You mean a lot to me. So please. When somebody comes in to give you your medicine, just take it. And remember that it's important to say please and thank you."

Candy listened quietly. But Tammy thought Candy respected her enough to do what she was asking, and the nurse would prove to be right.

Ø

Late Friday evening while Mark slept with the help of Demerol and Phenergan, his mother asked Darryl Barth if they could talk privately. He led her to the residents' office on the sixth floor assuming she wanted to discuss the chest tubes.

She wanted to discuss his future. "I understand that you're thinking of leaving medicine."

He did not know where she might have heard this but saw no point in denying it. "I don't belong in patient care," he said. "I get too involved and too upset. I'm not functioning the way I should around here, and I can't function in my life."

Ellen proceeded to give him a pep talk that lasted an hour. He couldn't leave medicine, she told him. His emotional involvement made him the doctor he was. If he left because he was ducking emotional pain, pediatrics would lose out. The kids would lose out. Learning to roll with the punches came with maturing, with putting in time. He was young yet.

The message Barth took most to heart as he listened to Ellen Price was more fundamental than the message Mark's mother had intended to deliver. He realized that the people he was playing cards with were seeing his hand. He hadn't appreciated how much was leaking, how much of his professional objectivity he was losing, how apparent his emotional flux had become. As Ellen talked, he realized that if he was transmitting unhappiness to parents, he must also be transmitting it to the children. He understood for the first time that if what a doctor feels as a person comes across, it could limit his effectiveness as a doctor.

Months later, Darryl Barth would look back on that hour with Mark Price's mother as a landmark of his internship.

Saturday, December 15

In a harsh wind, a young couple made their way slowly across the parking lot of Northwest Suburban Hospital. The man carried a suitcase and a shopping bag. Tom Gregory looked like a throwback to the '60s. His black hair hung to his shoulders, he was bearded, and he wore, along with jeans, a jacket, belt, and boots of black leather. Tied around his brow above silvered sunglasses was a folded red bandanna.

His wife supported herself on his free arm. With her oval face, willowy body, and long, straight brown hair, Robin Gregory bore a passing resemblance to the entertainer Cher. At twenty-eight she was two years older than her husband and a shade taller. She was also more conventional of dress. Proceeding toward their car, she took each step with care and effort. One week ago today, fully three months early and by emergency Caesarean section, she had been delivered of the Gregorys' third son.

The car was a run-down American model with tail fins. In silence Tom Gregory put the suitcase and the shopping bag in the trunk; in silence he helped his wife ease into the front seat. He became talkative only with beer in him. While there were things he might have liked to say to Robin this morning, they were things he had already tried to tell her without feeling she had understood him. He didn't know how else to prepare her. Nor did he know how to respond to her eagerness. She couldn't wait to see Brandon. She hadn't even wanted to go home first this morning to see Tommy and Keith, though on Sunday, one day after Brandon's birth, the twins had celebrated their first birthday without her.

As he drove out of the parking lot heading toward Children's Hospital, Tom felt Robin smiling at him. He tried to smile back.

To say the least, the pregnancy had not been planned. They had only ever wanted two children together. Finding themselves with two at once had stressed them financially and emotionally. The trailer was small, Tom's construction income was irregular, and Robin had awakened exhausted almost every day for months. The marriage had grown rocky. With his first wife Tom Gregory had had three sons. One had been born prematurely and died within a day. Even so, Robin had felt after the twins' birth that her husband had had enough children. He had agreed. In July he had had a vasectomy.

In September, losing weight and feeling unwell, Robin had gone for a checkup and been informed that she was three and a half months pregnant.

They had not seriously considered abortion. Having aborted two babies before marrying her first husband, Robin had had no desire to repeat the experience. The gynecologist had offered the possibility of adoption. The Gregorys had decided to postpone the decision until after the baby was born. Deep down Robin had always wanted a little girl. By the time she'd gotten used to being pregnant again, she'd become convinced that God was granting her wish.

Late one afternoon just two weeks after learning of the pregnancy, she had hemorrhaged into the toilet bowl. Tom had driven her—sobbing, certain she'd lost the baby—to Northwest Suburban, where Robin's gynecologist had assured them that she could hear the baby's heartbeat.

The bleeding had gradually slowed. The doctor had admitted Robin all the same. An ultrasound study done the next morning had revealed that the baby was fine. But the study had also shown the placenta to be lying directly over the birth canal, a condition known as placenta previa which carries the danger that the organ will detach itself and thus threaten the life of the fetus.

This condition, the hemorrhaging, and the fact that she had borne twins only months earlier identified Robin Gregory as a high-risk mother. However, both bleeding and placenta previa are rather common during pregnancy. In most cases the pregnancy proceeds normally so long as the mother takes precautions.

"You'll have to be very careful from now on," the doctor had told Robin, giving details. "You'll have to stay in bed for three weeks, and after that, until you deliver, you'll have to do just as little as possible."

Back home Robin had stopped caring whether the baby was a girl or a boy. It had seemed to her that the baby was fighting for its life. She had decided to fight for that life too.

They had hired a homemaker full-time. As they'd been eligible for government assistance, the woman's wages had been partly reimbursable by federal money. The arrangement had worked poorly. Someone different would come each time. None had seemed experienced. Feeling better, Robin had done more and more on her own. Though worried about doing too much, she had seen no alternative. The twins, nearing one year of age, had needed almost constant attention. The homemakers had begun working only half days and eventually had stopped coming at all.

On the Sunday before the twins' first birthday, the Gregorys had taken them to a Gregory family reunion upstate. Robin had accepted the invitation with mixed feelings. The doctor had told her not to travel. She had been on her feet a lot. Her water bag had been leaking a little.

On the other hand, Tom's whole family had not been together for many months. By this time Tom himself had been laid off. While the layoff had made them eligible for food stamps and medical assistance, it also meant that Robin would have to deliver through a clinic with a doctor she didn't know, and the loss of income was hard on them all. A family visit, Robin had thought, would cheer them up. She'd told Tom they could go if he would help with the kids.

He had agreed to help. Instead, upon arrival at his mother's, he'd started drinking and had stayed blitzed all day. Robin had come home from the reunion exhausted.

On the following Thursday after the twins had gone to bed, she had had a couple of drinks with Tom, which was unusual for her. When pregnant with the twins Robin had quit drinking and smoking altogether. During this pregnancy she'd had an occasional drink but rarely two. Suddenly she and Tom had found themselves on their bed in the living room, and he had begun to make love to her.

She'd pushed him away. The doctor had warned her not to have sex. But Tom had persisted. His passion, he'd said, was uncontrollable. Robin felt sure that his penis hadn't penetrated her cervix. Still, she had gone to sleep somewhat angry with Tom.

At 3:00 A.M. she had awakened wet, the sheet around her soaked with blood and fluid. She had wakened Tom. Since the bleeding had all but stopped, they'd decided not to call the clinic. Three hours later Robin had again awakened and, turning over, felt her bag pop. Warm fluid had gushed from her body.

Tom had driven her immediately to Northwest Suburban. She had been admitted for observation. An ultrasound study had shown that a small amount of amniotic fluid remained in her uterus.

Under optimal circumstances Robin would have been kept at Northwest long enough for doctors to ascertain that her condition was stable and would then have been transferred to one of several medical centers downtown that specialize in problem pregnancies and the care of high-risk infants. Instead she was told she'd be transferred if she went into labor. Meanwhile she was put on intravenous fluids and told to rest. "Sometimes the fluid replaces itself," the obstetrician had told her. "We want to see if yours will."

Once her membranes had ruptured, the chances that Robin would carry to term had become minimal. Most likely a woman in this situation will deliver within a week. Under optimal circumstances a doctor would have begun to educate the Gregorys about prematurity and its pitfalls, laying out likely prospects for premies of varying weights and thus affording the parents an opportunity to sort out in advance their feelings about proceeding with treatment for a baby whose prospects were poor. No such groundwork was laid for the Gregorys.

All day Friday Robin had lain quietly in bed and blamed herself for overdoing. Early Saturday morning a nurse helping her onto a bedpan had noticed a small segment of umbilical cord protruding from her vagina.

Ordering Robin to lie back, the nurse had yelled for the obstetrician, who had rushed in, glanced between Robin's legs, and repeated the order. "Lie down. I have to push his head back up in you."

There'd been no time for explanations. The umbilical cord had started down the birth canal. If the baby's head had also started down, it could be compressing the cord and cutting off the baby's oxygen supply. Treatment for a prolapsed cord is first to relieve the pressure manually and then to deliver the baby.

Brandon Gregory had been born a short time later weighing far too little to survive, if at all, without massive and sophisticated efforts on his behalf. Northwest Suburban was not equipped to make those efforts. Some community physicians, believing that the outcome in such cases often fails to justify the pain and suffering involved for either child or family, would decide not to transfer a baby as small as Brandon to a more sophisticated institution. In this case the obstetrician and a pediatrician who had appeared in the delivery room within minutes after the baby's birth had agreed between them to send the infant to Children's.

By coincidence the pediatrician had been a Children's Hospital fellow moonlighting at Northwest. He had arranged the transfer before consulting the parents. "Could not contact father and mother not sufficiently out of anesthesia at this time to inform of transport decision," the doctor had written in the baby's chart. Soon thereafter Tom Gregory had been located asleep in a waiting room. Told by the doctors that if the baby were to get what he needed, he would have to go to Children's, Gregory had signed the transport form. He could not have discussed the matter with his wife at this point even if it had occurred to him to do so. Robin would not really wake up until Brandon was two days old. By consenting to the baby's transfer by the Children's Hospital transport team, his father had in essence admitted Brandon to Children's and given permission for the treatment deemed necessary by the physicians involved.

Almost immediately upon his arrival in the Infant Intensive Care Unit at Children's, the baby had been put on a ventilator. In effect this decision had bound the ICU staff to sustain Brandon Gregory either until he was well enough to breathe on his own or until he was brain-dead. As a matter of policy, staff had proceeded to treat aggressively so as to lose no time with a baby showing signs of viability. Any delay in treatment under these circumstances can worsen the baby's prognosis.

On Sunday, one day following Brandon's birth, his father had visited him at Children's. After an hour's drive, he had been able to bear the sight of so many tubes in his son's tiny body for just twenty minutes. He had talked to a doctor but had found everything so confusing that that evening, back in his wife's room at Northwest Suburban, Tom Gregory had hardly known where to begin explaining.

"Maybe it's crazy," he had told Robin, "but I wanted to take all the tubes out and just let him go on his own. If he lived, he lived. If he didn't, he didn't."

She might have heard him differently had she not been on painkillers. Had she not still been in shock from all that had happened over the past few days, Robin might have registered that Tom was upset enough to say he was, which was very unusual for him. Instead she had focused on a comment made to her husband by a doctor at Children's: if Brandon got through the week, he'd probably live.

Groggy as she had been those first few days after delivering, the nurses taking care of Robin had given her regular reports from the nurses at Children's. As soon as she'd felt well enough, Robin had begun communicating with Brandon's nurses directly. To her their reports had seemed excellent. Brandon was on a respirator. Babies that little often forget to breathe, the nurses had told Robin, but the baby was breathing more on his own than he had at first. He needed less oxygen now than at first. From what Robin had gathered in these conversations, her baby really had no other problems.

During the entire week she had spent in the hospital after giving birth, Robin Gregory had spoken with a doctor from Children's only once. That doctor had called for permission to enroll Brandon in a study of vitamin E as a palliative for the eye disease that may develop in tiny infants requiring a lot of oxygen. Satisfied that the study couldn't hurt, Robin had told the doctor to go ahead. That no other doctor had called her from Children's the baby's mother had taken as a good sign.

She had glimpsed Brandon just briefly that first day. Right before he'd been wheeled out of her room in an incubator and rushed to the ambulance, somebody had guided her hand to a hole in the incubator, urging her to touch her son. Dazed and nauseated from drugs, she'd scarcely been able to open her eyes.

Nevertheless, she had gotten an impression. He hadn't seemed that small to her. Hard as it had been to focus, she'd thought he looked a little like the older twin. Later in the week when a girlfriend had said to her over the phone, "He must be so tiny and cute," Robin had replied happily, "Yes, and he's going to look like Tommy, too." For seven days Tom had been saying how small the baby was. His wife had heard small and thought cute. The image in Robin's mind now as she sat beside her husband in their car and watched the odometer tick off the miles to Children's Hospital was a picture-perfect little baby, all intact.

The Infant ICU at Children's is a world apart. Located off by itself in a corner of the fourth floor, it is isolated from casual traffic, difficult to find even on the second try, and forbidding from the outset. All three of the other critical care units on the fourth floor are entered directly from the hall through sets of double doors, partly glass, which ordinarily remain open. The entrance to the infant unit is a single windowless door which leads into a narrow windowless anteroom. That door never stands open. As it sighs shut under its own power, a visitor suddenly feels sealed off from the universe, a feeling not easily shed in this mysterious outpost.

On the right of the anteroom is a trough sink of stainless steel. On the left are a large canvas dump full of clean gowns in soft yellow and two smaller dumps for used gowns. A sign above the sink instructs all visitors to scrub carefully to the elbow, to don fresh gowns, and to refrain from touching a second baby without scrubbing a second time.

Beyond the anteroom and to the left is a small parents' lounge. To the right is the ICU itself. A sign taped to the glass door asks visitors to knock and wait. Inside, nurses and doctors talk, laugh, and work with babies, but not a sound escapes the unit. Within a moment or two the door is opened by a nurse or a clerk. Visitors must give their names and state their business. Though the door is not locked, one needs an invitation to get through it. By special arrangement the invitation may be extended to a grandparent or a sibling. Otherwise these and other visitors are asked to view the babies through glass from two hallways running alongside the unit.

The room is a large rectangle. In five glassed-in rooms that adjoin in an L along two walls, it can accommodate twenty patients. A few are enclosed in incubators. Most lie in open warmer beds which suffuse the patients in radiant heat from overhead and permit ready access and maximum surveillance. The nurses' station is a long table. Also contained within the rectangle are a supply room, a small room without windows for one patient needing isolation or special studies or protection from the stares of visitors, a nurses' lounge, and the head nurse's office.

Color seems next to absent. What strikes the eye at first glance is a Cubist impression of off-white, glass, stainless steel, read-out screens, tubes, dials, and vials—an overwhelming impression of technology. In other units color not only is part of the decor but is supplied by the patients themselves. Many children wear their own pajamas and nighties and robes. Beds are cluttered with books, games, dolls, stuffed animals. Get-well cards and paintings made in the playroom are taped up on walls. Little girls who get to feeling better might have bows in their hair.

In the Infant ICU most of the patients wear nothing. While a few of the bigger babies might wear diapers, the diapers at Children's, as everywhere else, are white. The full spectrum of skin shades does not begin to produce the splash provided by brightly patterned pj's. Toys are few and scattered—a small yellow bunny on this bed, a brown teddy bear on that, a red music box in another. No get-well cards. No accomplishments to show off. No hair bows.

The nurses do wear pale pink uniforms. The dresses provide some relief from off-white, glass, and stainless steel, as do the faded green surgical scrub suits worn by the residents and the pale yellow gowns worn by everyone else who enters the unit for any reason. Incubator bases are of pastel hues. But pastels cannot assert themselves in such surroundings. They soften the technology very little.

The effect of these surroundings on those who work in them is suggested by the way the nurses approach their bedmaking chores. Every morning a rack of freshly laundered cotton flannel sheets in miniature is left in the anteroom. Pastels dominate, not just solids but charming prints featuring happy children and animals. The sheets also come in white. Among the nurses, white sheets are the least popular. Faded as the pinks and yellows and blues and greens inevitably become, the nurses go after them on the linen cart, picking and choosing, coordinating colors, carrying off extras to tuck away for tomorrow. Making up a bed that looks nice is a minor but real source of gratification in the Infant ICU: a small act of sensual pleasure which, considering the sterility of the environment, considering what else the day might have in store for those taking care of the hospital's tiniest patients, seems wholly understandable.

Among the first of its kind in the country, the Infant ICU at Children's opened in 1962 to serve infants who had just had surgery. Today surgical patients are in the minority in this unit. One reason is competition. The services of pediatric surgeons are now offered by a number of hospitals in the region.

The other reason is abortion. Babies born with anomalies needing immediate surgical attention tend to be born to teenagers and to women over thirty-five. Since the Supreme Court declared abortions legal in 1973, these two groups have readily availed themselves, with the result that fewer babies are born needing surgery to survive.

Today the vast majority of patients in the Infant ICU are premature infants. Increasingly they are babies born to teenagers and to mothers who have had inadequate prenatal care. On an average they have entered the world twelve to fourteen weeks too early. Their mean weight is just over three pounds six ounces. In their fragile company, the occasional full-term, forty-week baby actually looks abnormal.

The tiniest of these patients may weigh just over a pound. Most babies that size don't live long enough to be admitted to Children's, or in any case they are rarely referred in, sometimes because they are the products of pregnancies known in advance to be high-risk and are thus delivered at hospitals having their own intensive care nurseries. The smallest infants cared for in the Infant ICU at Children's usually weigh in the near neighborhood of 750 grams: a pound ten ounces. They are, to a layperson's eye, appallingly tiny. Referred to by staff as 750-grammers, these patients take up little more space on their mattresses than centerpieces. They may not measure thirteen inches from crown to heel. Their heads are no bigger than large lemons.

Unless born with genetic anomalies, they are perfectly formed, at least insofar as can be seen. Yet they have been deprived of weeks of normal development, cast out of their natural environment long before they are equipped for life anywhere else. Except that they no longer draw sustenance from a mother's body, they are fetuses in every sense of the term. They bear less resemblance to Gerber babies than to specimens in glass jars.

Such a patient was Brandon Gregory. He had been admitted to Children's weighing 758 grams. In the week since, he had lost about an ounce.

The baby lay on his back asleep. Beneath him, on a sheet printed with little girls in sunbonnets, was a standard diaper that could have served him as a hammock. Over him, to minimize heat loss while permitting close observation, was a square blanket of Saran Wrap bordered in adhesive tape. His legs were splayed and drawn up sharply at the knees. His arms lay bent at the elbows, the tiny hands palm up, the tiny fingers curled into calyxes beneath the tiny ears. Brandon's eyebrows were two pale brown lines. His incipient hair was pale brown. His temples and much of the rest of his body were dusted with fine fetal down that would eventually disappear. Blood vessels showed in and under the translucent marbled skin of his abdomen as reddish-purple traces.

A green tube in the baby's mouth connected him to the respirator. The tube had been anchored with tape to his upper lip and cheeks from ear to ear. A clear tube had been taped into his umbilicus for painless blood sampling. Two more clear tubes had been inserted into his left foot and right wrist for medications and fluids in the form of intravenous feedings. Both those tubes were taped in place over foam blocks and rolled gauze which protected the baby's skin from direct contact with the adhesive.

A slim white wand had been taped to Brandon's chest to monitor his temperature. Three adhesive-backed "dots" had also been stuck on his chest and one thigh to monitor his heart and respiratory rates. Sheathed wires connected these leads to machinery just behind the bed. Red numbers, blinking red dots, and spiking or bouncing blue blips enlivened two readout screens behind the bed. No infant unit in the country was better equipped to treat a patient like Brandon Gregory, yet all the equipment and expertise available to him there could only provide him with an artificial environment that was at best a poor second to his mother's uterus.

The odds against his survival were very high. Based on weight alone he was three or four times more likely to die than to live, and weight was not the only strike against him. Most premies prior to delivery are perfectly normal fetuses. Were they to remain in the womb a full forty weeks, they would be perfectly normal babies. This could not be said with certainty of Brandon Gregory. The history of the pregnancy raised a question about the baby's normalcy in utero. The question had not been answered by Brandon's scores on a standard evaluation system one and five minutes postdelivery. Those scores had been neither very good nor very bad.

Furthermore, pressure on his umbilical cord in the birth canal could have deprived the baby of oxygen for longer than is customary during the birth process. Doctors could not be certain that he would grow up—if he grew up at all—with normal function intact.

To grow up intact or at all, Brandon Gregory would have to steer a path around obstacles that most premies his size do not manage to surmount. A host of hobgoblins awaited him. At their most malign, any one of them could kill him or leave him permanently disabled. They could be neither predicted nor prevented. The baby could have a massive intracranial hemorrhage. He could contract a fearful abdominal disorder known as necrotizing enterocolitis. He could become infected. Once off the respirator he would be at risk for both pneumothorax due to the immaturity of his lungs and for serious episodes of apnea, or lapses in breathing.

These were the hazards the child faced as a result of his immaturity. He could encounter additional hazards as a result of the high-tech treatment invoked to save him. From respirator therapy he could develop chronic lung disease and never get free of the machine. Oxygen therapy could blind him. Every tube entering his body from the outside world was a potential source of infection that could develop into fatal sepsis. Too little fluid could dehydrate him. Too much could stress his heart. Every drug he needed to correct one kind of problem could cause another. Of course treatment carries risks for patients of all ages and sizes. But few are as vulnerable as a patient weighing one pound ten ounces.

It would be difficult to overstate the fragility of a tiny premie. Babies the size of Brandon Gregory are so fragile that when they cry, they sometimes turn blue from lack of oxygen. They are so fragile that applying a stethoscope bell to their chests can make them turn blue. Their skin is so delicate that even the gentlest rub-

bing can irritate it, and tape can tear it if not pulled off with extreme care. Their constitutions are so delicate that they cannot
begin to tolerate ordinary percussion. When a premie's lungs need
clearing, a nurse will graze that baby's chest with an electric
vibrator.

Tiny premies are so fragile that it stresses them to be touched.
Their oxygen levels drop. They burn up calories they can't spare.

To avoid stressing these infants unduly, staff takes their vital
signs every four hours instead of every two. In between times the
nurses rely on the monitors and their own eyes. Though premies
are thought to need affectionate touching and stroking as much as
does any other baby, though infant bonding is considered important in this unit, though parental touch and holding are encouraged
when the babies seem able to tolerate those disturbances, most of
the time staff members think it best for the premies to be bothered
as little as possible.

Yet despite his exquisite fragility, despite the list of catastrophes
to which he might at any time fall prey, Brandon Gregory could not
be counted down. Premies his size had begun to survive in small
numbers around 1975, when neonatal medicine in general and respirator therapy in particular had reached a certain level of sophis-
tication. Data were still quite sketchy when Brandon was admitted to
Children's. What research had been done, however, showed that
some 750-grammers had apparently survived to be normal, or
nearly normal—at least so far.

Unfortunately, the prospects for any given baby that size were
unknowable. Virtually all that could be said with total certainty of
these infants was that they were wholly unpredictable. A tiny patient
who looked absolutely terrible could turn around and step out of
the woods. A great-looking patient the same size in the next bed
could crash irretrievably in the space of a few hours.

Still, while Brandon Gregory's prognosis as a 750-grammer was
particularly poor, while his likeliest destiny was to die or to survive
in a moderately compromised condition, his prognosis as an individual baby held more promising possibilities, one being that he would
grow up a normal child. He had already successfully defied some of
the heavy odds against him. Most premies his size die in their first
twenty-four hours of life. Brandon had made it through a full week,
and he had done so despite many problems. He couldn't breathe

without a respirator. His liver wasn't functioning properly. There were indications that his kidneys weren't functioning properly. He had a heart murmur. He'd had jaundice. Doctors had been concerned for a couple of days that the baby might have sustained a mild intracranial hemorrhage.

Serious as these problems were, they were neither unexpected nor unusual in a fetus born after only twenty-six weeks' gestation. All were attributable to immature organ systems. In theory those systems could reach maturity given time. The goal of treatment was to buy that time: to give Brandon Gregory the fourteen weeks of development he'd missed in utero; to support him until he grew big enough and strong enough to get along without medical help.

Even for the experts this was a towering task. In the old days of neonatology, a specialty which came into being in the early 1970s, success had been measured by survival rates. By the end of that decade the focus had changed from survival to quality of survival. Even today achieving quality is no mean feat. Getting a premie totally intact from 750 grams to 1300 grams remains a huge challenge in the 1980s.

"Like stepping on a roller coaster," one Children's neonatologist tells parents. A doctor can never let his or her guard down. A zillion problems lie just around the corner. The potential for a bad outcome is a specter on the horizon every minute of every day.

But if all goes well, the baby can conceivably go home to lead a normal life of seventy years' duration. It was this kind of future that the experts at Children's were hoping to secure for Brandon Gregory.

In the anteroom Tom Gregory showed his wife how to scrub at the sink. Each tied a clean yellow gown on the other. They approached the closed glass door. Somewhat tentatively, Tom knocked.

Robin began to feel shaky. Through the glass she caught sight of a baby who looked terrible, and suddenly she became afraid.

Someone let them in. Ordinarily the nursing staff prepares a parent visiting for the first time. Apparently no one realized that Robin had not been in before. The Gregorys proceeded on their own. Once they got past the baby she'd seen first, Robin breathed a sigh of relief. The other babies seemed bigger and not so badly off.

Ahead of Robin, her husband turned a corner and stopped. Still in his sunglasses, he faced her. "Here he is."

Rounding the corner herself, she glanced down, stopped short, took a step back, and felt her heart break.

She burst into tears. Tom led her out of the unit and into the small waiting room. There, a few minutes later, Brandon's nurse found them—a man, stocky and curly-headed, about their age. Robin thought he was an aide.

The nurse apologized. He felt so bad not to have been there when the parents came in. He'd been to lunch, he explained. If he'd been in the unit, he could have prepared Mrs. Gregory.

Robin shook her head. Nothing could have prepared her.

The nurse begged them to go back in with him. As if dreaming, Robin followed the young man and her husband back to Brandon's bedside. Speaking slowly and in everyday language, the nurse explained about all the equipment. Robin could not begin to keep up with the information he was giving her. She could not imagine how a baby who looked as Brandon did could possibly survive.

The nurse urged Robin to touch the baby.

She could not bring herself to do so.

The nurse then said he would lift Brandon a little so she could get a better look at his face. Gently the young man began to edge his hands under the tiny form. Had the baby not been so fragile, he could easily have picked him up in one hand. As the nurse gathered the baby into both hands, Robin felt so sick at the flimsiness of her son's body that she had to turn away. How could God have allowed a baby so small and weak to be born? Back in the waiting room, she wept in anguish.

Until now, no one at Children's had laid out the facts and implications of Brandon's condition for either of his parents. Ordinarily this task is undertaken by the neonatologist in charge of the unit, a responsibility that rotates monthly. That doctor is automatically the physician of record for every medical patient in the Infant ICU. Brandon's attending physician was Roger Forbes. Forbes came in for rounds on weekends, but he had not been on the scene when Tom Gregory had paid his first visit to Brandon, nor was he in today.

Instead, tipped off by Brandon's nurse, a second-year resident now joined the Gregorys in the ICU lounge—the same doctor who had talked with Tom Gregory during his visit on Sunday.

The resident had learned a lesson from that encounter. Gregory's getup and long hair had said "counterculture" to the doctor. The man had kept his sunglasses on, presenting the resident a view of his own reflection, and his responses had been versions of "Hey, man, that's something."

But just as the resident had begun to conclude that he wasn't getting through to Brandon's father, Gregory had calmly and quietly asked the most pertinent question the doctor had heard all day. At rounds the next morning the resident had urged his colleagues to assume nothing from this father's appearance, because the man was tuning in.

Talking now with the Gregorys in the lounge, the doctor had to remind himself of his own advice. The patient's father was polite but so composed as to seem absent. The resident had the feeling that if there'd been a magazine on the table, Tom Gregory would have picked it up and breezed through it.

His wife, on the other hand, gave every indication of being overwhelmed. The doctor knew she must also be exhausted from her surgery. It impressed him that she was nonetheless able to involve herself in intense conversation with him for the better part of half an hour. Robin Gregory had many questions. She asked repeatedly whether Brandon was ever going to come home.

The resident did not attempt to paint a rosy picture. There would be lots of problems, he told the Gregorys. A baby as small as Brandon had a minefield to cross. That field had to be negotiated with extreme caution. Success was not guaranteed.

Knowing that parents in distress can absorb only so much information at one sitting, the resident concentrated on the baby's main difficulty at the moment. Almost all babies born three months prematurely, he told them, had serious problems breathing. Their lungs were so immature that they collapsed in upon themselves.

Many lay people knew this condition as hyaline membrane disease. Perhaps the Gregorys would remember that President and Mrs. Kennedy had lost a baby from this disease in 1963? Doctors now referred to it as respiratory distress syndrome. RDS was Brandon's primary diagnosis, as it was the chief diagnosis of most premies. Actually he had a relatively mild form of the disorder.

The resident summed up by telling the Gregorys that right now Brandon had no problems the doctors felt they could not manage. He emphasized that the situation could change at any time. He said no more about the future than that Brandon would have to be in the hospital at least as long as he would have been inside his mother, and perhaps much longer.

Walking out the door of the unit moments later, Robin's one thought was that she and Tom should not get too close to Brandon. That way if he died, it wouldn't hurt as much.

In the car she made a different decision.

During her first few days in the hospital, Robin had pumped her breasts religiously every two or three hours around the clock. But keeping to this schedule had made her breasts sore and worn her out. She'd been discouraged to discover that Brandon couldn't even use her milk until she got off postop antibiotics. So on Thursday morning, in disgust, she had asked the nurse taking care of her to get the pump out of the room.

Now Robin knew that she would go back to pumping. She felt she owed that to Brandon. By overdoing she had been partly to blame for what had happened to him. As small as he was, he was going to need all the help he could get.

Sunday, December 16

Late evening. Darryl Barth sat alone in the Adolescent nurses' station. Tomorrow morning he would be starting a new rotation within Children's Hospital. Responsibility for the patients he had been caring for would be turned over to another first-year resident, Alan Cavanaugh, a competent, committed intern for whom his predecessor on Adolescent felt enthusiastic respect. Tonight Barth was putting a formal end to his term in the unit by writing off-service summaries in each of his patients' charts.

He left Mark Price's chart till last. For several paragraphs the young doctor made his points in straightforward clinical terms. But he could not maintain a dispassionate tone throughout. Too much had happened to Mark. Too much had happened to Barth himself. While reporting the good news without embellishment—"Finally total expansion was achieved, and today, Day 18, Mark is more comfortable with decreased respiratory distress and pain"—he was unable to refrain from adding a reference to the cost: "His comfort belies the misery he's been through in past weeks here."

Nor did the resident deny himself a few sentences that were purely personal.

"I hope Mark is on the way to improvement," he wrote near the end of his entry, an understatement born of the chastening he had undergone in conversation with the patient's mother; yet he concluded this paragraph on a celebratory note: "Today he was happy watching the Bengals play."

And below that sentence, on a line all its own, indented halfway across the page like the closing of a letter, Darryl Barth inscribed a farewell, a benediction, a five-word pronouncement that his successor could read only as a charge:

"He's a wonderful, courageous kid."

Monday, December 17

10:00 A.M. Cardiothoracic surgery resident Drew Cipriani stood at Mark's bedside explaining to the patient and to Darryl Barth's replacement on Adolescent what he was about to do.

"Mark, I'm going to clamp your two lower chest tubes. You've had the fourth tube in for three days now, and the x-ray this morning shows that the lung is still one hundred percent expanded. We think that tube is doing the job by itself. We'd like to get the other three out. The way we'll do that is to clamp them first so they stop functioning, then wait a day. If the lung doesn't go down, we'll pull those tubes."

Mark nodded, grinning. "So maybe I'll get home by Christmas!"

Cipriani couldn't promise. But the situation was certainly looking up, and the CT surgeon was glad to be able to give the boy good news for a change.

The fourth chest tube had added appreciably to Mark's suffering. About 11:00 Friday evening, hours after the insertion and despite the increased dose of Demerol, he had broken down and cried from pain. After receiving chloral hydrate for sleep, he had needed pain medications three times through the night. Yet he had refused the Demerol and Phenergan on Saturday morning. He had taken nothing until after lunch, telling the nurses he was trying not to use pain meds unless he really needed them because he didn't like being so groggy. He had refused them again last evening.

This morning Daniel Earnshaw had changed the orders back to codeine and Tylenol. So far Mark seemed reasonably comfortable. The nurses thought he might be tolerating his discomfort better now that his lung was up and he could look forward to going home. His spirits had also been lifted by the resumption this morning of his breathing treatments. No percussion yet, but he was getting Mucomyst every four hours and vibration on his right side. Not only would this help his breathing, but as a partial return to his regular routine it was also a psychological boost for Mark, making him feel on the road back to what for him was normal life.

"Okay, Mark," Cipriani said, "what I'm going to do here is turn off the Emerson. . . ." He rotated a dial to O and flicked a switch. Immediately the noise at the bedside diminished by half.

Cipriani showed Mark a small metal clamp. "Now I'm just going to slip this onto the tube. . . . Okay, there's the first one. . . ."

Dr. Alan Cavanaugh watched the patient watching the surgeon and thought that Mark Price was one of the sickest children he had ever seen. Cavanaugh was twenty-six, blond and clean-cut. He had grown up across the city from Children's and attended the university and medical school next door. His plan was to specialize in pediatric cardiology.

"Okay," Cipriani said, "that's all for today." One by one he had dropped the dressings from all four chest tubes into a wastebasket; on the way out, he would ask a nurse to come in and place new dressings over the insertion sites. "I'm going to order a chest x-ray," he told Mark, "and if the pneumothorax hasn't increased, I'll leave these two tubes clamped until tomorrow, and then if the x-ray's still okay, we'll go ahead and take them out."

Mark nodded soberly. "What happens if my lung collapses again?"

"Then we'll just unclamp the chest tubes."

"When you take them out, does it hurt?"

"You shouldn't feel anything more than just a pinch."

Ø

Downstairs in the Infant Intensive Care Unit, Brandon Gregory's day had begun far less propitiously than Mark's. The baby had developed his first serious complication of prematurity.

The problem lay in his circulatory system. A duct necessary to fetal blood flow had failed to close off as it should have within a few days of the baby's birth. Known as patent ductus arteriosis, this condition was almost unheard of until the mid-1960s, when small premies began living long enough to develop it. PDA plays havoc with newborn circulation. It congests the baby's lungs and overloads the heart. The effort of the heart to respond to the overload produces sounds of turbulent blood flow—a murmur—which can be heard through a stethoscope.

The murmur is not necessarily alarming to doctors, nor is the presence of a PDA in itself. The situation becomes worrisome—and life-threatening—only when the heart becomes dangerously overworked. This had happened with Brandon. Yesterday morning he had been a tiny premie with a heart murmur. By afternoon he'd begun to show signs of stress. A diuretic had not helped him. This morning he had suddenly developed the symptoms of significant PDA.

At one time doctors would send all such patients to the Operating Room. There a surgeon would cut into the baby's chest and tie off the ductus. But for a baby the size of Brandon Gregory, surgery itself was life-threatening. Blood loss amounting to just two teaspoonfuls could put him into shock.

In 1974 doctors had discovered that PDAs sometimes closed down spontaneously in patients receiving an anti-inflammatory drug called Indomethacin. To test whether this drug could be trusted as a safe alternative to the OR for babies who were otherwise sure to die, a group of experts had designed and launched a major research study that would ultimately enroll two thousand infants in thirteen centers. Among those experts was Roger Forbes, the neonatologist in charge of the Infant ICU for December and Brandon's doctor.

As of noon on Monday Brandon Gregory was a candidate for the PDA study, and Forbes wanted him on it. If Brandon got Indomethacin and was helped by it, he could avoid surgery. The doctor could not prescribe the drug precisely because it was still experimental in these circumstances. Only as part of the research did the patient stand a chance of staying out of the Operating Room.

Forbes needed the parents' consent. The person who placed the call was Elsa Montaigue, a nurse working as a full-time research associate on the PDA study at Children's, an attractive, dark-haired woman in her thirties who was herself a mother.

Robin Gregory was not expecting a phone call from Children's Hospital. From two conversations she had had with ICU nurses on Sunday and another this morning, she had received the impression that the baby was all right. As Elsa Montaigue explained who she was, Robin felt confused. Before she could get the situation straight in her mind, the woman had told her that Brandon had a heart murmur and that they were starting to worry about it.

Robin's own heart began to pound in fear.

As the nurse continued talking, however, the mother relaxed a little. The doctor who'd called her last week about the vitamin E study had said someone else might be calling about another study. Robin concluded that he must have been referring to the study she was now hearing about. She surmised that Elsa Montaigue had made Brandon's condition sound somewhat bad at first so the parents would be sure to sign the papers.

The nurse assured Robin that if the baby didn't improve, they would take him off the study and close the blood vessel in the Operating Room. Robin asked about the surgery. She gathered from the reply that it was a ten-minute operation.

But when the woman said, "If you'd like, I'll ask the doctor to call you," fear hit Robin like an avalanche. In the nine days Brandon had been at Children's, only one doctor had called them, and only to get their permission for the vitamin E study. It dawned on Robin now that something must really be wrong.

"Here comes Dr. Forbes now," the woman was saying. "Let me hang up and talk to him and have him call you right back."

Robin did not move from the spot. When the phone rang again, her hand was still on the receiver.

She had never heard of Dr. Forbes. He sounded young to her, though not as young as the doctor she and Tom had talked to on Saturday. Listening to him explain all over again what she'd just been told by the nurse, Robin realized for the first time that not every baby on the study got the drug. This confused her and frightened her further. If Brandon got the sugar pill and got worse, would it be too late?

The doctor assured her that they'd go ahead with surgery even if the baby got the drug and got worse. He asked if she would give permission to enter Brandon on the study.

Robin said yes feeling she had no choice. Was this, then, God's purpose in letting Brandon be born so early: had her baby been put on earth as a guinea pig to help the doctors learn more about how to care for babies as little as Brandon was?

Dr. Forbes told Robin that a decision would have to be made about surgery within forty-eight hours. He asked her when she and Tom could get to the hospital.

She told him they'd come in this evening, as soon as they'd gotten the twins settled down for the night.

He said he thought it was a good idea for them to see their baby this evening, in case he didn't get better.

Ø

Shortly after noon Mark's mother arrived on Adolescent bringing him a gift-wrapped package dropped off at the house on Sunday by a boy whose name was familiar to him. The present was an electronic game called Concentration. The enclosed get-well card had been signed, "From all your friends in woodshop class."

This morning he had received several Christmas cards from kids at school he didn't know. He speculated that they were friends of his brother's. The kids had written notes saying how brave he was and how proud they were of him. They hoped he was feeling better, they said. They were looking forward to meeting him when he got back.

This attention amazed him. He had thought none of the kids at his new school cared that he was in the hospital.

He'd thought he had been having problems making friends there. He hadn't taken this personally. When he'd first gone to school and been fairly healthy, the kids had gotten to know him and like him. At the next school, where he'd begun getting sicker, it had taken him longer to meet people. They'd noticed his skinniness. Or they'd noticed that his chest had started to stick out. Sometimes on the phone they had let him know that they thought he was nice. But his first weeks at this new high school had been the pits, a fact he attributed to the way he looked now.

There had been one uncomfortable incident. One day right after classes started had been very hot. Mark had been sweating, and his shirt had stuck to him so his pigeon breast had been quite obvious. In the cafeteria line, a boy had said to him, "What are you trying to do, grow tits?"

Mark had attempted to laugh off the comment. He'd noticed other kids watching, including a couple of girls.

"I didn't mean to hurt your feelings," the boy had said then.

Mark had told him not to worry about it. He really hadn't been hurt. He'd taken the comment as nothing more than a dumb statement. But it had embarrassed him, because he was sensitive about his masculinity.

He had long since given up girls. Back in seventh grade he had had a close friend named Melody Painter. When he was in the hospital, which wasn't often, she would come to see him. For a while after she had moved to Florida, they had exchanged cards. Then Mark had written Melody a letter which she hadn't answered. He had not written her again.

In eighth grade he had asked girls out—not the prettiest, and not the most popular—and they had refused him. That was even before he had started getting sick. He had understood that the girls might have refused him because he was small. After eighth grade, when the Prices had moved to a nearby town, Mark had made one more effort to get himself a date. When that girl said no, he had lost his confidence. He hadn't tried again. He didn't feel comfortable with girls in high school, where nearly everybody was miles taller than he was. He'd seen a couple of girls who were shorter, but they weren't skinny like he was.

So he wasn't looking for girlfriends now. Just friends.

Mark wadded up the gift paper and shot it into the wastebasket next to his bed. He counted his cards. Four of them. Four kids who might become his friends as soon as he got out of the hospital, plus how many were there in his woodshop class? Maybe ten more? Maybe fifteen?

He had told only one person at his new school that he had CF. A

boy in his English class had kept asking him why he kept getting
sick. Finally Mark had explained. Until now he had thought that
boy was the only friend he had.

Ø

Downstairs in the Intermediate ICU, play therapist Kay Mitchell,
one of Jody Robinson's many Children's Hospital friends, had unrolled a shag rug the color of cinnamon on the floor near Jody's
bed. Mitchell herself sat near one end of it. Jody sat cross-legged
beside her on a small white blanket laid over the rug, looking up at
her freckled face. Over his diaper he wore a white long-sleeved T-
shirt shot with red, blue, green, and yellow. He also had on a pair of
bright blue jogging shoes. His ventilator tubes went under one arm
and stretched back to the machine behind him like two curved jet
streams. For four days now the ventilator had been breathing for
Jody only once per minute. He had suffered no ill effects. He'd
recovered from the bronchoscopy without difficulty. His mother
had not been heard from since her phone call on Monday.

From a cart beside her, Mitchell produced two plastic cups. One
was empty. The other was full of little balls made from a claylike
substance she called bread dough.

"Okay, Jody, we're going to take the balls out of this cup and put
them into this one, okay?"

The exercise was meant to give him practice with his pincer
grasp, an element of fine motor control. As she proffered the full
cup, he reached for one of the balls and took it out between thumb
and forefinger. His remaining three fingers spread out like a fan.
Instead of putting the ball into the empty cup, he drew it to him for
a closer look.

"Squish it!" Mitchell urged him. She pressed his thumb and forefinger deep into the soft dough. "Squish it!" He looked startled at
first, then delighted.

"Okay, Jody, now put the ball into this cup. *In.* That's good. Now
take another one out of here . . . *out* . . . good . . . and put it *in* here
. . . good! Now another one . . ."

She spent an hour with him whenever she could. Her goal was to
help Jody make strides in all areas of normal child development.
Mitchell was not concerned that Jody develop at the same pace a

normal child would. She only wanted him to make progress at a pace that suited him.

Rummaging in a box on her cart, the play therapist brought out a fuzzy blue bunny puppet which she dropped over her right hand. She held the bunny close to Jody. He regarded the blue face in fascination.

The bunny nodded in greeting. Its ears flopped forward over its eyes.

"Hi, Jody! Hi! Hi there!" The bunny cocked its head first on one side, then on the other. The patient scooted even closer to Mitchell than he already was, digging his heels into the thick pile of the rug.

"Where's the bunny's nose, Jody? Right! Now what about his eyes? Where's his eyes? Good!" Her praise excited him. Shaking his hands in the air, he threw back his head and laughed.

"Now, Jody, where's his mouth?"

This was harder. The mouth wasn't a marking or a button; it was a big opening that gave the face two parts. Mitchell raised Jody's hand to the mouth so he could touch it. He pulled his hand away. Picking up a blue block, he offered the block to the bunny.

Mitchell smiled. She whisked the puppet off her hand and hid it behind her. When she'd first hidden a toy from Jody, he had simply accepted its absence. She'd wondered whether this was merely happenstance or a function of developmental delay. A normal child would ordinarily look for a plaything that had suddenly disappeared.

He reached for the puppet, craning around her to see what might have become of it.

She lifted him as close to her as it was possible for him to be, short of sitting on her lap. Guiding his arm, she helped him lean far enough over in just the right spot. Suddenly he whipped his arm back with the limp bunny clutched in his fist.

"Jody, you found it! Good boy! Good for you!"

He beamed.

She asked him to help her put some blocks back in a bucket. When they had finished, she slipped the puppet on her hand again and made the paws wave.

"Bye-bye, Jody." The bunny shook the child's hand. "Can you wave goodbye to the rabbit? Bye-bye? Bye-bye, Jody."

Raising his hand palm inward, he opened and closed his fingers

several times, a gesture more of beckoning than of farewell. His
Pope wave, the nurses called it. But he had the idea, and Mitchell
didn't press the point.

She was one of four staff members at Children's who made regular visits to Jody to help him develop as much as his condition
would permit. The others were a speech therapist, an occupational
therapist, and a registered dietitian.

The speech therapist was beginning to teach Jody sign language.
When first involved with him, she had tried and been able to desen-
sitize his gag somewhat, knowing it would hamper eating if the child
ever got to that point. More recently she had been working to increase his powers of comprehension. As he understood so much
more than he was able to say, the speech therapist expected him to
move very quickly into sign language.

At the same time she was preparing him for true speech.
Though most people with tracheostomies can make no meaningful
sound, a few can, depending on fluke combinations of individual
anatomy, muscle strength, trach tube placement, and body position-
ing. The speech therapist kept experimenting with different positions with Jody, hoping to hit on a key combination that would allow
him to emit words.

Meanwhile she was teaching him to form words even though he
couldn't actually say them. This effort drew on a skill he had already mastered: imitation. Sometimes having him just watch her,
sometimes having him place his hand on her lips or throat and then
on his own, the therapist would repeat vowels and consonants and
syllables for Jody and invite him to copy her as best he could. He
loved these exercises. He treated them as a game, which was exactly
what the speech therapist wanted: that the work be fun for him.

Of course she did not try to teach him to say any version of
"Mommy."

The occupational therapist was attempting to help Jody make
adaptations that would permit him to explore and enjoy as wide a
range of activities as possible given his limits. For a long time she
had concentrated hardest on getting him accustomed to lying on his
tummy and on building up the capabilities of his left hand while
decreasing his dependence on the right.

More recently the OT had also been working with him on standing up and sitting down. Because the child had never learned to crawl, he had never been forced to support his own weight, and his arm muscles were underdeveloped. Now he seemed on the verge of being able to stand without support, but he wasn't yet strong enough to pull himself up into that position. His arm strength was improving, however.

The OT had also been attempting to develop a protective reaction in Jody. When he lost his balance while sitting, he knew enough to put his arms out at his sides to keep himself from tipping over. But because he'd never learned to crawl or to stand unassisted, he'd never had the experience of falling forward. The notion of putting his arms out front to break a fall was something he had to learn. The OT's approach was to stand Jody on the floor and tilt him headfirst over a fat cylindrical bolster, encouraging him to take his weight on his hands and knees.

Like her counterpart in speech, the occupational therapist worked with the nurses as well as the patient. By teaching the nurses what Jody needed to learn, they surrounded the child with people able to provide therapy when the therapists weren't around.

At one time a physical therapist had also spent time with Jody. She continued to make suggestions to the others involved in his care. However, except that his knees locked and prevented him from sitting down from a standing position, he really had no specific muscle or movement problems. His body did almost everything he asked of it.

His problem was coordination. He was also saddled with his ventilator tubes. The feeding tube in his abdomen likewise interfered with his ability to play freely. These peculiarities made him a logical candidate for OT. While work with a physical therapist might also have benefited him, those involved had agreed it would be better to let the PT have input from a distance than to inundate the child with helpers.

The dietitian was one of the people responsible for making sure that Jody Robinson received proper nourishment. There had been a time when both she and the nurses had despaired of ever accomplishing this simple goal. For a period in his younger days, Jody had had terrible problems with his gastrostomy tube. Serious leakage at the insertion site had not been the worst of those problems. Sometimes when sneezing or coughing he'd pop the tube out entirely, and on more than one occasion he had actually splattered his stomach contents on the ceiling. They'd nicknamed him Old Faithful.

Amazingly enough, he had never had a severe nutrition problem. For that the dietitian credited the nurses. Part of her job was to check trays coming back to the kitchen to see how much was actually being eaten by patients well enough to have regular food. Some days tray after tray would come back with nothing gone. One did not have to have been at the bedside to know the story. The kids hadn't felt well enough to eat, their parents hadn't been in to help, the dietitian hadn't gotten up to encourage them, the nurses hadn't had the time.

The children of Intermediate, by contrast, rarely if ever missed a meal. Even during the long siege of troubles with Jody's gastrostomy, when the nurses had stuff flying all over them and were having to change the patient's bed for the tenth time, they'd made sure he got every feeding around the clock without ever skipping one, and they'd worked hard to give him the richest possible concentration of calories in the smallest possible volume. So smoothly had they worked together on this effort that it had almost seemed to the dietitian as if each shift of nurses in Intermediate was identical to the one it followed. They'd exemplified a philosophy that she had come to impute to the unit as a whole: the refusal to ever let anything slide.

These days she paid a formal call on Jody once a week. During those visits she would assess his caloric intake, do complicated measurements that would allow her to calculate his muscle and fat stores, look for changes in his height and weight, recommend modifications of his formula, and answer any questions a nurse might have. Extended consultations had long since ceased to be necessary. The child was growing beautifully. In terms of height, weight, and activity level, the dietitian judged Jody to be right where he should be for someone his age.

The attentiveness and the expert services of nurses, therapists, and the dietitian were of course reflected in a hospital bill for Jody Robinson that was growing daily by leaps and bounds.

Also reflected in that bill were twenty-one major or minor surgical procedures or evaluations; close monitoring by critical care

specialists and the coordination by those specialists of Jody's treatment and development programs; a bed in the ICU for 577 days,
as of today, December 17; heat, light, clean sheets, and towels;
hundreds or perhaps thousands of tests and studies of all kinds,
including x-rays; use of the ventilator and other equipment; medicines; adhesive tape, gauze pads, strings that went around Jody's
neck to keep the trach tube securely in place, soaps, creams, diapers, disposable syringes, and suction catheters; food; water; pacifiers.

Because his mother was on welfare, Jody Robinson was a Medicaid patient. The payments made by Medicaid for services rendered
to Jody Robinson at Children's Hospital represented state and federal moneys whose source was the American taxpayer. The difference between those payments and the actual cost of Jody's care
was made up by more generous insurers issuing reimbursements
for the children of their subscribers: men and women who were also
American taxpayers.

As reflected in the amounts charged to Medicaid, the price tag
for Jody Robinson's life in his nearly nineteen months on earth so
far had come to a grand total of $393,281—nearly $5,000 for every
week that Sabra Robinson's firstborn had spent at Children's.

That the child was alive to incur such expenses was due most
fundamentally to the decisions made about him in his first few
hours out of the womb and to the critical surgery performed on
him in his first few days at Children's. Those operations could have
been done by any of several general surgeons on Pierce Lynd's staff.
It so happened that they had been done by Herbert Russell. A
stocky man with white hair, divorced father of four grown children,
Russell had been at Children's for twenty-five years. He had undertaken all of Jody's surgery except the work done on the child's
larynx and would eventually perform, if the patient survived that
long, the very tricky colon interposition that would at last give Jody
Robinson a fully functioning digestive tract.

Day in and day out for nearly a quarter of a century, on countless children of all ages, Herbert Russell had performed operations
in accordance with unwritten policy of the surgical service under
Pierce Lynd that the surgeons at Children's Hospital would make
every effort to save the life of every child brought into the institu-

tion with problems susceptible of repair in the operating room unless the child was irrefutably and irretrievably dying.

Russell knew that certain people in other hospitals, seeing a newborn with multiple anomalies, might say some version of "Well, let's just throw it in the wastebasket. These problems are too complicated to fix." For much of Herbert Russell's long career, pediatric surgeons even in centers such as Children's had understood that if a baby needed to go to the OR more than a couple of times, the child was probably not going to make it.

By the time Jody Robinson was admitted to Children's, this was no longer true. Support systems had so improved—respirators, intravenous feeding, intensive care—that a child needing multiple operations stood a good or even excellent chance of surviving them. Surgeons at Children's had found that if they immediately took care of the life-threatening problems in such cases and then gradually attacked the child's other problems one by one, very often they would have a good result.

Unless the patient was clearly dying, the surgeons never approached a case on the premise that the best treatment might be no treatment. The tacit policy of the institution and of the surgical service molded by Pierce Lynd was that if the family or anyone else wanted to send a patient to the surgeons at Children's Hospital, the child would get the full works.

It was Herbert Russell's considered opinion that in choosing this course, he and his colleagues might very well be guilty of a head-in-the-sand attitude. In the first place, when a baby was admitted from another hospital, the surgeons at Children's presumed that the decision to transfer represented conviction on the part of the referring physician and the parents that surgery would serve the child's best interests. In fact, Russell believed, a transfer sometimes or even often represented the desire of a community physician to ship the child out and let the problem be someone else's.

In the second place, the surgeon had doubts that saving the lives of certain patients was in the best interests of either the child or the family. Experience had shown Russell that technological improvements had caused a number of babies who probably would succumb eventually anyway before their time to live longer than perhaps they might have otherwise, and therefore to suffer longer than they would have otherwise.

The parents endured that suffering and suffered in other ways when a child with significant defects lived, in Russell's opinion. Bad anomalies ruined marriages and destroyed families. He had seen it over and over. They all had. There was no question in Russell's mind that raising an imperfect child was a stressful business from beginning to end.

Among the patients whose lives Herbert Russell had saved over the years were a number of children with Down's syndrome. All Down's babies are destined to be retarded, though no one can say at birth just how retarded they'll be. A certain percentage of those infants are born with intestinal obstructions that are incompatible with life. In some hospitals parents are offered the option of with-holding treatment. Not at Children's.

Russell had in his desk drawer several letters from the mother of a Down's patient whose gut he had repaired. The mother had writ-ten to say how wonderful the whole experience had been for her whole family. The mother herself was involved in Down's counsel-ing. Her husband had become active in Girl Scouting. An older daughter had decided on a career in social work. None of it would have happened, the mother wrote, had this little retarded child not lived among them.

The surgeon was quite prepared to concede that what the mother said was so. He had heard it said many times that defective children brought out the best in families. He had seen situations that bore out this view.

But he remained unconvinced that the family was better off with the child alive than it would have been had the child died. Russell had also observed that when people had no choice but to accept a certain situation, they managed to drum up good things to say about it. In his opinion, any family of a defective child that was pursuing worthwhile activities would have done so anyway. The ac-tivities might have been different, and perhaps they would have been even more worthwhile. Maybe the family members would be making an even greater contribution to the community if they were not tied down to that abnormal child. Just because they were doing something good didn't mean they were doing the best of which they were capable.

Furthermore, it seemed to Russell that having an abnormal child kept some parents from going on to have a subsequent baby or two, a baby or babies who would very likely be normal. The possibility of certain deformities repeating themselves is virtually nil. But many parents don't want to take the risk. So by saving badly damaged infants, Russell reasoned, the surgeons at Children's might actually have kept one or two perfectly healthy babies out of the world.

Nobody ever worried about that part of it, the surgeon felt. Nobody ever worried about the effect of the damaged child on potential children who would have been fine. Nobody talked about the harassment of the mother, the father, the siblings, and the grandparents as they attempted to care for and adjust their lives to the defective child in their midst. Nobody ever talked about the total ramifications of the abnormal child, including and perhaps especially those in a position to know best. Unless she shared the information, no one knew what went through a mother's head as she bathed and dressed and fed a deformed offspring who hadn't a prayer of ever being normal.

That society had not called a halt to the saving of children with significant defects indicated to Herbert Russell that those lives were a burden society was willing to bear, however great the purchase price. He understood that less affluent societies approached such matters differently. On a visit to China Russell had learned that children with colon troubles serious enough to require that those patients be sent forth into the world with a colostomy were not sent forth into the world at all. In Africa, he'd heard, physicians who did a colostomy on a child never saw the patient again. For one reason or another, the child never returned for follow-up visits.

Russell certainly did not applaud these practices, if practices they were. But looking at the efforts expended at Children's and elsewhere to salvage children so defective that in the spectrum of their dysfunctions a colostomy was merely one inconvenience, he sometimes wondered whether perhaps Western society had become too sophisticated and affluent for its own good.

Yet while he had reservations about treating in all but the direst circumstances on the premise that life should be saved whatever its potential or lack thereof, Herbert Russell would have had reservations at least as strong about proceeding on any other premise.

The surgeon in chief for most of Russell's tenure at Children's had believed that withholding support from abnormal infants was a form of murder which in principle differed little from genocide. For Pierce Lynd, nontreatment was justified only when death was inevitable. His rejection of any other approach was interpreted by his white-haired colleague as a refusal to yield the eighth of an inch that others might then construe as a mile and a half, thus releasing from Pandora's box the seeds of the destruction of a moral society. On this subject there were people in and out of Children's who thought Lynd had gone off the deep end, as Lynd himself was well aware.

Herbert Russell wasn't one of them. He himself did not subscribe to the Pandora's box theory. Russell believed modern civilization to be capable of making reasonable judgments about when to intervene on behalf of life and when to let well enough alone. He felt confident that denizens of today's world could preside over such discriminations without falling prey to excess.

Nonetheless, Russell shared certain of Pierce Lynd's fundamental concerns. By coincidence, the two surgeons had visited Auschwitz together after lecturing in Poland one year. Auschwitz had had a profound effect upon them both. The stark reminder of how successfully Adolf Hitler had been able to seduce the German intelligentsia had been staggering to Russell. Though he saw no parallels between Hitler's Germany and contemporary America, could not imagine happening here what had happened there, Herbert Russell nonetheless knew enough history to be cognizant of society's tendency from Roman times forward to rid itself of undesirables, however a given culture chose to define that term. A society had to be very careful, in Russell's view, that it did not delegate responsibility for life-and-death decisions to people who lacked the scope to make them.

This, the surgeon knew, was far easier said than done. Unfortunately, those who had the scope didn't necessarily agree with each other. Pierce Lynd had been in a good position to make decisions of this nature. He'd had a lot of knowledge and a lot of experience. But he had reached one conclusion while Herbert Russell, who also had a great deal of knowledge and experience, had reached another.

The issue was too complicated to be served by a single solution, in Russell's opinion. It could not be reduced to one answer. Since it could not, the surgeon believed it best for doctors to err on the side of conservatism. It was far better for them to make a mistake by saving a child than the other way around.

This approach was especially important, in Russell's mind, for physicians with high public and professional visibility. Children's Hospital had an excellent reputation both locally and internationally. On any given day Russell's professional counsel might be sought by pediatric surgeons in such places as Liverpool, England; Colombia, South America; and Kansas City, Missouri. If prominent hospitals such as Children's relaxed their dedication to saving lives, they would surely be mimicked. They had to be extremely careful about the precedents they set. This was one factor behind the tone Pierce Lynd had set for his associates, and Russell respected him for it.

So if by taking a conservative approach the surgeons at Children's were guilty of a head-in-the-sand attitude, it was nevertheless an attitude they could live with, in Russell's view. It also had a certain practical value. When one started with the premise that virtually every child should be saved, one did not have to get involved in prickly, time-consuming arguments over theology, philosophy, or cost-benefit ratios. One simply operated.

Had he felt wholly bound by this premise, Russell believed he would long since have left Children's Hospital. But Pierce Lynd for all his strong convictions had not been a dictator. There was leeway in the system he had forged. What Russell did as a surgeon he did by choice.

He had no doubt that if he decided to ship a patient back to the referring hospital without operating, he was "big and ugly enough" to handle any trouble he might run into with his peers, which in any case would amount, he thought, to little more than a flurry. He had always tried to avoid such trouble because he didn't think the gain was worth the cost. Russell could acknowledge that this was a way of keeping peace with his boss. Or, as he put it on one occasion, "If you know your father doesn't like you smoking, you don't smoke in front of him."

Under Pierce Lynd's successor, Herbert Russell anticipated feeling more freedom. Meanwhile he had accepted the stance of the Division of Surgery as the best one for him to take in that institution at that moment in history, and he had continued to perform surgery he might wish withheld from a grandchild of his if he had grandchildren.

About a grandchild, of course, he would not have had, nor would he have wanted, the authority to make the decision himself. But if a daughter or daughter-in-law of his were to give birth to a child with certain combinations of significant anomalies, Russell would offer the parents a very detailed description of the pros and cons of treatment as he saw them and would make very sure before the baby was transferred to Children's Hospital or anywhere else that there was a hell of a lot of discussion and soul-searching and sorting out.

However, if Jody Robinson had been born into his family, Russell would have recommended all the surgery that was ultimately done on the child. As a grandfather he would have felt the same way he'd felt as a surgeon when first confronted by Jody: that this baby should be supported. This baby had a chance to surmount the obstacles fate had laid in his path and to lead a relatively full life.

The child had a lot going for him now, in Russell's opinion. He had a functioning rectum, a functioning urinary tract, genitalia that would work, legs that would walk him around, a functioning brain. Eventually, if all went well, he would be able to swallow food. Perhaps he would have a moderately good speaking voice. If nothing catastrophic occurred in the meantime, Jody Robinson would grow up to be an independent, self-sufficient individual.

Russell would have opposed the enormous effort exerted on Jody's behalf had he felt that by assigning this child a bed, the hospital was denying care to a patient with an even better prognosis who needed the expertise that Children's offered. But the surgeon couldn't imagine that the hospital would ever be confronted with such a choice. Society in its affluence had made a place for Jody Robinson and was providing for him there. Herbert Russell saw no sign that society was about to disavow that commitment.

When the play therapist had left Intermediate, Jody was lifted back into his crib by a young nurse who was learning his care. Suddenly he began to gag. His eyes bulged and became teary. He wheezed hard. Sweat broke out all over his face. Secretions poured out the side of his neck, drenching the four-by-four gauze pads that

covered the opening of his esophagus, drenching the T-shirt underneath. His color darkened slightly.

But as Jan Haver came up to see if the young nurse needed
help, the gagging stopped. With eyes still full, Jody gave Jan a big
smile.

"Okay, turn it off," Haver teased him. She tossed a towel over
his head, covering his face. "Turn off that gagging, Jody!"

He yanked the towel away.

"There he is!"

Kicking with excitement, he put the towel back on his head. This
time it hung down over his eyes Madonna-style. The nurses
laughed.

"He's been gagging," the young nurse told Peter Crossin, who
had just walked into Intermediate and come over to greet Jody. "He
soaked everything!"

Leaning on the raised side rail, Crossin watched the patient
closely for a moment. By now the activity around another bedside
had absorbed the baby's attention. He seemed perfectly fine.

"He recovers fast, doesn't he?" said Crossin in a tone intended to
twit the nurses. He chucked Jody under the chin. The patient gave
his doctor a dazzling smile.

Haver rolled her eyes. "No wonder everybody thinks we're big
liars around here!"

Ø

Roger Forbes had a quick supper in the hospital cafeteria and
went back to his office. While waiting for Brandon Gregory's parents, he would catch up on desk chores. The doctor worked with
his sleeves rolled up. Though he wore a jacket only for meetings,
Forbes dressed more formally than many physicians at Children's:
no sport shirts, and he never loosened his tie at the hospital.

He was forty, with boyish features and dark blond wavy hair cut
shorter than was fashionable. A trim forty, considering that his only
sports were summer fishing and occasional squash with his teenaged
daughter. There were two younger daughters. His wife was a former teacher who these days devoted herself to a child abuse program in the Junior League.

Forbes, too, had changed fields. By training a pediatric cardiologist, he had become a neonatal specialist when asked in 1970 to take over the Infant ICU. He'd run the unit until this year, when he'd become too busy with his other responsibilities. Currently he held two titles at Children's: Director of the Division of Neonatology and associate physician in chief of the hospital. He would not have given up his rotations in the unit every fourth month even if staffing had permitted. Forbes enjoyed administration, but he had no desire to forsake the practice of medicine.

The call came about 9:00. Slipping into his suit jacket, the doctor walked through the deserted third-floor hallways, took the stairs to the fourth floor, where there was much more activity, and proceeded to the Infant ICU. He found the Gregorys in the small waiting room. Research associate Elsa Montaigue, who had also stayed late to see them, was drawing diagrams to show Brandon's parents the problems in blood flow that resulted from patent ductus arteriosis.

Forbes introduced himself and sat down. For some minutes he and Montaigue went over the diagrams with the Gregorys. The doctor again explained the study. He told the family that Brandon now met the criteria for surgery within forty-eight hours if he didn't improve, sooner if he got worse, that the baby had a fifty-fifty chance of surviving the operation, and that the next few days would be hairy. To make sure they grasped his meaning, Forbes told the young couple across from him that it would be important for them to stay in close touch.

He had heard about the Gregorys, of course, so Forbes was not surprised that the father left his sunglasses on and seemed very reticent. When Tom Gregory began to respond, however, Forbes saw that his responses were appropriate to the situation; and his questions, though phrased in a kind of shorthand with no apparent emotion, were clear and to the point.

The mother seemed mainly frightened. Forbes had been impressed on the phone with her this morning that she had not wanted to leave her other children until they'd gone to sleep. A good, solid citizen, the doctor had thought at the time. Now Robin Gregory seemed unable to express herself. Whenever Forbes asked her if she had questions, she'd simply look at her husband, as if she had questions but was trying to pass them on by ESP.

Nonetheless, it was the doctor's impression that the family was holding up very well.

When he felt persuaded that the Gregorys understood the full extent of their son's peril from the overload on his heart, Roger Forbes planted a note of hope. He told Brandon's parents that their baby might possibly be one of those tiny premies who tolerate PDA surgery with little difficulty. However, the doctor emphasized, even if Brandon had the surgery and tolerated it very well indeed, he would by no means be out of danger. He would still be subject to all the other hazards posed by extreme prematurity, any one of which could claim his life.

Forbes went through them: his "laundry list," as he called it, of immature organ systems that were ill prepared for the tasks just handed them; the risks that imperil all premies.

Not wanting to overwhelm the Gregorys, Forbes attempted to portray their son's situation in broad strokes and simple language. Because odds are not necessarily relevant to a specific baby, he did not cite odds. Because of Brandon's difficult birth history, the doctor was somewhat more pessimistic in this conversation than he would have been otherwise. He emphasized the unknowns and told the Gregorys in essence that he and his colleagues would do everything they could to help Brandon get across the minefield intact.

It never occurred to Roger Forbes to ask the Gregorys whether they *wanted* everything done for their son. Such a question at this juncture would have been unthinkable to Forbes. If Brandon had arrived at Children's blue, shocky, and flaccid, if over his nine days in the unit he hadn't moved a muscle, had made no respiratory effort, and had developed signs of severe intracranial hemorrhage, if he had been unresponsive to resuscitation, then Roger Forbes might be preparing to discuss with the Gregorys at what point in their baby's terminal illness they might wish to have therapy discontinued.

But Brandon had arrived at Children's pink and kicking and showing clear signs that his heart was pumping blood effectively, his activity and alertness a sign of viability. He had lost weight since, but this was to be expected. While possibly he had suffered a mild intracranial hemorrhage, there was no indication of a major bleed, though he could have bled severely without exhibiting clinical symptoms.

His vital signs had been stable all week. Until his circulation had become a problem, he had required only minimal levels of artificial ventilation. He remained active. Though the baby was in real danger from his PDA, so far there had been no disasters. That Brandon had made it through nine whole days suggested he was a good deal tougher than most babies his size and could use well the assistance provided him.

Furthermore, Forbes's own principles demanded that he treat Brandon, and treat him aggressively. The baby was more alive than dead. As Roger Forbes understood the law, a doctor who took steps to effect the death of a live baby, by either omission or commission, was performing premeditated murder.

Forbes had grown up steeped in Catholicism. Though he now felt distaste for much of organized religion and deplored the "authoritarian crap" of the conservative church, and though he sent his own children to public schools, Forbes nevertheless continued to attend mass regularly and considered himself a good Catholic. He felt comfortable with most of Catholicism's spiritual tenets, among them reverence for life. Like Pierce Lynd, he believed in treating all patients who were not indisputably dying. He would not turn his back on an infant who was wiggling or digesting food or looking up at him.

Also in common with Lynd, Forbes was viewed within the hospital and beyond as a "pro-lifer." He disliked the label. To him the charge implied that he was blindly keeping babies alive no matter how dead they were. In fact once death began, Forbes firmly believed that it ought to be allowed to proceed. Always with the parents' knowledge and consent, he himself had had, on many occasions, the dubious privilege of turning off a respirator or of deciding to withhold from a patient all further medical interventions except for comfort measures. He did not cherish the notion of life at all cost.

But he would pull a plug only in very carefully defined circumstances. Forbes had to see evidence that the baby had suffered brain or heart or lung damage from which recovery was clearly impossible. He would not pull a plug merely on a suspicion of irreversible damage. Nor would he withdraw support from or fail to institute therapy in a patient who seemed likely to survive but with mild, moderate, or severe handicaps. He would not withhold treatment from any baby just because the child might turn out badly. Regardless of prognosis, if the patient was not indisputably dying, Roger Forbes would treat aggressively, giving the baby every chance at whatever kind of existence lay ahead.

Sometimes the Infant ICU staff is confronted with a patient too sick to demonstrate much life but not quite sick enough to be pronounced hopeless. Forbes's approach was to treat until the baby declared his or her intentions. Knowing he must inevitably be merely prolonging death for some of these patients, he took no pleasure in it.

But Brandon Gregory's doctor had learned a humbling lesson quite early in his career. A premie had come into the old Children's weighing 690 grams on her first day of life. By the end of her second week in the hospital, she had looked like a baby bird fallen from the nest. Her weight had gone down to 500 grams—one pound one ounce. She had seemed barely alive. At the age of five months the child had been discharged in good shape. At eighteen months she'd been walking, dancing, and singing nursery rhymes. Forbes had last seen her in her ninth year. The girl was normal, the message unambiguous: no matter how bad a premie looked, the outcome was not a foregone conclusion.

Another doctor might have outlined his or her philosophy of treatment to the Gregorys and, if the parents considered it incompatible with their own, offered to help them find for Brandon a physician with whose beliefs the family would feel more comfortable. Roger Forbes's instincts did not lie in this direction. Though he would have answered honestly had Brandon's parents asked him direct questions about his philosophy, in essence Forbes saw no option for the Gregorys any more than he saw one for himself. Studies had shown that a 750-grammer could thrive and prosper with proper care. The parents had willingly sent their baby to the Infant ICU at Children's. Brandon was alive and should thus, in Forbes's opinion, have every chance, no matter what the odds against his survival as either a normal or an abnormal child.

While she could not trust herself to speak, Robin Gregory sat listening to Roger Forbes feeling impressed by him. So far he was the oldest doctor she had seen in the unit. It was obvious to her that he knew what he was doing. She felt confident that he understood her desire to have Brandon taken off the study and sent to surgery if he got worse. For these reasons the baby's mother was perfectly willing to sign the papers.

Tom Gregory, too, felt confidence in Forbes. He had faith in all the doctors and nurses at Children's. Tom had first heard of the hospital when his first wife had borne their premature infant. That baby had lived only twenty-two hours. He had never become stable enough to be transferred to Children's. But there had been talk of transferring him. The baby's father had gathered from the talk that children were flown into this hospital from all over and that it was the best place a sick child could be.

So he, too, was ready to consent to anything the people at Children's wanted to try with his son. If their experiments didn't work with Brandon, perhaps they would help some other child. Gregory had said this to his wife in the car, hoping to make her feel better.

He himself expected Brandon to die. The other baby had died, and he had been twice as big as this one. That had been five or six years ago. Dr. Forbes had said the technology was much more advanced now. But Tom Gregory simply could not imagine a technology advanced enough to save a baby this small.

Proceeding to their son's bedside, the Gregorys were horrified to see that the baby's right arm and hand were reddish-purple and swollen. A term entered Robin's mind that she hadn't heard in years: elephantiasis. To her the arm looked dead.

There was a nurse at the bedside, a young man who introduced himself and welcomed the Gregorys by saying he'd be happy to answer any questions they had. Robin asked him if they were going to have to amputate the baby's arm.

The nurse assured her that they would not. The blood vessels were very fragile in a baby as small as Brandon, he explained. Bruising and swelling caused by the IV needles were common.

"It looks like there's no circulation."

The nurse assured the parents that blood was circulating in the arm.

The mother could not see how. "Does he feel pain?"

The nurse had worked in the unit more than two years; yet he gave an answer that would have won the disapproval of most of his colleagues there, an answer the baby's mother did not believe. "They don't feel pain like we do," the nurse replied.

Robin wondered how he could know what Brandon felt.

As she and Tom stood looking down at their son in silence, the nurse watched them with sympathy and concern. He was sure that had the baby been his, he'd be feeling just as frightened and leery and distant as the Gregorys seemed to be feeling. Though they had brought in a musical bunny and a little stuffed dog, neither parent seemed to be bonding with Brandon.

"Why don't you touch him?" The nurse spoke softly. He lifted the Saran Wrap at the baby's toes.

After a moment, Robin slipped her hand in. Her fingertips accidentally encountered the discolored arm. Its hardness scared Robin. She pulled back, directing her fingers carefully to the only part of the baby's body that was relatively free of equipment: his tiny chest. She stroked him, barely touching him.

Without opening his eyes, Brandon kicked his right leg. It stretched straight out at a wide angle from his body, then snapped back into a V. The limb was so elastic that the movement seemed without purpose and slightly crazed, like the kick of a marionette in the hands of an amateur.

His mother let her fingers come to rest on Brandon's skin. Lowering her head, she prayed to God for healing power.

The nurse asked her if she would like to hold Brandon.

She looked at him startled. "I don't think so."

He tried to convince her that even though the baby was very sick, his condition was stable enough that he could tolerate being held by his mother.

Still she resisted, and so did Tom.

But when the nurse asked her a third time, Robin began to think that maybe she would hold Brandon in case it was the last time she ever saw him alive.

The nurse found her a chair. He gave her a blanket. It took him a few minutes to make the necessary adjustments in equipment and to wrap the patient in blankets, but finally he lifted the tiny bundle from the warmer bed and laid Brandon, tubes and all, in his mother's arms.

She couldn't get over how much smaller he felt than the twins had felt. In fact, he was so light and so wrapped up that had she not been able to see his little head, Robin might have sworn that she was holding an armful of blankets. Preoccupied with those thoughts, she was not aware for several seconds that he didn't seem to be moving.

"He's not breathing," she said to the nurse.

He bent over Brandon. "Yes, he is. I can tell by the color of his skin."

But Robin felt panicky. "Maybe we should put him back."

She was still attempting to get this point across when the baby's heart rate dropped suddenly, and his color got very dusky. Immediately the nurse put Brandon back to bed and began to give him extra oxygen through a balloon device called a Mapleson. Though he could see that the baby's mother was frightened, though he himself had been a little frightened momentarily, Brandon's nurse felt he had the situation well under control.

This was not the Gregorys' impression. Although they could see the baby's chest rise when the nurse squeezed the bag on the Mapleson, it seemed to Brandon's parents that when he wasn't squeezing, their son's chest didn't move.

Robin stood frozen at the bedside thinking that if God had been helping her in any way, she had just ruined it.

Beside her, Tom tried to decide whether he should hit the nurse. Stopped only by the thought that if he did level a punch, he would stop the nurse from helping Brandon, the baby's father walked out of the unit in a fury.

The nurse sensed a problem. As to the proportions or the cause, he hadn't a clue. He felt bad about Gregory's sudden exit. Brandon needed love from his father too.

By this time the baby's heart had kicked in strong again, and Robin could see by the monitors that Brandon was okay.

"I think the excitement of being moved was just too much for him," the nurse said. "But he'll get used to it." And then Robin understood him to say, "He'll just have to."

She looked at the young man in disbelief. He'll just *have* to?

Not as far as his mother was concerned. As far as Robin was concerned, she was never going to hold him again until he got to be good-sized and had most of his tubes out.

Before leaving Children's that night, Brandon's mother bent down and kissed her baby for the first time. "If he dies, at least I held him," she kept thinking in the car as Tom drove the long dark miles back to their trailer park. "I didn't enjoy it, but at least I held him once. At least I kissed him."

Not far from home they stopped at a bar where, feeling utterly drained, Robin Gregory ordered the first drink she had had or wanted since the night before Brandon's birth.

Tuesday, December 18

Candy Rudolph was still in the hospital. Her face and head had remained unusually swollen on Saturday and Sunday, and yesterday the swelling had actually increased. Obviously the cerebrospinal leak in the membrane covering her brain had yet to resolve itself. Candy could not be discharged until the doctors were certain that the fluid that was continuing to accumulate under her scalp would resorb into her system.

Their plan as of rounds this morning was to take some of the CSF out from below by tapping Candy's spine today and again tomorrow. Ideally this would help relieve the pressure in her head. With the pressure reduced, the leak in her dura would have a chance to seal itself off spontaneously. Moreover, a puncture in the base of the spine would permit excess fluid to leak out there and be absorbed into the surrounding soft tissue, thus further decreasing the pressure in the skull. If the taps worked and fluid did not reaccumulate, the patient could probably be discharged on Thursday.

At 9:45 Candy's nurse was alerted by phone that the neurosurgeons were on their way up. As gently as she could, the nurse informed the child. Candy screamed so hard and so fearfully that the nurses decided to give her a sedative. When neurosurgery resident Nate Pontiac finally arrived with a junior resident about 10:30, his patient was sound asleep.

As he carried her into the treatment room, she woke up and began to cry all over again. All Candy knew of the situation was that two doctors she'd never seen before were about to put a needle in her back. Terrified, she fought them with all the armaments at a six-year-old's disposal, yelling and kicking and screaming at the top of her lungs. In the end it took the junior resident and a nurse to hold her down.

Over the weekend she had actually begun to feel rather cheerful. In large part this was because her left eye had begun to stay half open by itself, permitting Candy to be on her own again for the first time in nearly two weeks. She had painted, colored, played with other patients in the playroom, gone to the Children's Hospital Sunday school, and received a visit from her little sister. The nurses had encouraged this, thinking that Amy's presence would boost Candy's spirits, which it had.

The delay in discharge had come as a big disappointment to the whole family. Yet at least over the weekend, Candy's mother had been able to accept it with some equanimity. Bill had driven in from Long Island on Friday evening. His presence throughout the weekend had lifted some weight off his wife's shoulders. Furthermore, fed up with feeling torn between her two children, and missing Amy terribly, Yvonne had retrieved her younger daughter from her in-laws and would now keep the child with her at the Brandts' until Candy was well enough to return to Long Island. A family friend would stay with Amy during the day.

More at peace with herself, then, Yvonne had been able to take the long view on Saturday and Sunday. The surgery had been a year in the planning, she had reminded herself. Another day or two didn't make that much difference.

But when Yvonne and her mother had arrived at Children's Monday morning to discover that Candy would have to stay until Wednesday or Thursday, the child's mother had been nearly distraught. By this time Rolfe Lorimer had left the country on a business trip that would extend into a brief vacation. In desperation the two women had gone in search of Guillermo Perez. He, too, had been out of town. But the secretary in Neurosurgery had taken note of the distress in the women's faces and had asked Perez's colleague, neurosurgeon Colin Kendall, to see them. They had left his office feeling somewhat better.

Back upstairs they had found the child in tears. She had bumped her head in the playroom. Though it hadn't been enough of a bump to worry the nurses, Candy had sobbed her heart out.

Yvonne had understood. She herself had cried at the breakfast table.

She had tried to console Candy with a new blue nightie, but it had not fit over the child's head.

Ø

As of this morning, Tuesday, the two chest tubes going into

Mark's back had been clamped for twenty-four hours. An x-ray done just before noon showed a small recurrent pneumothorax at the apex of his lung. He and his mother got the news from Kate and Alan Cavanaugh.

Though Mark didn't want to cry in front of Dr. Cavanaugh, he couldn't help it.

Kate bent over him, holding him.

"I wanted to be home for Christmas!"

"I know. Maybe you still can be." But she didn't see how.

Dr. Cipriani came in. "I'm going to have to unclamp those tubes, Mark," he said. "I'm sorry." He turned on the Emerson. He lifted the patient's pajama top.

Mark sniffed and dried his tears. "Then what?"

Cipriani had been in the OR all night with two big emergencies. He was weary of questions from Mark and about him to which he didn't have answers. Saying only, "Then we'll have to see," he unclamped the tubes and left the room.

Ø

All over the hospital were patients who yearned as Mark did to get home for Christmas. Staff members taking care of them were doing everything in their power to make these wishes come true, or at the very least to make the holiday as enjoyable as possible for patients who couldn't get home. This always happens at Children's in December. When possible, surgery is postponed. When possible, therapy is stepped up or modified to help the kids feel as well as they can for the season that more than any other celebrates childhood in our society. For children who are dying, staff and parents alike may wage fervent campaigns, conscious or unconscious, to get those youngsters through one last Christmas.

As elsewhere, the season has a mystical aspect at Children's. This would be difficult to prove. But one hears stories. Most typically they involve mothers of children in desperate straits, a special breed of mothers who refuse to accept either the doctors' predictions or the weight of the evidence, who stand over the bedside willing a glimmer that should be impossible but does occur, who pull their children through, some speculate, by *wanting* to, by the sheer force of their loving energy. For some reason such miracles often seem to occur at Children's around the twenty-fifth of December.

Wednesday, December 19

Trial A of the research study into which Brandon Gregory had been entered Monday evening provided that he receive three intravenous doses of the "study medicine" twelve hours apart. For each dose given, the chances were two in three that the patient would get a placebo and one in three that he would get Indomethacin. When it worked, the drug could close down a life-threatening patent ductus arteriosis within a few hours.

Brandon had received his last dose of study medicine at 11:00 Tuesday evening. Now, some twelve hours later, Roger Forbes and PDA research associate Elsa Montaigue had met at the patient's bedside to evaluate the baby's condition and determine his immediate fate.

His condition was not good. If Brandon had received Indomethacin, it hadn't helped him. The heart murmur was continuous now, which hadn't been true before. The position of the liver indicated congestion around the heart. Through a stethoscope sounds resembling a waterfall nearly obscured the infant's breath sounds. The PDA was beginning to tax his breathing. His kidneys were barely functioning.

Had the baby shown real improvement, he could have been granted a grace period of forty-eight hours before further decisions were made about him. But a grace period was out of the question for Brandon Gregory. He now met the criteria for entry into Trial B of the research study.

Elsa Montaigue handed Roger Forbes a white envelope the size of a party invitation. The envelope had been numbered and sealed. Inside was a card bearing one of two words: SURGERY or INDOMETHACIN.

Forbes opened the envelope and groaned.

Ø

In the Intermediate Unit on another part of the fourth floor, meanwhile, Jody Robinson had spiked a fever—the fourth child in the unit to do so in as many days. The others were also manifesting heavy secretions and diarrhea. Jody had no diarrhea, but the secretions issuing from his esophagostomy had been thicker than usual all morning, and he was refusing to drink out of his beloved green cup. Though he would dip his hands into the water, he wanted no part of swallowing.

The reason for the children's malaise had yet to be determined. Thick secretions often point to respiratory infection. All the kids had such flare-ups periodically. Because their pulmonary function was impaired, they could not clear their lungs as well as would have been ideal. Pseudomonas bacteria which in a normal physiologic environment would be washed out by secretions remained in these children's lungs and colonized. The bugs were closely monitored in Intermediate. Secretion samples from every child were cultured twice a week. If the cultures showed the presence of high numbers of the bacteria and the patient exhibited troublesome symptoms, the child was treated with antibiotics.

However, none of the patients' trach secretions had yet grown pseudomonas, nor had their stool cultures. It was possible that they simply had common colds. They had so little resistance, the children of Intermediate. Exposed to germs brought in by doctors, nurses, technicians, cleaners, therapists, parents, and a host of other people with business at the hospital, the kids were sitting ducks. Those to whom an infection would surely be life-threatening were placed in isolation. There was no practical way to protect all the others.

Ø

Shortly before 1:00 Roger Forbes, Elsa Montaigue, and a surgeon met with Brandon Gregory's parents in the Infant ICU waiting room to review the situation with them and attempt to answer their questions. Tom Gregory was concerned about bone pain. By friends who had served in Vietnam and by his own brother, who had had a hip operation, Tom had been told that the pain resulting from cut bones could not be relieved. The surgeon assured the baby's father that only flesh would be cut.

The baby's mother could not begin to focus her thoughts on such detail. She was trying hard to get her bearings. When the subject had first been mentioned on the phone Monday morning, Robin had gotten the impression that the surgery was of no great consequence. Despite the meeting with Forbes and Montaigue on Monday evening, Brandon's mother had arrived at Children's this afternoon under that same impression.

"The other day they talked to us about the surgery as if it was a ten-minute operation and there was nothing to it," Robin said finally, addressing the surgeon. "You're making it sound like it's a matter of life and death."

The surgeon replied that while the procedure might take ten minutes in a bigger baby, Brandon's size made it much more difficult.

Robin turned to Roger Forbes. "You're saying that without surgery he's going to die in a matter of days?"

Forbes affirmed that this was so. He added that even if Brandon survived the surgery, he was still a very sick baby with many serious problems to overcome. Tom Gregory wondered briefly what the doctor meant. Forbes, of course, had spent the better part of an hour on Monday evening laying out what he meant. But with the best of intentions and with nearly a decade of experience behind him, Roger Forbes had not succeeded in getting that message through to either Gregory, perhaps because Brandon's young parents had been too dazed by shock or sadness to have either grasped or retained what the doctor had attempted to convey.

But they now understood the stakes involved in the surgery. Without the operation Brandon would die. With it he might die. Listening to the doctors, Robin Gregory put her son's chances for surviving the surgery at one in a million. She could not understand why God would permit Brandon to survive his birth three months early only to die from an operation eleven days later.

When Forbes handed her the consent form, Robin passed it immediately to her husband. They had both given permission for the PDA study. But parental consent required only one signature, and Robin did not want her name on a piece of paper she thought of as her baby's death warrant.

Brandon was wheeled out of the Infant ICU to the Operating Room at 2:00. Down to 685 grams, he was one of the smallest premies ever to be sent for surgery at Children's Hospital. He was so small that when the operation was over and an observer who had glanced away from the table momentarily looked back to discover that the patient had been taken away already, the observer was told to look more closely. The baby had not been moved. He was simply hidden from view by an OR sheet tossed casually across the operating table between the observer and the patient.

That tiny person came through surgery like a trooper.

The Gregorys got their first hint of this from the smiling faces on the doctors who wheeled the baby back into the ICU at 4:15. One of them was Roger Forbes. Catching sight of the parents, he gave them a big grin and raised his thumb and forefinger in a circle.

Forbes was very pleased. The murmur was gone. The baby was nice and pink, a sign that his blood was now circulating properly. His kidneys were functioning properly. His temperature had picked up. His ventilatory status had improved. Considering all the possibilities, this patient had returned from the OR in fine shape.

Brandon had been paralyzed for surgery, Forbes explained to the Gregorys, so he wouldn't be moving for a while. But as they stood talking at the bedside, the baby's nurse said suddenly, "There goes an eye!" Sure enough, to his mother's great surprise, the baby was beginning to blink. A short time later he moved an arm. Robin caressed it. She stroked his tiny head. She couldn't get over how good it made her feel to see him start to wake up.

Watching the baby, watching his wife, Tom Gregory began to feel a little hope about Brandon. Or, as he put it to himself, "That dude is really hanging in there."

Thursday, December 20

Making rounds very early, plastic surgery fellow Kevin McCoy was forced to conclude that the taps performed on Candy Rudolph on Tuesday and Wednesday had not resolved the problem of fluid accumulation beneath the child's scalp. Her face and head were still very swollen. McCoy could feel tension on Candy's incision.

As Guillermo Perez was still out of town, the fellow called

Neurosurgery and formulated a new plan with Perez's colleague, Colin Kendall. First, McCoy would apply a pressure dressing, a turban much like Candy's original bandages but above the eyes, not over them, and wrapped more tightly to obliterate the space into which the fluid was leaking. Ideally this would force the CSF to seek routes into the body, where it would be absorbed. To encourage this downward flow of fluid, the patient would be kept on her feet and as active as possible.

Meanwhile additional spinal taps would be done today and tomorrow, providing a total of four holes in the lower spine through which fluid could drain off into surrounding tissue. The child would be discharged in any case on Saturday but would remain in the city for observation.

Ø

Instead of confronting complications, Kevin McCoy would undoubtedly have preferred to be among the dozen doctors and nurses gathered for rounds this morning at Brandon Gregory's bedside in the Infant ICU. As they stood looking down at the tiny soul who would by now be midway through his seventh month in his mother's womb, the faces of the people who had followed the baby's fortunes most closely over the past twenty-four hours were all but beaming.

He was lying naked and apparently comfortably on a striped blanket. A sheet of Saran Wrap covered him. As he had developed jaundice again, he was being treated with phototherapy lights which shone down on him from either side of his warmer bed. To protect his eyes from those lights, he was wearing a miniature gauze mask. His right arm was still purple and had turned scaly. A spot of skin on the baby's abdomen had reddened, apparently the result of his sensitivity to the adhesive on the monitor leads.

The person responsible for presenting the patient for discussion was second-year resident Logan Sadler, a tall, hefty woman of twenty-six with a thick brown braid down her back. Rounds customarily begin with a spate of numbers. Logan Sadler gave a victory speech of sorts.

"Seeing this baby this morning," she began with a big smile at Roger Forbes and the others around her, "I'm really amazed by him! He's so vastly improved! The transfusions they gave him in the OR resulted in his having a marvelous hemoglobin last night, probably the highest one he's ever had in his life, which must be one reason he looks so fantastic today! He still has a long, long way to go, but he's shown us that he can go through a lot without falling by the wayside. He's done beautifully!

"In fact," said Sadler, grinning, "when the radiologist saw the films this morning, she demanded to know what had happened to this baby yesterday. When I told her he'd gone to the operating room, she said, 'Oh, that explains it! I couldn't figure out why everything was getting better all of a sudden!'"

Forbes noted that the baby's respiratory status had improved faster than was usual after surgery. He interpreted this to mean that the lung difficulties Brandon had manifested right before the operation were primarily or entirely related to his PDA difficulties. Forbes was finishing this thought when suddenly the baby stirred. His tiny feet began to pedal hard, determination plain in every thrust.

"*Look at him!*" cried Elsa Montaigue. "*He's kicking his Saran Wrap off! He's kicking his Saran Wrap off!*"

The faces looking down at Brandon Gregory lit up with admiration. From Roger Forbes's side a fellow spoke, a Midwesterner and a mother who had completed her pediatrics residency and was now specializing in neonatology. Because a fellow is the person responsible for the unit when the attending physician is not present, the woman's words carried the weight of a pronouncement.

"He seems like a good baby," she said with a special smile at her listeners. "We want to give him every chance."

"A 'good' baby?" Logan Sadler had suddenly become a lioness defending her cub. "I'd say the fact that he went to surgery weighing 685 grams and came back looking like he looks now means he's a remarkable baby!"

This enthusiasm came from two people who ordinarily had reservations about treating premature infants the size of Brandon Gregory.

Logan Sadler's reservations were new and rather tentative. As a medical student she had known almost nothing about premies. Asked occasionally by friends, colleagues, or family members what she thought of nurseries known to support the very tiniest new-borns, Sadler had invariably given an answer informed by her re-gard for modern technology: "They're wonderful." To Logan Sadler the student, keeping these infants alive had seemed a very interesting medical challenge.

Logan Sadler the resident still felt this way to some extent. Only by going after such babies aggressively, she knew, could doctors find out how far the frontiers could be pushed back. This inquiry had human as well as scientific value: untold numbers of parents went home happy with babies who might otherwise have died. Sadler had met some of those parents. She herself had taken care of some of those babies in other units at Children's after they'd left the ICU. After they'd been discharged, she had continued to follow them in clinic. So Sadler knew firsthand now the kind of progress some tiny premies were capable of making.

But she also knew firsthand their limitations. Sadler had taken care of infants the size of Brandon Gregory who had died or who had gone through such rough times that even though they had sur-vived, it was hard for Sadler to imagine that they could be doing well at home. She had a better grasp of the data now than she'd had in medical school. She knew that if the success stories were encour-aging, they were still exceptions to the rule. Thus had Logan Sadler begun to question the wisdom of treating every tiny premie ag-gressively.

The fellow's reservations were more profound. She actually felt biased against babies weighing less than 1,000 grams at birth. Though she rooted for them and took good care of them, her feel-ings about them were primarily pessimistic. Looking at a baby the size of Brandon Gregory, the fellow thought of all the things that could go wrong and all the things she had seen go wrong in other tiny premies. She remained unpersuaded that the effort and cost of saving many of those infants was justified by the outcome that could be anticipated.

The fellow was concerned not only about the babies themselves but also about their families. She and her husband had a seven-year-old daughter. The child was normal, healthy, and wonderful. Even so, the fellow was not finding it easy to lead a professional life around that little presence. Imagining life if the child had been se-verely damaged, the doctor could think only that it would be a disaster. She was well aware that faced with tough situations, most people can call on resources they've never known they had. The fellow had seen parents cope beautifully with abnormal children. She herself would never have wanted to be in those parents' shoes.

There was no point, in her opinion, in life for its own sake. The fellow had worked in Intermediate. She knew Jody Robinson and found him just as attractive as everybody else did. Yet she considered the incredible investment that had been made in the child—an investment that had failed to make Jody healthy enough even to go down the hall, let alone leave the hospital—to be a misuse of society's resources. All over the city were ghetto kids getting too little to eat and receiving minimum health care, or none at all. Why weren't pro-life groups worried about the sanctity of those lives? In the fellow's opinion, the pro-lifers had closed their eyes to society's realities.

She also felt that too many doctors had turned their backs on their own responsibilities. Too many supported life out of a conviction that to withdraw support was to play God. But one played God just as much by saying yes to every life, the fellow believed. Hard as the decisions always were, sometimes somebody had to say no. She herself was prepared to say no in her own practice when the situation warranted.

About Brandon Gregory, however, the fellow was enthusiastic. In fact, she felt as much enthusiasm about this patient as she had felt about any tiny premie in some months.

Roger Forbes joined in the rejoicing without saying what else he was thinking. He knew he didn't have to. The others were just as aware as he was that this baby was very far from being home free. Brandon Gregory remained one of the three sickest patients in the Infant ICU. His condition was critical. He was actually no further ahead than he had been five days ago before the PDA had started acting up. He was still a very tiny and immature baby. Almost all the problems of extreme prematurity still lay ahead of him.

Ø

Yvonne Rudolph spent Thursday morning with her younger daughter and did not arrive at Children's until nearly noon. Tammy Torrence grabbed her as she passed the nurses' station.

After telling Yvonne about the pressure dressing and the doctors' intentions, she walked with Candy's mother into Candy's room. There Yvonne saw that because of the pressure bandage, fluid had descended into Candy's eyelids and so increased the swelling there that the child who had been unable to see out of her right eye since surgery now could not see out of her left, either.

Candy was distraught. "Mommy, hold me! I want to go home!"

Yvonne turned to Tammy. "I want to see a doctor up here within the next three minutes."

The nurse greatly sympathized with the mother's frustration and felt a lot of her own. She found craniofacial cases emotionally wearing under the best of circumstances. This child had been in so long and suffered so much distress that Tammy, who gave her patients everything she had even when they weren't in such distress, had herself begun to take Candy's setbacks very hard.

"I know how you feel," she said to her patient's mother. "I don't blame you. I'll call somebody right away."

A doctor came immediately, a bearded neurosurgical resident whom Yvonne had never met. He observed that the pressure dressing didn't seem to be doing much good. To the great relief of both Rudolphs, he began to take it off. While he worked, Yvonne pumped him about the doctors' plans. Perhaps out of inexperience, the resident chose to cite the worst possible scenario. If they couldn't control the fluid with the spinal taps, he said, they might have to take Candy back to the operating room and open her head up again and repair the leak in her dura surgically.

Yvonne tried her best to control her reaction in front of Candy. But as soon as the doctor had finished, the patient's mother escaped into the hallway in search of Tammy and collapsed in tears in Tammy's arms.

Ø

Afternoon found almost all the children in the Intermediate Unit to be a little under the weather. Like Jody Robinson, they were feverish and had diarrhea and problems with their secretions that were suggestive of respiratory infections. When the last nurse had returned from lunch, the staff decided on the spur of the moment to try to cheer the children up by having rhythm band.

Five patients including Jody were old enough and well enough to participate. They were gathered on a faded bedspread near Jody's bed. One child sat on his mother's lap, another on a nurse's, the rest on the spread. The nurses handed out instruments: a seed-filled gourd, a bell, a pair of cymbals, a Tinker Toys box with a wooden drumstick, a tambourine for Jody. He liked to be King of the Drums, but the nurses liked to give everyone a chance at everything.

"Okay, now is everybody ready for 'Jingle Bells'?" Dressed in slacks and a cotton shirt, head nurse Jan Haver sat cross-legged on the blanket poised over a toy xylophone. She was twenty-four, a vital person who rarely bothered with makeup. Her cheeks were flushed.

"Okay, ready? This is 'Jingle Bells'! Come on, we have to practice for our Christmas party! Here we go! One! Two! Three! Four!" She brought down her stick on the multicolored bars. On real instruments, Haver had real talent. As a high school student she had played piano for weddings and parties and had turned down a bassoon scholarship at one college to study nursing at another.

She sang to her own accompaniment. The other nurses joined in. "Jingle bells! Jingle bells! Jingle all the way! Oh, what fun it is to ride . . ."

Rhythm band had become an institution in Intermediate. Noticing one day that a child's interest in a xylophone was waning, Jan Haver had picked up the instrument herself and had tried to entertain the baby with her own rendition of "When the Saints Go Marching In." Several other nurses had grabbed instruments and chimed in. For a while rhythm band had consisted of nurses giving concerts to the kids.

But when half a dozen of the children got old enough to play the instruments themselves, someone got the idea of sitting them down together on the floor and letting them have jam sessions. It couldn't happen very often. The timing depended on the right confluence of schedules and mood and, most important, on how the children felt. When it did occur, it was always a special occasion. The kids loved it.

Of those now playing instruments, only Jan Haver observed the beat. The kids took their cues not from the tune she was playing but from each other or from whim or from the nurses who called out encouragement. "Come on, Scotty! Good, Demetrius! Let's hear it, Elizabeth! Keep it up, Jody!"

Jody's eyes were watery, and his face looked even puffier than usual, but he slapped away at his tambourine with a big grin on his face. One-legged Demetrius was so absorbed in watching the others that he completely forgot about the cymbals on his own hands. The only consistent player was Scotty, a child nearing two with chronic lung disease, who banged away with his drumstick like a workman hammering a nail that never reached its destination.

Haver led her group from "Jingle Bells" to "You Are My Sunshine" to "Do Re Mi" from *The Sound of Music*. As the patients played, their antics made the nurses laugh, which egged the kids on to more antics. Sensing, finally, that the children were reaching a pitch that, compounded by fevers, could easily tip over into tears, Haver decided it was time to stop.

"Okay, everybody, now how about if we do our favorite as the last number, and then everybody can do something else for a while. Scotty, are you ready? Craig? Elizabeth? 'When the Saints.' Here we go! One! Two! Three! 'Oh, when the saints go marching in . . .'"

A few minutes later, when rhythm band was over and the nurses had put the children back in their beds, Jan Haver walked over to the west bay of the unit on an errand and was greeted by a broad smile on the face of the mother of one of the short-term patients.

Haver grinned. "You must think we're all loony-tunes up here!"

"Yes," the mother admitted, laughing, "but I also think it's really nice!"

Ø

If Yvonne Rudolph had known about rhythm band, she might have taken Candy downstairs to see it as a way of keeping her out of bed and on her feet as much as possible, per doctors' orders. Yvonne was finding this directive difficult to carry out. Candy kept saying she was too tired, which her mother interpreted to mean disgusted. Drained and apprehensive, Yvonne lacked the strength to push the child and was also a little afraid to push her. The afternoon wore on. No one came up to perform the scheduled spinal tap.

Finally at 3:30 Candy's mother made her second trip in four

days to the Neurosurgery Department. She found Drs. Kendall and Perez standing in their outer office. Upon learning why she was so distressed, the neurosurgeons reassured Yvonne that more skull surgery was extremely unlikely. At most Candy might need a tube inserted into her spine that could drain off fluid continuously. The doctors speculated that this minor operation would not be necessary. They still planned to release the child on Saturday unless something went very wrong in the meantime, to keep her active over the weekend, and to see her early next week. Then if the swelling persisted, the doctors would consider bringing her back in and placing a shunt.

Yvonne left Neurosurgery feeling vastly relieved. But her relief did not survive the afternoon. Alone at a Children's cafeteria table at suppertime, she succumbed to tears of despair. Had they done the right thing for Candy?

It came down to this, in Yvonne's mind: Candy had had to go through so much because people couldn't accept differences. If someone couldn't walk and went through life in a wheelchair, people stared. If a child's face was a little different, people stared. On many occasions Yvonne had thought of putting a sign around Candy's neck saying, SHE'S A PERFECTLY NORMAL KID. BUG OFF.

Instead she and Bill had signed a permission form for craniofacial reconstructive surgery.

Had it been worth what it was costing all of them, Candy most especially?

Yvonne did not honestly know. Sometimes she wondered whether she would ever take home the little girl she'd brought into Children's on December 2.

Back on Six, she found her father and her daughter skipping hand in hand down the hall. Her father's face was flushed above his clerical collar, and he was calling out "Beep-beep!" as in a Road Runner cartoon, and Candy was laughing. *Laughing.* Pastor Brandt told his daughter that he was doing his part to solve the child's fluid problem. A moment ago, he said, puffing for breath, they had almost literally run into Dr. Kendall, who had put his fingers on the minister's pulse and asked him if he thought he was really up to that kind of activity!

Candy was tugging at her grandfather's hand. "Come on, Poppa! *Come on!*"

Friday, December 21

Yvonne Rudolph arrived at Children's about 9:30 braced for bad news. But for once there was only good news. The swelling in Candy's head was no worse. In fact, her condition so pleased the neurosurgeons that they had decided to skip the fourth spinal tap! She was to be discharged on Saturday as scheduled.

Ø

The Oncology Clinic waiting room had been decorated for Christmas with tinsel and paper cutouts. Both secretaries' desks were laden with holiday goodies homemade by parents and brought in to share: doughnuts, cookies, candies, nuts, dried fruits, a real gingerbread house. One of the doctors came out from the back with a box of mints he'd just received from a patient. Letting his eyes wander over the sweet buffet, he finally helped himself to a frosted doughnut.

"Watch out, you'll get fat," warned Ellie, the secretary who did most of the Clinic billing. "I've really gained weight on this job!"

Ordinarily Marie DeRose was alert to the secretaries' banter. Often she joined in, glad for the distraction. This morning she sat in a corner by the windows, working on her *Star Wars* rug as if she were alone in the crowded room.

Gina was not feeling well. A few days after her clinic visit on December 7, she had become extremely tired. The next day she'd complained of feeling sick at her stomach. That night she had sat down for dinner saying she was starving, then suddenly had lost her appetite and eaten nothing. The following day she had begun to vomit mucus.

Her disposition had changed. Ever since she'd started to feel better, Gina had been behaving more and more like herself. Now she was moody and withdrawn, like someone depressed. Things annoyed her. Obviously tired, she'd insist on going to school but would come home in the afternoon and go to sleep on the couch.

She'd make her mother promise to wake her at seven so she could do homework and then be angry if Marie chose instead to let her sleep. About many things she simply didn't want to be bothered.

At first Marie and Tony had not been terribly concerned. Some seven weeks had passed since the child had completed radiation. The doctors had told the DeRoses that six to eight weeks after the last treatment, Gina might experience a reaction lasting seven to ten days. As the symptoms they'd described were precisely Gina's symptoms now, her parents had at first assumed that radiation explained them.

Marie had called Children's one night just to make sure. The doctor had assured her that her assumption was probably correct. As the child would be coming into Clinic soon anyway, he'd told her mother, there was no need to make a special appointment.

Marie had hung up feeling much better. In one way Gina had been very lucky. She had never gotten sick with any of her medicines. Marie had actually worried about this at one point. The doctors had prepared her for such side effects as high fever, sore jaws, mouth sores, vomiting, ulcers, nosebleeds, abdominal pain, constipation, and convulsions. Gina had gotten a little tired that first week home and had run a small fever. Every day Marie had looked in vain for one of the other problems to develop. Finally one day in Clinic she had grabbed a doctor and said to him, all upset, "What's the matter with Gina? Aren't the medicines working?"

"Why do you ask?"

"She has no symptoms. No side effects."

He had smiled. Kindly. "Are you complaining? We said 'might,' remember?"

Of course the child had lost her hair. Yet hair loss that was temporary and radiation aftereffects that were also temporary seemed to Marie and Tony DeRose a very small price to pay for their daughter's health.

But while the phone call to Children's had told Gina's parents that she was probably all right physically, her behavior continued to disturb them. In essence she had shut them out. Asked how she felt or what was wrong, she'd reply, "I'm just tired. I'm all right. I don't want to talk about it." Both Marie and Tony had tried to tell Gina that if something was really wrong with her, they needed to know and to bring it to the attention of the doctor. Her response had

been to give them a look that said, "Leave me alone." It had occurred to Marie that perhaps the medicines were having some permanent effect on Gina's personality.

And then last night, along with throwing up mucus, she had run
a temperature of 102 degrees, for no apparent reason.

Maybe it's just a little fever, her parents had told themselves.
Kids were always getting fevers.

"Hi, Mrs. DeRose." Dr. Silver had come up beside her. He was
carrying a chart with a name on it that wasn't Gina's, and he remained standing. "I just ran into Gina back in the lab. She doesn't
seem too perky." He added after a moment, "You're upset, aren't
you."

"She hasn't been feeling well, and . . ."

"I heard. I was away for a few days last week, but when I got
back, the doctor you talked to on the phone told me. What's going
on?"

She gave him the details. He felt certain that what she was describing was either late effects of radiation or the beginnings of a
cold.

"I'll give her a good thorough check," Silver told his patient's
mother, "but I don't think there's anything to worry about."

"I was afraid that the cancer might . . . might be . . ."

"Might be coming back?" He put a hand on her shoulder. "No.
It's really too early for the cancer to come back."

Even that was hard to hear.

"Do you think she's frightened?" Silver asked.

"Maybe you could get that out of her. I can't. She's not talking to
anybody at our house. I can't tell you how she feels. It's like she
takes everything in stride." She blew her nose. Her eyes were full.
She was as upset as Sam Silver had ever seen her.

He thought he could understand why. Leukemia could be handled with medication. No known pill could make a child open up to
her family if she didn't want to.

"Do you want me to try to talk with her?"

"I wish you would. I've said to her, 'Gina, go over to your aunt's
house. Talk to *somebody*.' She doesn't talk to anybody. Maybe I'm
making more out of it than I should. Maybe she's just little, where a
teenager might want to sit and talk. But try. Maybe she'll talk to
you."

She sat on the examining table in patchwork jeans and a pale blue T-shirt bearing a picture of Snoopy and a caption that read: I'M NOT PERFECT, BUT I'M PRETTY PERFECT. MAGNA CUM LAUDE. Usually Gina liked being teased about her funny T-shirts. Not today. She answered her doctor's questions in monosyllables.

He gave her a very thorough examination. When he had finished, Silver stuffed his stethoscope into his back pocket and sat down on the desk corner nearest her, dangling his foot. He was dressed in a plain green shirt, green corduroy trousers, and loafers. His shirt pocket was full of pens.

"I wanted to talk to you a little," he said nonchalantly, fiddling with a pen. "I know you're not feeling well, and your mother said you haven't really been yourself since last week."

She met his eyes without answering.

Silver made guesses. Peds training had taught him that while ill teenagers think a lot about what is going to happen to them ultimately, younger kids tend to have more immediate concerns. The whole issue of body image is very important to these children, especially to girls. Gina was just reaching the age when girls begin to talk endlessly about dresses, about hair, about appearance in general. This child had no hair. Prednisone had conferred chubbiness upon a body that had been plump to begin with.

"I wondered if maybe your wig was bothering you."

She shrugged.

"I wondered," he prompted, "if maybe your wig had fallen off at school and somebody made fun of you."

She could have told him how afraid she'd been, wearing her wig to school that first time, that the kids would make fun of her the way they called the kids with glasses Four-Eyes. She could have said that she had only told Christine and Michelle and a few others but hadn't shown them—no way!—and that some of the kids still didn't believe that all her hair had fallen out. Instead she said only, "No."

Silver waited. When the child didn't elaborate, he tried a different tack. "The other thing I was wondering about was whether you think you're not doing well and we're hiding that from you. Is that what's upsetting you?"

She shrugged again and dropped her eyes. On one finger was a ring she had gotten from the dentist at Children's, a dime-store ring with a green stone. Twisting the ring, she replied, very quietly, "No."

But Dr. Sam addressed the shrug. "Gina, when we found out you had leukemia, we told you. Remember?"

She nodded without looking up.

"Well, if you weren't doing well now, we'd tell you. You're doing very well. Your blood counts are just fine. The reason you've been so tired is that you've had radiation. This sometimes happens to people six or eight weeks after radiation. They get tired and don't feel like eating and aren't themselves. It should go away within a few days."

She sat quite still.

"Do you want to ask me anything?"

A pause. "No."

"The only other thing I wanted to say to you was that if you're worried about having to go back in the hospital, I want you to know that there's a good chance you'll never have to be in the hospital again because of your leukemia. I can't absolutely promise you, but there's a good chance."

Although she said nothing, the change in her demeanor was perceptible to him.

"Don't forget," he told her, "if you ever have questions, you can call me or your social worker whenever you want to." The worker was the young graduate student Gina had met her first day at Children's, and the child was crazy about her.

"I do have one question."

"What is it?"

Suddenly she giggled. "When you use that stethoscope and write stuff on paper afterwards, what do you write down?"

In conversation with the child's mother a few minutes later, Silver tried to be sensitive to the possibility that Marie DeRose was in a period of emotional letdown. The intensity of the past few months was over now. Gina was in remission and on maintenance therapy, or close to it. When a crisis is over, the adrenaline inevitably subsides. All the DeRoses knew for certain about the future was that they could not know what it held. They could only wait.

Silver emphasized to Marie that sooner or later Gina would settle into a routine. Once she did, he said, the DeRoses would see that the patterns of their lives were not drastically altered by her leukemia. In fact, he added, one goal of treatment was to help families return to normal patterns. Clinic staff members were not simply trying to buy time for Gina, Sam Silver stressed to her mother. They were aiming to cure her. In the meantime they wanted her to live as normally as possible so she would continue to develop normally from one stage of growth to the next. As the family made these important transitions, the doctors told his patient's mother, the staff stood ready to help in any way that seemed useful.

Sam Silver never felt more challenged as a doctor than when confronting the emotional impact of cancer on patients and families. The technical aspects of his job demanded relatively little of his talents. Most leukemics whose care was being managed at Children's were part of a research study under way in some thirty institutions all over North America. Treatment protocols had been worked out by study designers in fine detail. The only real test of medical skill arose when a child being treated became ill. Then the doctor had to figure out whether the illness was caused by the disease or by the medicine. Once this had been established, however, the physician's course was ordinarily clear.

The greater challenge, in Silver's mind, was not scientific but human. His wife's mother had died of cancer. Though he had never met her, Silver knew that she had felt abandoned by her doctors, who had spent virtually no time with her. She had faced her dying feeling herself to be just another number in their files. Silver had known such physicians. His own instinct was to be the kind of doctor who helped people through their trials to the best of his ability. In fact he had chosen his field in part to give himself that opportunity.

Sam Silver could not say exactly why he had wanted to enter medicine. As a kid he'd been very fond of a cousin who, asked what he wanted to be, would always say "A doctor." At some point Silver had begun to copy his cousin's answer. He could not recall a specific moment of decision.

He was clearer on why he had wanted pediatrics. He loved children and had a low tolerance for working with sick adults. He had become interested in oncology as a senior medical student. The dynamism of the field had intrigued him. A disease that had once killed everyone it touched had lost its invincibility. Significant leaps were being made in almost every form of childhood malignancy. The technology of treatment was all new. Yet a major question loomed on the horizon. Now that many cancer patients could anticipate long-term survival, what would happen to those patients years down the line as a result of the very chemicals and radiation therapies that had gotten them that far? Oncology was an important field and a changing one.

Silver had been drawn to it for those reasons and one other: the potential it offered for close relationships with patients and families. Cancer doctors have a captive audience. If a child with asthma sounds okay, the parents might skip the medications. Children with cancer do not miss appointments. When they do well, they see their doctors often. If they begin to do poorly, they see their doctors even more often. A physician inevitably learns a great deal about the problems faced by these patients and their families, not just medical problems but emotional problems as well. Ideally, Silver had thought, a physician who loved kids could help solve some of these problems.

Asked by relatives or friends how he could stand working with children who had cancer, Silver would sometimes reply that cancer was not necessarily the most terrible disease a child could have. He had formed this opinion as a pediatric resident. During that period Silver had met any number of children with cystic fibrosis. He had been struck by the extent to which their illness affected them.

They couldn't breathe. They couldn't eat. They couldn't run around. They spent much more time in the hospital than did kids in remission with cancer. When Silver's patients were doing well, they were out leading normal lives. The CF kids could not lead anything like a normal life. Not one of them would be cured. Many or even most of Silver's patients would grow up to have careers, spouses, children, and probably grandchildren.

The research study in which Gina DeRose was a participant represented a new era in cancer inquiry. For years investigators had concentrated on the crudest of questions: how can people with cancer be salvaged? This focus still obtains with those forms of the disease showing least improvement in survival rates. But by the time Gina had her first appointment at Children's Hospital, the focus in acute lymphocytic leukemia, the commonest of childhood cancers, had changed rather remarkably.

By this time doctors could distinguish at the time of diagnosis between patients who were likely to do well or very well and the minority who were likely to do poorly. Except in the latter group, oncologists also knew by this time how to treat ALL successfully. That is, they knew how to effect a remission that was likelier than not to last. Patients were by all appearances being cured. Thus the attention of researchers had shifted from survival per se to a far subtler matter: the quality of survival, or, more specifically, the long-term effects of treatment.

Remission is achieved and maintained in acute lymphocytic leukemia as in other cancers by drugs that are toxic to humans. While these chemicals destroy malignant cells, they also harm normal cells. The cranial irradiation used in tandem with drugs in ALL is likewise injurious to normal tissue. Known side effects of these therapies in the short run include brain, heart, lung, and liver damage; dysfunction of the reproductive organs; altered immunity; memory and learning problems; secondary cancers; crippling; and death. The implications for patients now being saved to live for many years are not yet known and may not be known for decades.

Nowhere in the field of oncology are late effects of greater concern than in pediatrics. If children have the most to gain from aggressive cancer therapies, they also have the most to lose. They are growing organisms. Treatment may interrupt growth and prevent normal development. The child who suffers permanent impairment at an early stage must bear that burden for an entire lifetime.

When the alternative is certain early death, such impairment may be considered a small price to pay for survival. But is it small enough? Is it as small as it can possibly be? These questions began to assume importance in pediatric oncology as more and more children began to live longer and longer. By the mid-1970s pediatric oncologists all over the country had begun to ask themselves an unusual question about acute lymphocytic leukemia and other curable forms of childhood malignancy: Can we do as well with less? Can we treat the disease successfully without putting the patient at risk for serious problems down the line?

This question could be answered in no single institution. Cancer in children is rare. No one center can accumulate enough patients for a reliable analysis of any major issue in pediatric oncology. Such issues are customarily explored through collaborative research projects overseen by one of two umbrella organizations that exist for the purpose, each representing a number of different hospitals.

Late in 1978 one of these organizations, the Children's Cancer Study Group, inaugurated the largest study of acute lymphocytic leukemia ever undertaken. The broad purpose of the research is to find out how to cure more children with the fewest possible ill effects. Final results may not be tabulated until the late 1980s. The project comprises three arms: one for patients with the best prognosis, one for patients who stand an average chance of doing well, and one for patients whose outlook at the time of the diagnosis is poor. In the latter study, the focus is the basic issue of survival. What treatments will permit these children to grow up, or even to be alive five years from now? The patients in this group receive a variety of treatments, all aggressive.

The children most likely to be cured are treated least aggressively. Divided into subgroups, they get either standard leukemia therapy or standard therapy with certain elements subtracted. It is of these children that researchers are asking in its purest form the question "Can we do as well with less?"

Of the children with average chances the researchers are in a sense asking the flip side of that question. These children receive either standard treatment or standard treatment with something added. The results of this study will show whether a child's outcome can be improved with a little more therapy of this or that kind at this or that point. It was this study into which Gina DeRose was entered, with her parents' written permission, on her first day at Children's Hospital.

Because malignancy is rare in childhood, every child who becomes part of an oncology research project contributes important information to the adults attempting to conquer cancer in all children who contract it. Each child studied is a tributary flowing into a large river of knowledge that changes constantly and that may one day answer the last question ever to need asking about the disease.

By the time the CCSG leukemia study was closed to participants in 1981, 2,386 children had been entered into its regimens. More than half of them—1,220—fall somewhere in between the children likeliest to be cured and those likeliest to die. Those 1,220 children

will help researchers determine how the commonest form of childhood cancer is ideally treated in patients with an average prognosis—a question that could not begin to be answered without the
children. One/1220th of that answer will be provided by honor student and former cheerleader Gina Marie DeRose.

On the day after Christmas, five days after his talk with Gina's
mother in Clinic, Sam Silver would call the DeRose residence to give
her the results of the latest blood tests done to determine enzyme
elevation. Unfortunately, the enzymes would be back up. Silver
would have to say that he was going to take Gina off Methotrexate
completely for the second time. Though not viewing this as particularly bad news, he would certainly have preferred to call and say
that the enzymes were fine, especially since Marie DeRose had recently been so upset about her daughter. Silver would dial with his
fingers crossed that by now Gina at least felt better.

The phone would be answered by a child sounding busy and
breathless, as if she had snatched the receiver off the hook while
tearing through the house. Silver would imagine her in her jeans
and one of her funny T-shirts racing outside to play.

"Hi," he would say. "It's Dr. Silver. How are you?"

"Oh, Dr. Sam! I'm fine! I'm myself again!"

That much would be obvious.

Ø

While Sam Silver was attempting to reassure Gina DeRose's
mother in the Oncology Clinic on the Friday before Christmas, a
nurse in the Infant Intensive Care Unit was attempting to thread a
long, slender feeding tube into Brandon Gregory's small intestine
through his minuscule right nostril.

The infant was making slower progress on his ventilator settings
than his condition at rounds on Thursday morning had seemed to
promise. However, with ductus surgery now two days behind him,
Brandon had continued to gain ground in other ways. His color was
good, he seemed quite comfortable, and he was beginning to keep
his eyes open much more than he had before. In fact, he was even
trying to look around a little. His caregivers were hoping to start
him on tube feedings before nightfall.

With the PDA crisis over, the matter of feeds was now of paramount importance for Brandon Gregory. His weight was down to 660 grams. He had been getting some nourishment in the form of hyperalimentation, a substance rich in calories that was being administered intravenously. But a baby on hyperal for prolonged periods can develop liver problems. Furthermore, in a patient with veins as infinitesimal as those of this baby, the substance must go in greatly diluted. The support it provides is inadequate to the patient's needs. Brandon had to be fed by mouth or he would die of starvation.

Feeding a tiny premie by mouth is one of the trickiest challenges in all of neonatology. To begin with, infants born after only twenty-six or twenty-eight weeks' gestation have virtually no digestive enzymes. Introducing nutrients usually stimulates the production of enzymes, but at rates impossible to predict in any given premie.

The machinery, furthermore, is extraordinarily small. The stomach capacity of a baby weighing 750 grams may not exceed a couple of cubic centimeters—a fraction of an ounce. Too much formula can rupture the organ. Since the rate of absorption is unknown in any given patient, however, caregivers have no good way of knowing how much is too much.

Had Brandon Gregory been able to nurse at his mother's breast, he would simply stop taking milk when he'd had enough. But a baby born three months early can neither suck nor swallow reliably. Breast-feeding is out of the question for tiny premies. They must be tube-fed. This approach has the advantage of conserving the patients' strength. However, the amounts of formula administered through a tube cannot be limited by the natural governor of the baby's own desires. Staff has to guess and judge how much the patient can tolerate.

A wrong guess can result in air buildup, diarrhea, cyanosis, bloody stools, or the baby's demise. Death can occur from the aspiration of vomitus if a tiny premie is fed too fast. Or the infant can succumb to a catastrophic case of necrotizing enterocolitis, an inflammation of the immature gut that afflicts bowel tissue with gangrene.

Among the hobgoblins of prematurity, NEC is one of the most treacherous. Its specific cause is unknown. A definite connection with feeds has never been proved. But the disease follows frequently enough upon the introduction of feedings that neo-natologists cannot consider it a coincidence. NEC can kill an infant in a matter of hours. Infant ICU nurses watch constantly for signs of it in their patients.

If detected early, some cases of the disease can be treated suc-cessfully. Too often the disease can be diagnosed only after it has progressed far enough to put the patient in immediate danger of dying. At this point the only hope is surgery. But of all premies needing surgery for NEC, only half are destined to survive.

Thus doctors and nurses walk a tightrope when feeding tiny premies. They must continually challenge the patient to eat without pushing him or her over the brink. If they advance feeds too slowly, they court the consequences to brain and body of prolonged caloric insufficiency. Feeding too fast risks aspiration and NEC. Achieving the proper pace for any given premie is a task demanding less tech-nology than art. It must be done by simple trial and error. It rarely goes smoothly. Increasing a baby's weight from a pound and a half to three pounds often takes months.

With Brandon Gregory as with all tiny premies about to take nourishment by mouth, then, the Infant ICU staff would proceed with enormous caution. The first thing Brandon would get once his feeding tube was in place was a single cc. of sterile water: a scant quarter teaspoon. This would test his ability to handle any fluid at all in his digestive tract. If within the next few hours he showed no ill effect, he'd be given a cc. of sterile water mixed with a bit of glucose. If he had no trouble with the low concentration, he would be tried on a slightly higher concentration of glucose.

Assuming he tolerated this without difficulty, he would then be-gin to receive very small amounts of quarter-strength formula: a blend of predigested protein and very simple sugar. As the hours passed, he would be watched very closely for adverse signs. If none appeared, he would gradually be increased to half-strength for-mula, to three-quarter-strength, and finally to full-strength. If he continued to do well on full-strength, he would start on breast milk. Roger Forbes thought it possible that Brandon would be on breast milk by Monday.

If he did all right on small amounts of breast milk, staff could begin building up the volume. The more calories the baby got by mouth, the fewer he'd be given intravenously. As soon as he was taking through the feeding tube the optimum number of calories required for growth, the hyperal would be completely discontinued. When this might occur was anyone's guess.

Brandon's parents had no concept that their son was about to be launched on so precarious a journey. They knew he was soon to be fed, and Robin Gregory in particular was very pleased that he was. She'd been concerned about his nutrition. She was extremely concerned about his weight. These concerns had gotten temporarily lost in her fears about the baby's heart problems. Ever since the surgery, however, the nurses' reports to her on the phone had greatly encouraged Robin. She had the impression that the worst was behind Brandon, and that now all he had to do was eat.

Ø

The pains taken to nourish a premie at Children's are unique. No other class of patients requires the fine calibrations and extreme caution necessary in the feeding of beings who are physiologically unready to be fed. However, good nourishment is important for all hospital patients. It can be difficult to achieve, obviously, because people who are sick may not feel much like eating. Adults may try because they know it's good for them. Children often need encouragement to try. In its own way, the effort made at Children's to tempt patients' palates almost rivals the pains taken with premies.

Five different diets are available to youngsters able to take food by mouth: house, junior house, soft, low-sodium, and low-sugar. Within those diets, many choices are offered. A child on the house diet may choose breakfast from these selections: orange juice, apple juice, a banana; Cream of Wheat, cornflakes, Cheerios, oatmeal, Froot Loops, raisin bran; pancakes, scrambled eggs, bacon, hash browns; white toast, wheat toast, English muffin, bagel, honey bun; whole, skim, or chocolate milk, hot tea, coffee. Three hot entrees are offered on every diet at every meal.

As indicated by the presence of Froot Loops on the breakfast menu, diets are tailored to children's likes and dislikes. Hamburgers are offered for lunch every day. Hot dogs are offered for supper every evening. Every three months a "satisfaction survey" is conducted, which gives patients a chance to list their favorite foods, and the menus reflect the kids' strong preferences for chicken, pizza, spaghetti, corn, rice, French fries, ice cream, and cake. Consideration is also given to ethnic tastes. For example, black youngsters may order collard greens and gravy with their rice.

Children who see nothing appealing on the menu may order anything else they want so long as it's within their dietary restrictions. There are many special requests, and food service workers make many extra trips to the store. If a parent says a child will eat only Chef Boy-ar-dee Ravioli, the child will have it. If a cancer patient requests Count Chocula for breakfast, a box of that cereal will be delivered to the patient's bedside. Especially for long-term patients who are not eating well, the dietary staff does its utmost to get those children what they want.

The staff does all this and weekly "specials" besides. Specials fall into three categories. They may take the form of a treat added to the menu: croissant sandwiches, for example, or a choice of homemade muffins for breakfast, or an extra dessert. The favorite in this category is a banana split offered with a selection of candy or cookie toppings.

A second kind of special involves the distribution of afternoon snacks from carts: for example, fresh fruit from a watermelon boat, giant chocolate chip cookies, holiday cupcakes. Once a food service employee dressed up as a clown and passed out cotton candy. Another time an employee dressed up as a pirate and passed out chocolate coins. When black astronaut Guy Bluford visited Children's, the kids were given ice cream rockets. Alternative snacks are always offered to patients who can't eat ice cream or cookies—an Italian ice, perhaps, or a piece of fruit.

For the third kind of special, a theme is observed in menus for an entire day: Italian Day, Soul Day, E.T. Day, Pac-Man Day, Smurf Day, and Hawaiian Day, to cite a few. When the food itself cannot be made to conform to the idea, staff members simply name it appropriately. On Michael Jackson "Thriller" Day, the kids were offered "Beat It Beets" and "Pretty Young Thing Potatoes." Trays were dispensed from carts bearing Michael Jackson posters by employees wearing Michael Jackson T-shirts. Though not hired for showmanship, the workers are said to enjoy these events almost as much as the children do.

Once in a while a parent will register a complaint about the food offered to patients at Children's. Some parents object to sweetened cereals. Others object to hot dogs. The hot dogs available are all beef, but they do contain some nitrites. Believing that the parents have a point, the director of dietary services is rethinking the wisdom of offering hot dogs every night. Similarly, the chief dietitian intends to offer a sweetened cereal only every other morning.

To an outsider sensitive about good nutrition, the wide range of foods available to patients at Children's may seem unduly heavy on sweets of all kinds. Hospital experts point out that when a child is sick, normal dietary principles may be superseded by broader concerns. Many patients at Children's are eating poorly because they are recovering from surgery. Many others have been hospitalized for failure to thrive, a diagnosis descriptive mainly of failure to gain weight. All those youngsters need high-protein, high-calorie diets. Sweets are offered because the children will eat them.

Ø

Candy Rudolph was still picking at her food nearly three weeks after her operation, but her mother had every intention of insisting on well-balanced meals as soon as she got her daughter home. Several times on Friday Tammy Torrence assured Yvonne that Candy would start eating well again as soon as she felt well.

When the day shift was over and Tammy had finished up her work, she went into Candy's room to say goodbye. The nurse had tomorrow off. She would not see Candy go home. But she made the child promise to visit when she came back for checkups, a promise not difficult to extract.

Candy gave Tammy a big hug, several kisses, and a bottle of perfume with a card she had signed herself. Inside the card Yvonne had written, "Thank you for being so nice to our little girl." Hugging Tammy herself, Yvonne said warmly, not for the first time, "You're the best nurse on the floor."

Tammy drove home feeling great. Sometimes she would say to people that as the world understood the word, she had no real talents. She couldn't play an instrument, dance, or do anything of that sort. Her strong point was her ability to get along with people, especially children. If a child looked for her in the morning, as Candy always had, if a mother told her what a good nurse she was, Tammy could feel she had accomplished something important and done it well. In this case she had helped a whole family through a particularly difficult hospitalization. Knowing herself capable of that gave Tammy a confidence she knew would make things a little easier for the next family.

Saturday, December 22

Candy's mother and father arrived on Six Surgical at 10:00 A.M. bringing warm clothes for their daughter. They found her in the playroom. Though somewhat subdued, she had been promised a surprise at her grandparents' house and was eager to get there. She was wearing the new blue nightie that on Monday had not fit over her head.

High on her brow was a Band-Aid from the most recent fluid tap. Her left eyelid was slightly more open today than yesterday. The right was still swollen shut. However, the puffiness had decreased, and the bruise color had faded from red to tan. Maroon-black scab covered most of the incision across the child's skull. The rest of her scalp was dark with a scrub growth of hair. From days of being lain on, the longer fringe hanging down the back of her neck went every which way. She had been at Children's for three whole weeks.

Back in the room, Yvonne slipped the nightie off. Raising her arms, Candy winced. Her chest incision was a bit red at one end but otherwise looked fine. On her back were two small brownish bruises from two of her spinal taps. A Band-Aid covered the third and most recent wound. Yvonne helped Candy into underpants, a flowered undershirt, a white sweater with red stripes, red pants to match, white socks, red shoes. The process went slowly. Candy was sensitive about her head and leery of raising her arms. When the sweater went on over the plastic identification bracelet on her wrist, the child scolded her mother. "Don't cover that up!" She refused to take the bracelet off until Amy had seen it. When Yvonne tried to put a soft brush through her fringe, Candy winced and stopped the brush with her hand. "Ow!"

While Bill went down to the business office, Yvonne packed Candy's things, then filled a plastic basin with books and toys belonging to the hospital and returned them to the playroom. When she returned, Dr. Whitehill was waiting to talk to her. The chief resident in plastic surgery was smiling.

Briefly he went over the discharge orders. Candy was to remain up and about as much as possible. For mild discomfort she could have aspirin. If she had severe discomfort or if the swelling in her head increased, the Rudolphs were to call the hospital. The ointment given them by a nurse was to be used on Candy's right eye until it opened. She could have tub baths starting immediately. She was to return to Children's on Monday to see neurosurgeon Guillermo Perez.

Back from the business office, Bill Rudolph joined his wife in thanking the doctor for everything that had been done on their daughter's behalf.

Yvonne bundled Candy into her navy coat. As Bill helped the child with the buttons, his wife put a cap on Candy's head over Candy's protests. Nurses clustered in the doorway. "Where's my hug and kiss?" one asked.

The patient grinned and went toward her with arms open wide.

There were more grins and more hugs. Telling Candy how happy they were that she was better, the nurses urged her to come back and see them.

"You won't have to stay," they were careful to assure her. "Just come and visit us, okay?"

The Rudolphs took the elevator down to the underground garage and got in the car. They drove up the ramp and paid the parking lot attendant. When they drove out into daylight, Yvonne knew that their ordeal was finally over. They were going home— home to grandparents Candy adored and a little sister she had sorely missed, home to a new seven-room dollhouse with sliding doors, home to a normal diet, normal habits, a normal schedule, a normal family life. Home. For a new beginning.

Ø

Home. Where Mark had planned to be long before now.

In his room in the Adolescent Unit, he pretended to doze. He was curled on his right side against the cranked-up mattress with rolled pillows at his back for support. For more than three weeks this had been one of the few positions his body had been able to find that allowed him to get breath without squishing any of his chest tubes or putting direct pressure on any of his incisions. He found it hard to believe that in a few days he would probably be able to lean his whole back against the mattress.

He was down to one chest tube, the fourth, the tube just below his left armpit. His pain had decreased substantially. Since Wednesday, when the first tube had come out, he had needed codeine and Tylenol only four times. The three incisions were still sore, and he was still having pain at the site of the remaining tube; but for the first time in three weeks he was not preoccupied by pain. For the first time in three weeks he could see that it was not going to last forever. He could see that one morning he would wake up and feel no pain whatsoever, because the chest tubes would all be gone and the incisions would all be healed.

He knew now that this would not happen before Christmas. The third tube had come out this morning. Afterward his lung had collapsed about five percent. Thinking the fourth tube had become clogged again, as it apparently had on Wednesday too, Dr. Cipriani had irrigated it for the second time in four days: unhooked it from the Emerson and squirted some sterile saline solution into it. Just for good measure, he had also changed the connection between the tube and the Emerson. Another x-ray had been done. Mark was waiting now for the results.

However, Dr. Cipriani had told him that as long as the lung was unstable for whatever reason, the fourth tube would have to stay in. Once the lung became stable, it would have to remain stable for several days before the surgeons could consider taking the tube out. Then they'd have to clamp the tube and watch him for at least a day and maybe more. So there was no way he could get home by Christmas. There wasn't even a chance.

He was very depressed. He had refused his A.M. care and had hardly spoken to his mother or the nurses all morning. "Gee, you're grouchy today," the x-ray technician had teased when she'd come up to do the second x-ray. "You'd be grouchy too," he had snapped at her, "if you had to be in the hospital for Christmas." This afternoon his mother was out getting him a tree for his room. Mark didn't care whether he had a tree or not. He wanted to go home.

He had had such plans. He had all kinds of money—money he'd saved from his allowance and his birthday, money he'd won off Bob or other people playing cards or pool, Christmas money he'd been receiving from his relatives and from people at church. The first thing he wanted to do when he got home was take his whole family to Widow Brown's Restaurant for dinner. Then he wanted to buy his parents either a microwave oven or a digital clock-radio for their bedroom. A microwave would be nice for him too. He could use it to make the baked potatoes he liked for a snack in the afternoons. He hadn't decided yet what to get for Randy and Denise. He knew he'd buy a metal detector for himself. He'd been wanting one for a long time.

He lay wishing that Children's Hospital weren't so far from home. If it were closer, his parents wouldn't have that long drive back and forth, and maybe his mother wouldn't be so tired. If he were in a hospital closer to home, he could see more people more often. Maybe he could even see his dog. He missed Taffy so much. He missed everybody, including his sister.

"Honey?"

He had fallen asleep. His mother was standing in her coat at the foot of his bed with a small fake Christmas tree in her arms.

"Look!" She held the tree out toward him.

He nodded.

"And look!" Setting the tree on a chair, she opened a paper bag and took out several boxes of shiny miniature balls. "Aren't these nice? What if I put the tree right here on your bedside table, and we'll decorate it together?"

He hung one ornament and refused to hang any more. Ellen finished the tree herself. Her son closed his eyes and appeared to sleep. An hour passed, and then about 2:00 Dr. Cavanaugh came in to tell Mark that once again his lung was fully reexpanded.

The patient's spirits improved somewhat.

Ø

Two floors down in the Infant ICU, Brandon Gregory had begun receiving half-strength formula at the rate of 3 cc. an hour. It was being pumped into his feeding tube by a small boxlike machine at his bedside. The baby had tolerated quarter-strength formula without difficulty. On the ventilator he had made no progress at all over the past twenty-four hours. However, he remained stable, and the staff members taking care of the infant had no immediate worries about him.

They were far more worried about his resident. Logan Sadler had developed a blood clot in her leg and been hospitalized next door with phlebitis. She was to be away from her patients for two weeks.

So Brandon had a new resident as of this afternoon, a dark-haired woman who was, like Sadler, in her second year of training at Children's. Though on occasion this doctor had taken night call in the Infant ICU, she had yet to serve a full rotation there. She had assumed her new responsibilities feeling very nervous. She was most nervous about Brandon Gregory, not because he was the most acutely ill of Logan Sadler's patients in the unit presently—he wasn't—but simply because he was the smallest. He was so small that he scared her.

Ø

About 4:00, when she had done her last chore for the day, Adolescent nurse Carol Buchanan walked toward Mark's room summoning cheerfulness. She found it easier to go into his room now that three of the chest tubes were out and he was feeling more comfortable. But he still looked terrible, and she hated to face him knowing he knew he'd be at Children's for Christmas.

Mark and his mother were reading when Carol came through the door.

"I just came in to say goodbye," she said brightly, adding an apology for interrupting them. "I'm leaving the city tonight to spend Christmas with my parents, and then I'm going skiing. I'm really sorry you have to be in here, Mark, but I know you'll be out before I get back in ten days, and I hope I won't see you now for a long time."

Looking up from the latest issue of *Psychology Today,* he gave her a grin. "Thanks a lot!"

She caught Ellen's eye, delighted at this sign of life in him. "You know what I mean!"

"You can't leave right this minute," he said, "because I didn't give you my Christmas present yet." He picked up one of several small packages, identically wrapped, from his bedside table. "Here. Merry Christmas."

"Thank you!" She shook the package close to her ear. "I can't imagine what's in it!" Her surprise was phony and calculated to make him laugh. He returned the favor. "Same thing I gave everybody else!"

The card attached to the package read "Love, Mark." Removing the ribbon, Carol tore the paper and drew from a box a tree ornament inscribed with her name.

"Oh, Mark!" She hugged him. "Thank you so much."

He looked pleased. "My Mom went and got them."

"But you paid for them," Ellen corrected, "and you told me what to get."

"Carol, maybe you can tell me," Mark said without warning, "why everybody I'm giving Christmas presents to won't take care of me anymore."

Her heart skipped a beat. "What?"

"All my favorites aren't taking care of me anymore." His manner was puzzled. "Are they afraid to take care of me? You're not afraid to take care of me, are you?"

Looking from his face to his mother's, Carol saw that these questions had taken Ellen, too, by surprise.

She lied to him. "Of course not, Mark. You know this room is between two districts. Sometimes the nurses in front take it, sometimes the nurses in back take it, depending on who's busiest." That was true except in special cases. She was sure he knew he was one. Yet he seemed to accept her explanation.

Minutes later, saying goodbye to Ellen Price at the elevator, Carol confessed in tears to Mark's mother.

Ellen hugged her. "Don't be hard on yourself for that, Carol. You've all been wonderful to him. You're like his big sisters. I know you feel close to him. I know that his pain hurts you just as much as it hurts me. There are times I have to get out of that room myself."

After dinner at home that evening, Daniel Earnshaw returned to Children's bringing with him the football player who had just become engaged to his younger daughter.

From the underground parking lot the two men took the elevator to the sixth floor. The spacious car was crowded with parents. Among them Earnshaw's future son-in-law was a mammoth presence. Standing well over six feet tall, weighing nearly three hundred pounds, he carried himself like the star he was—a first-string linebacker for the professional team headquartered a few miles from Children's, a man known to telecasters, sportswriters, and fans all over the nation as one of the toughest defensive players in the league. Parents stole glances at him as the elevator ascended. It was clear from their faces and their whispers that several of them recognized him.

After depositing their coats in Earnshaw's office, the physician and his guest set out for the Adolescent Unit. The visitor had never been to Children's before. As they walked, Earnshaw pointed things out to him and answered his questions.

Inside himself he was anticipating Mark's reaction. Mark knew of his doctor's connection with the football player. Earnshaw had been promising his patient for some months that one day he would bring the man in. But the pneumothorax had pushed him to ask his daughter's fiancé to name a day. More specifically, the boy's depression had pushed him. Earnshaw hoped that a visit from a football star would cheer Mark up, would shatter his depression, would interrupt the slow nosedive into despair that had hastened the death of Perry Smith.

They entered the Adolescent Unit, passed the nurses' station, approached the door of Mark's room. Earnshaw had prepared his companion for what the man was about to see. He hoped he had prepared him enough.

Mark was alone when they entered. He was sitting cross-legged reading with his pajama top unbuttoned. Hearing them, he looked up. In the split second that passed before introductions were made, Daniel Earnshaw saw Mark Price's eyes grow huge, causing the doctor to realize for the first time in his life that the term "eyes as big as saucers" had literal meaning; and he saw the linebacker who was going to marry his daughter respond to the sight of the boy in the bed by turning away, so overcome that he had to look at the wall to get himself together before he could go up to Mark and talk.

Months later these images would remain vivid in Earnshaw's memory. He would remember the linebacker turning away, and he would remember the patient's eyes. However long he lived, Daniel Earnshaw thought he would never forget the look in Mark's eyes when the football star walked in his door.

Christmas Eve

Brandon Gregory did so beautifully on his tube feedings over the weekend that by 6:00 Sunday evening he had been receiving full-strength formula at 6 cc. per hour. Long after midnight the patient had given every evidence of being just fine.

But the doctors gathered at Brandon's bedside for rounds the morning of Christmas Eve saw a baby who did not look fine at all. His belly was distended. His liver was enlarged. His color was the pale grayish-red of uncooked sausage. He was lethargic. Whether the patient's condition related to feeds was impossible to prove. But the suggestion of a connection was strong enough to prompt Roger Forbes to tell the residents that "in retrospectroscope," it had probably been a mistake to increase Brandon to 6 cc. quite so fast.

Forbes ascribed no blame. Brandon had shown himself able to tolerate full-strength formula at 4 cc. per hour. A baby who did well on 4 cc. could reasonably be tried on 6.

Nonetheless, the deterioration in Brandon's condition left his caregivers no choice but to stop feeding him temporarily. Assuming he improved, he'd have to start all over again on quarter-strength formula and build up slowly. Ideally his system would need only one day of rest.

Even so, these developments constituted a definite setback for Roger Forbes's tiny patient. Brandon was now more than two weeks old. He had yet to regain his birth weight. Every day he went without adequate calories was a step in the direction of greater problems. Furthermore, the baby had now identified himself to be a premie who could not tolerate feeds very well.

This worried Forbes for more than one reason. When the feeding process is long and fraught with as many reverses as were likely to occur in Brandon's case, parents often get very discouraged.

They come in week after week to see a baby who not only still has tubes everywhere but who is also putting on weight so slowly that the gain is almost imperceptible. Unless they get to know the baby, to bring in mobiles and teddy bears and interact with their tiny offspring as much as the infant's condition permits, parents sometimes find it hard to regard that infant as a member of their family.

Forbes considered it important that they do so. Whether Brandon Gregory lived or died, his doctor believed it was important for Brandon's parents to think of their son as a member of the family who had done his best to survive. Forbes had not seen the Gregorys in the unit much. He knew the nurses would encourage them to come in as often as they could. When rounds were over, however, just to fortify the message, Forbes mentioned his concerns to the social worker attached to the Infant ICU, who promised to call the Gregorys before the day was out.

Ø

Mark Price also suffered a setback the morning of Christmas Eve, albeit a small one. Films taken after breakfast showed that his lung had gone down slightly.

This finding did not particularly upset the patient. In fact the pneumothorax was less than five percent. Kate thought Mark could tolerate this slight collapse now that he was down to one tube; and now that that tube was attached not to an Emerson but to a Pleurevac, he saw himself as getting better.

He certainly felt better. In the past twenty-four hours he had asked for codeine and Tylenol only twice. Though still quite weak, he was doing part of his own A.M. care again. His appetite had improved. He seemed to be enjoying his visitors more. His mother could leave the room for longer than five minutes without his sending somebody to bring her back. Though he remained somewhat down about having to be in the hospital over the holiday, he had adjusted to the disappointment surprisingly well. There was no doubt in Kate's mind that meeting the football player Saturday night had given Mark a big boost. He talked about it to anybody who came in the room, inviting everybody to look at the autographed photograph he had propped against an empty cola can on his bedside table.

While Kate was giving his roommate a bed bath, Mark asked her why the nurses had made no plans for a floor Christmas party.

"Because Carol and a few of the other people who are good at organizing those things were going to be away, and the rest of us didn't get our act together," she answered, to which he replied cheerfully, "I think that's terrible!"

Kate thought it wonderful that he felt well enough to care how Christmas was going to be celebrated on Adolescent.

Ø

The phone rang in the Gregorys' trailer just as Robin was about to stop wrapping presents and start fixing lunch. The caller was a social worker from Children's. The social worker said she had been told by one of the Infant ICU nurses that Brandon's parents hadn't visited in about a week. If this was true, the social worker wondered, was there any particular reason?

The baby's mother was offended. In the ten days that had passed since her own discharge from Northwest Suburban, she and Tom had gone into the hospital four times. Robin had been making daily notes on her calendar since Brandon's birth, so she was able to give the worker dates and times. They hadn't visited more often, she'd said, because they couldn't afford to. Their income from Unemployment was sixty-one dollars a week. Behind in their bills, they were having trouble just paying for rent and food for the four of them. There was very little money available for gas.

The social worker apologized. She said the nurses in the unit had probably just forgotten to record the visits in Brandon's chart. She suggested that the Gregorys might be able to get money for gas and parking from Welfare or some other program.

"Call your own social worker," she urged Robin, "and if you have trouble, get back to me."

Robin promised to make the call.

In a longer conversation, the social worker might have learned of other ways to be helpful to the Gregorys, who were under considerable pressure. They'd been fighting about money. Hating to let bills go unpaid, Robin would chide her husband about having no job; then in the next breath she'd turn around and say it was just as well he wasn't working because she was still tired from her own surgery and needed him to help her with the twins. Either way Tom hardly knew how to respond. As Robin was well aware, if he found a job now, they'd lose the medical assistance that was paying Brandon's bills.

The Gregorys were also reacting very differently to the tiny infant who was struggling for his life at Children's Hospital. Robin had become committed to the child. Though still reluctant to get too close to a baby she might lose, she was no longer horrified by the sight of Brandon. In fact, she now thought he was rather cute. She was beginning to see him as her son. His dying would hurt much more now, Robin thought, than had he died in the birth room. But she expected now that he would live. The nurses' reports since the operation had all seemed good to Robin. She thought of Brandon now as a fighter who could take anything.

In a way his being in the hospital was actually something of a relief to his mother. This way she was getting a chance to recuperate. By the time he got home, she'd be on her feet, and the twins would be that much older. It would still be rough, but they'd have had a chance to prepare for him.

Nevertheless, his absence from her daily life felt very odd to Robin. One night she had cried herself to sleep thinking, *I've gone through another Caesarean and all the difficulty since, and I can't even have my baby with me. I can't even hold him.* She wondered what poor Brandon must be making of all that had happened to him. Being unable to visit him every day made her feel terrible. To compensate she called the unit every day and sometimes twice a day.

Her husband, on the other hand, maintained a good distance between himself and his new son. Tom Gregory had never developed the commitment to the pregnancy that his wife had, and although he could admire Brandon's grit and was concerned about his condition, he lacked strong feelings for the baby. His strongest feeling *about* Brandon was that sooner or later he was going to die.

Tom Gregory visited Children's because his wife wanted to and because the nurses said it gave a baby more support if parents came. In one way, Tom could see their point. In another way, he couldn't understand how a baby who wasn't even supposed to be born yet could realize that his parents were supporting him, or even that they were there. Seeing Brandon with his tubes and his bruises always made Tom Gregory feel worse. As the baby's father, he would have preferred to come in only once in a while and the rest of the time take the nurses' word for it that the baby was or was not doing well.

As his wife's husband, Gregory worried about whether he was giving Robin the right support. His own way of handling situations that troubled him was to try to keep his mind off them as much as possible. Yet he was finding it hard to help Robin keep her mind off this situation when he could hardly stop thinking about it himself. In any case he had the impression that she didn't think much of his way of trying to support her. So if he couldn't support her now, what should he say to her if the baby died?

The social worker from Children's did offer on the phone to help the Gregorys any way she could. She did not offer specifics. The parents did not press for any. Neither suggested a face-to-face meeting, and none was to take place.

Ø

Ellen Price arrived back at Children's Hospital right after lunch. She had gone home Saturday evening to spend Sunday with Bob while Mark's natural father visited his son. Now she had returned with her overnight bag to stay through Christmas Day. Later this afternoon Bob would be in to see Mark before going home to spend Christmas Eve with Randy and Denise and his own son. In the morning they would all come to the hospital. On Christmas Day the whole family would be together for the first time since Mark's admission to Children's on the twenty-ninth of November.

Ellen found her son sitting on the edge of his bed, legs dangling. He was counting his money. He had plans for her.

"I don't understand this hospital," he said. "Here it is Christmas Eve, and they're playing the same old stuff over the intercom. No Christmas carols."

"Don't you imagine they're doing that out of sensitivity to the Jewish people who don't celebrate Christmas?"

"Yeah, but not playing them is insensitive to Christians! It's ridiculous, Christmas Eve without Christmas carols! First," he said, handing his mother some bills and two quarters, "I'd like you to put this in the collection plate at church on Sunday."

She looked at him with surprise. At other times while hospitalized he had given her dollar bills for church. She was now holding $13.50.

"It's ten percent of what the people at church have given me," he explained. "Now, the next thing is I'd like you to do is take this other money to Sears and get me the best portable radio you can buy, AM/FM, weather band, everything. Just tell them you want the best."

Ellen, who hated shopping under ideal circumstances, headed out through holiday traffic to a Sears store in the middle of the city feeling overjoyed that he wanted something she could give him.

In her absence, as planned, Mark kept a special appointment with the recreation therapist. When it had become clear to Mark that he would not get home for Christmas, when he had told Joe Noyes of his disappointment at not being able to buy things for his family, Joe had responded with an offer. Every year people and organizations from all over donate unwrapped presents to Children's to be distributed to patients hospitalized during the holiday. The gifts are collected in the play therapists' offices. Usually the nurses go down and choose presents for each child. But in light of the fact that Mark had been in the hospital so long, and because he was so concerned about having something to give his family on Christmas morning, Joe had proposed that he bring up a boxful of donated presents and let Mark choose among them.

So while his mother was at Sears, Mark stayed in bed and did his Christmas shopping. And as Mark finished his shopping on the sixth floor, Candy Rudolph settled onto a chair between her mother and grandfather in the hall outside the Neurosurgery Department three floors down and waited for her name to be called.

Ø

Several other young patients sitting nearby sneaked looks at Candy whenever she was not looking their way. Though adorably outfitted in patent-leather shoes and a dusty pink dress with a lace yoke and lace-trimmed long sleeves, the child still had no hair to speak of, she had an ugly if healing gash from ear to ear, and her right eyelid was still swollen shut. Though the swelling in her head had diminished substantially, her face looked decidedly odd.

Guillermo Perez emerged from his big corner office, greeted the children waiting to see him, walked toward Candy, and touched his fingertips to the top of her head. "Ah!" He smiled. "I see you got cured without me!" He nodded at Pastor Brandt, then smiled at the patient's mother. "As far as I'm concerned," he said, "she's cured!" He turned, called another name, and disappeared with that family back into his office.

Yvonne looked at her father in astonishment. "I hope that wasn't our appointment!"

Candy's mother was in excellent spirits. She could feel no fluid at all now under the child's scalp. Each day a little more bone was visible. The right eye opened much more easily now when Yvonne applied ointment to it. In the two days since her discharge from Six Surgical, the child's spirits had improved almost miraculously. Back in the familiar surroundings of her grandparents' house, Candy was freer and more relaxed than Yvonne had seen her since the day of her admission to the hospital. While the child continued to warn her sister to "Be careful of my head," this morning Yvonne had discovered both girls turning somersaults on pillows on the floor.

Candy was not yet her old self. On Saturday night and again on Sunday night, she had awakened tearful half a dozen times. She cried when being helped to dress, complained of pain in her back, legs, and chest, and was very jumpy when anybody went near her.

She was still fussy about food and still spoiled. This morning when offered more pancakes by her grandmother, the child had been downright rude. In other circumstances she would have been spanked. Yvonne was now insisting that Candy Land be played by the rules. As a result, Candy preferred playing the game with Amy, who was too young to fully understand the rules and let her sister cheat to her heart's content. Yvonne had every hope that these patterns would change as soon as the Rudolphs rejoined under one roof and began to function as a family again.

Guillermo Perez came back into the hall. "Okay, Candy, you can follow me, and bring your mother and grandfather if you want to."

They sat down in his office. "Come over here, Candy," the doctor urged.

Sitting on her grandfather's lap, she buried her head in his shoulder.

Perez shrugged sadly. "Okay, be that way. Well," he continued, looking from Yvonne to her father, "the cerebrospinal fluid leak got healed. It must have been a very small leak. I usually find that the best treatment is to send the child home!"

Pastor Brandt shifted Candy on his knee and pointed to a slight bump on the child's left temple. "Is this swelling?"

Perez walked over and touched it. "Well, that's the end of a bone graft. That's the frontal bone advancement you're seeing there. More than likely that spot will be tender for a while, but the tenderness will go away. The only thing we have to worry about now is those gaps in her skull." He returned to his desk. "We'll talk about those when we start to discuss the jaw surgery a year from now."

Yvonne mentioned that Candy had been waking up several times a night. As she started to add that this was very unusual, Perez interrupted.

"If anyone had done to me what we did to her, I'd have nightmares for the rest of my life!"

Yvonne had another question. "She says her head hurts sometimes."

Perez nodded. "When there are many little pieces of bone fusing, it's painful, unfortunately. That will get better."

"She also mentions pains in her legs," said Pastor Brandt.

Perez shrugged. "She had several spinal taps, and she's been in bed not using her legs for a long time."

"So that's natural too."

"Yes."

"Is there any reason she can't wear a wig?"

"Not at all." Perez picked up a pen. "Make it tax-deductible. I'll give you a prescription." He began to write. "Do you want a swimming pool too?"

Even Candy smiled.

"So unless something new develops, when of course you'll call me," Perez said, "I'll see you on the twenty-fifth when you come in to see Dr. Lorimer. Come on, Candy," he said as the child stood with her grandfather, "give me a kiss goodbye."

Again she hid her face.

"All right, be that way." He managed to sound both desolate and in full sympathy with her wishes. He asked her what Santa Claus was going to bring her, but she wouldn't answer him.

Moments later, on the way to the garage, Yvonne asked her daughter, "Why didn't you like Dr. Perez today?"

Candy looked up at her and said simply, "I was afraid he was going to hurt me."

Ø

The trip to Sears and back had taken Ellen Price more than two hours, but Mark was thrilled with the radio she had chosen. He found a station playing Christmas carols and turned up the volume as high as he dared, sending his mother to the door to make sure the music wasn't too loud in the hall. A number of nurses came in to see Mark's new toy, as Kate was calling it, and as he showed it off to them, Mark was all smiles. "Now it sounds like Christmas in here!"

He couldn't wait for Bob to see the radio. When Bob arrived, Mark glowed in his father's enthusiasm for the new purchase.

Bob had a surprise for Mark—a tall can of cold beer which he had sneaked in in his big coat pocket, drawing from the boy a loud "Yee-haw!"

"I asked Dr. Earnshaw if I could bring that in to you," Bob said, laughing, "and he said he'd pretend he didn't hear the question!" Mark drank beer rarely, but he liked it once in a while, and because it provided some calories, his parents did not discourage him.

When the day shift was over, Kate came in to wish the Prices a Merry Christmas. She was leaving within the hour to spend five days with her family and her boyfriend back in her hometown.

Mark handed her the one remaining small square box from his bedside table, saying almost shyly, "I saved yours till last. You'd better open this first, because you probably won't like it after you see what my parents are giving you."

She laughed. "Mark, you know I'll like anything you give me, even if you are a rotten kid!"

Kate never gave presents to patients or parents because she couldn't afford to give to all of them and didn't want to give to only some. But she opened her gift from Mark wishing she had made an exception in his case.

"Oh, Mark, this is beautiful! I love these. I even thought of getting one for my mother and sister. I don't care if you are only a teenage boy," she said, replacing the ornament and setting the box on a chair. "I'm going to kiss you anyway!" She hugged him. "I love your present, Mark. Thank you so much." He accepted this fuss with embarrassment.

Bob handed her another small box, this one flat and narrow.

"We wanted to get you something special because you're part of the family," Ellen said.

Kate lifted from the box a sterling silver necklace with a cluster of four little green stones at the center. "It's an Irish necklace!"

"For our favorite Irishperson!" said Ellen.

"I can't believe you went all the way to Ireland to get me a necklace!"

"Only for you," Bob said.

She thanked them, hugging them. "It's beautiful. Thank you. Both of you. All of you. I really appreciate it."

"Before everything gets too soppy around here," Mark said, "why don't I open up this beer . . ."

"Shhhhh!"

He grinned. "Why don't I open up this b-e-e-r," he continued in a whisper, "and everybody can have a little s-i-p!"

He popped the top, spraying beer on himself and the bed. Just as he was about to put the can to his lips, Allyson Fay walked in the door, a dark-haired nurse Mark had gotten to know during this admission. Seeing the can, she put her hands on her hips and said sternly, "Just what is going on here?" A second later she burst out laughing. "Wait till I report this! Is this how you think you're going to get out of here for Christmas? Kicked out for drinking beer?"

Mark shrugged. "It was worth a try! Want some?"

"I do not! I've got work to do." She held up a rolled sheet of paper.

"What's that?"

"The results of your chest x-ray this afternoon."

He sobered instantly. "What does it show?"

She didn't answer. Instead, finding a blank spot on the wall where all his cards were taped up, unrolling the paper in front of her so that none of the others could see it, she stuck it on the wall with tape peeled from her wrist, then stood back.

In one corner of the paper she had drawn a Santa Claus smiling. Across the top she had written, in bold characters of bright red, "100%!"

Ø

"Braaan-don. Braaan-don."

Christmas Eve. Children throughout the land awaited Santa Claus. Robin Gregory bent over her baby's warmer bed until her long hair nearly touched the Saran Wrap covering him. "Braaan-don. Are you awake? Mommy's here to see you."

He was lying froglike on his back. His head was turned to one side. When his mother spoke, however, he made an effort to move his head and look at her, which was difficult for him because of the weight of the ventilator tubes going into his mouth. But he had obviously heard her and tried to respond. Robin was thrilled.

Continuing to talk to him in low tones, she wondered if he could distinguish her voice from the voices of the nurses. One nurse had suggested that she try to see Brandon with no one else around. That way he wouldn't associate her with pain or discomfort, and he could get used to her voice and her scent. This evening, not thinking, Robin had put on perfume before leaving for Children's. In the car she'd realized that the odor might be too strong for a tiny baby, so before coming into the unit, she had washed it off. Now she wondered whether it might be a good idea to find a perfume with a very light scent and wear it every time she came in so Brandon could associate it with her. She would try to remember to ask someone about this.

They had come in this evening with an Instamatic camera and a Christmas present to Brandon of several jars of his mother's breast milk. Robin was now off antibiotics. This meant that her son could now be nourished by her, or at least maybe he could in a couple of days. A nurse had told Robin on the phone this morning that Brandon had had problems feeding over the weekend and would have to start over again on quarter-strength prepared formula.

This news had distressed the baby's mother. His weight continued to distress her. The nurse had also said that as of this morning, Brandon weighed only one pound seven ounces. Robin did not think he could afford to lose any more.

Slipping her hand under one side of the Saran blanket, she curled Brandon's tiny fingers around the tip of her own forefinger. With her thumb she stroked his tiny knuckles. It seemed to her that he was beginning to look like a combination of the twins: Keith's nose, Tommy's hair. After a while she began to take some pictures of the baby.

Tom waited for her in the parents' lounge. Robin knew he'd been ready to leave the hospital almost since they'd arrived. He had spent only a few minutes with Brandon. As little as Tom spoke about his feelings, his wife was well aware that seeing the baby still bothered him.

She herself felt encouraged by Brandon's condition. It was Robin's understanding that he was getting along rather well. What impressed her in the nurses' reports these days was their comments about how active the baby was. His mother had noticed that too. She noticed it again this evening. Brandon moved around constantly. He was always kicking, causing Robin to comment to him now, while taking snapshots of her youngest son, that he seemed full of spunk. That the ICU staff had thought him lethargic all day she had no inkling.

She knew that since morning he'd been receiving a blood transfusion. But in explaining the reason—that the baby's color had turned poor—the nurses had transmitted to Robin Gregory only a fraction of the concern expressed about Brandon's appearance during rounds this morning, or, for that matter, the concern his caretakers now felt about his feedings. Yet Robin had specifically asked to be told if her son's condition grew worse in any way at all. Though breaking such news is actually a doctor's responsibility, the nurses had promised to let her know. But if they had tried to convey the concern of Monday morning, they had failed. Robin left her baby's bedside Monday evening not realizing that his situation had grown more worrisome. She hadn't noticed that his skin was dusky.

As she said good night to him, she wound up the little musical bunny she had brought in on one of her first visits and laid it next to Brandon. The bunny played a nursery rhyme. Soft notes rose into the air. The baby's eyes seemed to be trying to identify the source. His mother thought he liked the sound.

Christmas Day

It was tradition in Mark's family that gifts were opened after breakfast on Christmas morning and that before breakfast everybody dressed for the occasion.

Waking early on December 25 at Children's Hospital, Mark announced to his mother as she was folding up her bedding that he wanted to get dressed.

When his A.M. care was done, Ellen and his nurse got Mark into a shirt and trousers. They let the shirt hang out a little on his left side around the chest tube. The clothes camouflaged his thinness and made him seem less sick than he looked in pajamas. His blond hair had grown so long in the nearly four weeks he had spent in the hospital that the nurses had begun to tease him about it. After he had combed it out of his eyes, Ellen took a number of pictures of him. He smiled for all of them.

The rest of the family came, and they exchanged presents. Mark had gotten his main gift, his watch, before coming into the hospital. He had received most of his other gifts over the past week, an attempt on his mother's part to take his mind off his troubles. But he opened a game called Family Feud, and he exclaimed over *The Book of Lists,* which he had also been wanting. The things he gave included record albums for his sister and brother, cologne for Bob, and string art for his mother.

The Prices spent the day talking, playing games, kidding with each other and the nurses, and feasting on Children's Hospital Christmas fare and on cookies brought from home. When supper was over and Bob said reluctantly that they'd better be starting back, there was a general rush to pick up the room and pack the things to be taken to the car, and with everybody talking and laughing, several moments passed before they realized that Mark had been trying to get their attention.

"Can you all be quiet just for a moment?" He was sitting in bed still dressed, except for his bare feet, and smiling. But his tone was serious. "I want you all to come here, everybody, and listen. I have something I want to say."

They gathered around him waiting, wondering.

Still smiling, he looked at each face in turn and said, "I want to thank every one of you for making this a very beautiful Christmas. It's been a wonderful day, one of the best Christmases ever. I just want to thank you all very much."

Ellen thought he looked as happy as she had ever seen him.

Bob left Children's that evening with his optimism restored. Gone were all thoughts of his recent conclusion that Mark might be better off if he died; gone was all memory of his and Ellen's conversation with Dr. Earnshaw about no heroics. Bob left Children's Hospital Christmas night convinced that Mark would come home soon and that everything would be all right again, at least for a while. At least they'd have him two or three more years—not a long time as measured against a normal human life span, but certainly far better than losing him here and now.

JANUARY

Thursday, December 27

Sirens screamed into the gathering dusk, disturbing momentarily the peace of everyone within earshot for blocks around. With all the speed possible at the onset of rush hour, the ambulance raced through the streets of the city toward Children's Hospital.

In the rear lay a nine-year-old boy in a coma. He was covered to his chin by gray-green sheets. His brown body had been immobilized by leather straps, his head by strips of wide adhesive tape across his brow which were anchored above each shoulder to the sheet pulled tight over the stretcher pad. Beneath the strips a bandage covered the child's left temple. Both eyelids were swollen; the left was especially swollen and purple. On the boy's right cheekbone was a small, fresh scrape. In one nostril was a slim tube inserted to drain his stomach contents so he wouldn't vomit and draw that substance into his lungs. In his mouth was an oral airway, a plastic device inserted to prevent him from biting down on the tube that connected him to a respirator. He was being tended in the ambulance by a nurse, a resident, and a doctor training as a specialist in critical care.

Freddy Eberly. Frederick Patterson Eberly, his mother's sole offspring, her reason for rising at six each morning to fold linens in the laundry of a hospital ten miles from home, from the doll's house she had so recently bought after years in a tiny apartment, years of scrimping and saving so that her growing son might have more space.

He was big for nine. Not fat, but taller and sturdier than most boys in fourth grade. He had dreamed of becoming a professional linebacker. In fact he had given himself the nickname Pro. Other sports interested him too. At church day camp this past summer he had received certificates for swimming and miniature golf and an award for being "most athletic" among his peers. He had also received a clock-radio for being good. His mother proudly showed off these and other records of her son's achievements: a certificate awarded him for attending day camp, another for his participation in the school district pen-pal program, still another signed by the school principal commending Freddy for outstanding citizenship. His report cards showed C's and B's in subjects, mostly B's in work habits, mostly A's in behavior. He had always liked school.

On weekdays when there was no school, he stayed with a woman he knew as Grandma Baker. Since he was now on Christmas vacation, he had been on his way to her house this morning. Usually he was dropped off there by his uncle, a security guard at the hospital that also employed his mother. Last night, however, his uncle's car had broken down.

So this morning, on the way to catching a bus herself, the child's mother had put him on a bus that would take him to within a few blocks of his destination. She had done this feeling some concern. When Freddy got off, he would have to cross a highway. Yet he had made the trip a number of times alone and many times with her.

Always before Sharita Queen had asked the driver to let the boy know when he should get off. This morning Freddy had insisted that he knew where to get off. He had seemed to want to show her that he could do it. She had wanted to let him.

But he'd become confused, apparently. He'd gotten off one stop too soon. Had the unfamiliarity of the landscape disoriented him so that he was looking for landmarks instead of watching for cars? Had he turned to wave goodbye to the bus driver? Or had he simply bounced down the steps and onto the street too excited about vacation to remember about crossing highways?

He had started to cross in front of the bus. An automobile had been coming up alongside too fast to stop. The car had slammed into the child and propelled him through the air. He had landed on the pavement in a heap.

He had been taken immediately to the nearest hospital, Springfield Community. It happened to be where his mother worked. Examined in the emergency room, he had been found to be critically injured: in shock, gasping, flaccid from the nipples down, bleeding internally from a ruptured spleen and lacerated liver, and suffering from a serious head injury. He also had a broken leg, a bruised lung, and a variety of cuts and bruises. Doctors evaluating the patient had felt he was in imminent danger from loss of blood. Rushing him into the operating room, surgeons had removed his spleen and sewn up his liver. These efforts had stabilized the child's blood pressure; keeping him on a ventilator postoperatively had stabilized his breathing.

But as morning had passed into afternoon, Freddy's neurological condition had begun to deteriorate. Physicians had noted posturing, or intermittent rigidity, in the boy's limbs. While upon his admission both his pupils had reacted to light, they had been unequal in size, and one pupil now appeared to be fixed. These signs suggested a worse brain injury than the doctors had appreciated earlier. The patient obviously needed a CAT scan to determine whether surgery was necessary.

Unfortunately Springfield's only CAT scanner had just broken down. For this reason and because they had become convinced that the case demanded the expertise of neurosurgeons specializing in pediatrics, the physicians caring for Freddy Eberly at Springfield Community had made arrangements to transfer the boy to Children's.

The whine of the sirens diminished suddenly and ceased. Cutting a close corner off the boulevard into the circular driveway outside the Children's emergency room, the ambulance driver deliberately overshot the entrance, then backed up to park so that the distance between the rear doors of the vehicle and the doors into the hospital was a short, straight pathway.

He jumped to the pavement and opened the ambulance doors. With his help, the nurse and the two doctors quickly removed a small cart from the back of the ambulance, then several pieces of equipment which they loaded on the cart, and then the respirator and the wheeled stretcher holding the patient. A bystander whispered, "Oh, Lord have mercy!"

Accompanied by a security guard who held doors open for them, the transport team and the ambulance driver moved patient and equipment through the Emergency Room and down a hall toward a waiting elevator. Their pace was brisk, but they did not run. In his condition, the boy needed as little jostling as possible. Since his vital signs had been stabilized at Springfield, chances were strong that his life was in no immediate danger. Minutes were important, but not as important as getting the boy upstairs without further injury to his brain.

They were waiting for him in Acute. The afternoon there had been quiet enough that the mood now was dominated by the sky darkening outside the big windows, making the artificial light in the unit seem increasingly brighter. The calm was shattered when the transport team came through the double doors from the hall and rolled the stretcher to a stop alongside the empty bed in front of the nurses' station.

Instantly the patient was surrounded by medical personnel. Someone unbuckled the leather straps holding him immobile. Someone else drew off the sheets that covered him. Two pairs of hands unhooked the child from transport equipment and rehooked him to Acute equipment. On either side of him, nurses rolled the sheets he was lying on up against his body. Eight people prepared to lift him from the stretcher to the bed.

"We must assume a fractured spine until we know for sure," said one of the transport doctors. "What I'd like to do is lift fast to make sure nothing is dangling. Okay, ready? One . . . two . . . three . . . *lift!* Move that leg over! Okay, set him down. Good. Very nice." As someone pushed the stretcher aside, the silver bells of three stethoscopes went down on the patient's chest.

He lay naked and still, his face and form reposed as if in natural sleep. This apparent peacefulness was violated by evidence all over his body that the boy had been badly hurt. On his abdomen were a freshly sutured incision about six inches long and a much smaller hole cut by the surgeons to drain his belly. His broken right leg, which had not been set, was in a plaster splint wrapped thickly in Ace bandages from thigh to ankle. Patches of his left wrist and shoulder and the knuckles of his left hand were scraped raw. In the fluorescent glare of the unit, the purple of his swollen eyelids seemed deeper than it had in the ambulance. Beneath the endotracheal tube connecting him to the ventilator, the boy's tongue protruded slightly. He had a catheter in his penis and an intravenous line taped into his left ankle.

A blood pressure cuff was unwrapped from his arm. Electrocardiogram leads, backed with adhesive, were positioned on his chest. Meanwhile, standing a step or two back from the bed, anesthesiologist Stuart Leith was getting a rapid rundown from one of the two transport doctors, who referred occasionally to notes. Leith was beginning his last hours of a four-day rotation as physician in charge of Acute. He was in shirtsleeves, a relatively short man, but muscular, with olive skin, wire-rimmed glasses, and shiny brown hair.

Childhood polio had left him with a malformed left leg and a significant limp. When called upon to run, Leith gathered speed by hopping several steps at a time on his good foot. The man's life spoke for itself: he had a wife, two kids, a medical degree from Harvard, and a prime position in his field.

Leith could feel his adrenaline gearing up. His job was to coordinate care: to make sure the child got everything he needed in the proper order. The first priority in this case was to get a reading on the pressure inside the patient's cranium as soon as possible. This had become obvious to Leith within moments of the child's arrival. The decision had been made easy by the doctors at Springfield who had already operated on the child's belly.

Leith might have wished that they had not. The arrangement of notes in the chart accompanying the boy from the other hospital suggested that the neurosurgeon had not even laid eyes on this patient until after the surgery had been completed. Apparently the doctors had taken the patient into the OR without knowing the full extent of his head injury. If they'd been convinced that the boy would die without an operation, they'd been right to go ahead. Yet if the child had had a blood clot in his brain, the anesthesia could have killed him. The stress of the surgery and the delay in diagnosis and thus in treatment could very possibly have exacerbated the patient's head problems.

Whether appropriate or ill-advised, however, the patient's belly surgery was behind him. Leith did not need to waste time deliberating about the dangers of internal injuries. The boy's vital signs were stable. He had been properly ventilated. While there were indications that he might still be bleeding internally, he wasn't about to die from blood loss. Though Children's neurosurgeons would have to confirm the findings, spinal x-rays had shown that his neck was not broken. The fractured leg was the least of Leith's worries.

His major worry was the child's brain. Like any other tissue, the brain responds to injury by becoming swollen and inflamed. While edema is of no great consequence in the rest of the body, it is of tremendous consequence in the cranium, because the structure is a closed container. Too much swelling in that rigid box can cut off blood flow, depriving the brain of oxygen. Failure to control the swelling can lead to physical and mental dysfunction or to death. Adults who suffer severe head trauma die most often from blood clots or direct injury to the brain tissue. The most common autopsy finding in children who die after bad head injuries, however, is a very swollen brain.

Leith was still getting the transport doctor's report when the neurosurgeons walked into the unit: Nate Pontiac, the tall, dark, bearded, and very serious senior resident, and Scottish-born Colin Kendall, compact, wiry, dimpled, and puckish, a renowned expert on head trauma. As Pontiac quickly scanned the chart, the anesthesiologist shifted his weight on his good leg and briefed his colleagues from Neurosurgery.

Kendall listened with his eyes following the activity around the crowded bedside. As a child, he had needed surgery on a finger broken in a rugby game. The doctor had given him lollipops. Kendall had gone into medicine because the doctor had given him lollipops, or at least he had begun thinking of it then. He was dressed casually in plaid trousers and a striped shirt open at the throat. Every so often he interrupted Leith with a question in marked Scottish accents.

"When he got there, was he in shock?"

"Affirmative." The anesthesiologist offered the few details he had. Shock is the collapse of circulatory function. The child's early blood pressure readings at Springfield had been rather low.

"And there's been no evidence of leg movements since he got here?"

Hearing this, a nurse looked up from the patient and answered, "He's had periods of movement if you tickle his feet."

"That's right," Leith agreed, "but I haven't seen any spontaneous movement."

Kendall walked around the bed, squeezed in between a nurse and the respirator, and, under the close observation of the neurosurgery resident standing just across the bed, began to examine the child. Very gently he lifted the bandage off the boy's forehead. He touched the puffy skin around a short gash. A superficial injury unrelated to the chief cause for concern about this patient.

Grasping the boy's nearest hand, Kendall raised the arm free of the bed and shook it. He felt resistance. Flaccidity would have been the worst prognostic sign, but the arm did not behave like wet spaghetti. It had some tone. Kendall gave the patient's left nipple a sharp tweak. In response the boy's body flinched and seemed momentarily about to curl into fetal position. His arms actually came up off the mattress. Good signs. The child was not so deeply in coma that he could not react to pain.

As the nurses and residents made way for him, the neurosurgeon moved down the bed and lifted the patient's left leg. He flexed the leg at the knee. He extended it. He laid it down. He flexed, then extended, the boy's toes. The toes did nothing on their own. Kendall ran his fingernail hard along the boy's left instep. No visible response, but the foot seemed to stiffen slightly in his hand. So did the right foot after the same provocation.

Kendall returned to the head of the bed. Easing open the child's swollen left eyelid, he peered into the eye with a small high-intensity flashlight, then said to Leith, who was standing nearby, "He didn't get any narcotic?"

"Unknown to me."

The boy's pupils responded sluggishly and abnormally—an indication that the damage had penetrated below the hemispheres to the midbrain—but they were not fixed.

Kendall was pleasantly surprised by the patient's condition. The child was badly hurt, no question. Staff at Children's sees only a few patients a year as massively hurt as this boy was. He had a significant head injury of a kind to which young children are particularly prone. Teenagers and adults tend to drive into trees, walls, or other cars going sixty miles an hour and receive direct blows to their skulls. Children are more likely to be hurt running out into the street in front of cars going thirty miles an hour. The force of impact produces a shearing injury, which was what this boy had. When the automobile had hit him, the child's neck had snapped first one way and then another, dashing his brain against the walls of his cranium. The mild analogy Kendall used with parents was jello being shaken in a bowl. A shearing injury could be far worse than a direct blow. It could sever the spinal column from the brain stem. While that had not happened in this case, the child could be in a coma for weeks.

Yet a phone conversation with one of the doctors at Springfield had left Kendall with the impression that the child was much worse off, that he had suffered severe shock as well as severe head trauma. For some reason this is a terrible combination. But the boy's circulation had been stable from the time of surgery. Shock was behind him; it was not going to play the major role the neurosurgeon had feared it might.

So the youngster was not as badly off as he might have been, in Kendall's judgment. Unless something unforeseen occurred, the boy would not die. Without knowing how high the intracranial pressure was or what the CAT scan would reveal, the neurosurgeon was optimistic that the brain would make a good recovery: that the patient would get well enough to go back to school and would grow up to lead an independent life.

Kendall felt optimistic in part because a good outcome was favored by the odds. Most youngsters with severe head injuries get better. Despite a rather desperate appearance upon admission, a child is likely to improve and to regain more function than an adult who upon admission looks similarly desperate. For an adult with a bad head injury, the chances of ever being normal again are rather minimal. But a child can lie in a coma for two weeks and wake up completely alert without any loss of mental capacities. Though full reintegration into normal life may take a year or even longer, if these youngsters get over the hump of the initial injury, they usually do well.

At least this has been the experience at Children's. At Children's these patients are treated quite aggressively, and the number who die or remain severely disabled is significantly lower than in institutions where head trauma is approached more pessimistically. For most who recover, the consequences are relatively minor: problems with attention span, visual perception, short-term memory. If the child spends a year in classes for students with learning disabilities, these problems are often largely resolved. Only rarely is IQ affected.

Kendall's biggest concern about the patient from Springfield was the child's legs. Though both did react slightly to pinpricks, no one had seen any spontaneous or voluntary movement in the leg that was not broken. This raised troublesome questions about the condition of the spinal cord and the brain stem. Though there was no evidence of broken vertebrae, a shearing injury inevitably affects the nerve tissue protected by these bones. When the head snaps back and forth, its pivot is the top of the spine. The upper spinal cord controls everything below it. When it is badly impaired, the result is full or partial paralysis.

Or the lack of movement in the child's legs could be explained by damage to the brain stem, the innermost structure of the brain, the part responsible for breathing and motor control. The boy was unable to gag. Loss of gag response could mean brain stem involvement, as could the involuntary posturing and the patient's respiratory difficulties. He had arrived at Springfield gasping for air. Either spinal cord or brain stem damage could land the child in a wheelchair for the rest of his life.

These were problems to be faced when the patient regained consciousness and the extent of his injury became clear. The immediate task confronting Colin Kendall was to ascertain the nature of the injury in order to begin appropriate treatment. The first step was to get a bolt into the child's skull, a stainless-steel monitoring device that would measure his intracranial pressure. The next step was to send the patient for a CAT scan. Most likely that study would rule out surgery. Kids rarely incur the kind of head trauma that can be fixed in the operating room.

Instead this boy would probably receive the kind of medical treatment that has become routine at Children's in such cases. It had been the experience of Colin Kendall and other experts in pediatric head trauma that some of the damage occurring to a child's central nervous system at the moment of impact is reversible so long as it is not compounded by the intracranial pressure that results primarily from the swelling brain. The goal of treatment is to minimize that secondary damage: to control the pressure, and meanwhile to support those critical functions that might have been knocked out temporarily at the time of the accident—breathing, for example—until the brain recovers enough to regain command.

In times past, physicians sought to control pressure by taking the top of the patient's head off. Doctors practicing in the 1980s accord space to swelling brain tissue by reducing the amount of blood flowing into that organ. This is accomplished mainly by hyperventilation. The patient is put on a respirator and forced to breathe more rapidly and deeply than usual and thus to exhale or "blow off" more carbon dioxide than is expelled in normal breathing. Getting rid of CO_2 causes the blood vessels in the brain to constrict, thereby slowing circulation into the head.

A few times a year, when a patient's intracranial pressure is too high to be controlled by the usual measures, doctors at Children's resort to extraordinary measures. They induce paralysis, administer large dosages of barbiturates, and lower the patient's body temperature, in effect putting the child into a state of hibernation. The idea is to slow down metabolism, to so decrease the brain's demands for oxygen that blood flow can be reduced to a minimum without disastrous effect. The "barb coma" is maintained for at least seventy-two hours, until the danger from pressure has passed.

This is the theory. In fact the results of the treatment have been mixed at Children's and elsewhere. The notion of subjecting children to such radical therapy remains controversial in pediatrics. Doctors who employ barb coma have reservations about it, and the suspense is exceedingly hard on parents. For three days or longer, the child looks dead. No one can promise that he or she will be normal upon waking.

Enough patients have awakened in good shape, however, for doctors at Children's to think it better to try barb coma in extreme cases than to let those children die, as would surely be their fate. The critical need whenever intracranial pressure threatens the brain is to ascertain as soon as possible whether the child needs barbiturates and, if so, to get them started as soon as possible. However, since inserting the bolt involves drilling into the skull, the neurosurgeons didn't want to go ahead with the procedure on the boy from Springfield until repeat spine films had confirmed that the child's neck was not broken.

"Okay," Kendall said to his senior resident, feeling the child's head for bony landmarks that would dictate placement of the bolt, "let's get a STAT x-ray of his neck." "STAT" means the study needs to be done in a hurry yet is not an emergency. Kendall had seen no evidence of a broken neck, but many physicians at Children's repeat all x-rays from other hospitals to be absolutely certain that nothing important is missed.

Chief surgical resident Jerry Solomon arrived in the unit. Upon learning of the neurosurgeons' plans, he promptly expressed opposition to them. An ex-football player who wore his hair clipped short as if the Navy still had hold of him, Solomon was against sending the patient for a CAT scan until the boy had been checked out by a urologist and an orthopod. Getting a scan would be no small undertaking. Children's lacked the equipment. The boy would have to be taken next door to the university hospital, pushed in and out of elevators and walked through tunnels for a trip amounting to more than a quarter of a mile. An anesthesiologist and a neurosurgeon would have to go along. They'd have to take drugs and equipment for any emergency. The patient would be at risk every step of the way.

If the boy went now, Solomon pointed out to Leith and the neurosurgeons, it was conceivable that he'd have to go back later for a second test. An x-ray accompanying the patient from the other hospital suggested that one kidney was out of commission. However, the film was of such poor quality that the urology residents felt it needed to be redone. If a repeat study confirmed kidney dysfunction on one side, the child would need an arteriogram to determine whether or not the problem lay in decreased blood supply. As Children's had no facilities for arteriography, that study, too, would have to be done next door. There was no point in sending the patient over twice. Furthermore, Solomon argued, the boy had an immobilized fracture. He shouldn't be moved until an orthopod had determined whether or not the immobilization was adequate.

This reasoning proved persuasive. Leith and the neurosurgeons agreed to wait for the other consults.

Solomon made two phone calls, then went to the bedside to change the nasogastric tube that had been inserted to drain the patient's stomach contents. He was assisted by Angie Bremness, a blond nurse in her mid-twenties who had been assigned as the boy's primary nurse on the three-to-eleven shift. Two other nurses had also been working steadily on the patient since his arrival, suctioning him, taking his vital signs, tending his lacerations, calculating his medications, and mixing intravenous fluids.

The crowd around the child had thinned down momentarily. Taking advantage, Stuart Leith asked the critical care fellow, an anesthesiologist training to be an intensive care specialist, to put in an arterial line: to thread a narrow tube into an artery through the patient's skin and tape it in place, giving the doctors ready access to blood samples without having to stick the child each time. It was by way of the A-line that the patient's carbon dioxide levels would be measured. The boy was already being hyperventilated on the assumption that pressure had begun to compromise the circulation in his brain.

An x-ray technician arrived pushing a portable machine. She

took the spine films and stood by to take the kidney films. Residents from Urology and Orthopedics arrived within seconds of one another. The urology resident injected a red substance into an intravenous line now taped into the patient's right wrist, a double dose of dye which would show up as contrast on x-ray and provide a good picture of the kidneys and ureter.

Leith began to feel that progress was being made. Hoisting himself onto a stool behind the nurses' station, he surveyed the scene in front of him and checked off in his mind the chores that still lay ahead. Assuming that the child didn't need brain surgery or barbiturates, the leg would probably be set later tonight or sometime tomorrow. Also later this evening, assuming the boy did not need head surgery, they'd get a couple more monitors into him, and there would be odds and ends to finish up that would keep Leith and several other people busy with the patient well into the night. Had anything been forgotten? Leith could think of nothing. Everything that should have been done for the patient had been done or arranged for or could wait till later.

The anesthesiologist looked at his watch. It was 6:15. The boy from Springfield had been in Acute a little over an hour. Leith felt the admission had gone rather smoothly.

Some minutes later the x-ray technician handed films to the urology resident and to Colin Kendall. The news was good. Both kidneys were functioning. The patient would not need an arteriogram and would require no further attention from Urology. As anticipated, the repeat x-rays of the child's spine showed no broken vertebrae.

"The neck looks perfectly stable to me," Kendall said, passing the films to Jerry Solomon and nodding at Nate Pontiac. "Let's get the bolt in."

At that moment Angie Bremness put her hand on Leith's arm. "Mom's here."

He gave the young woman his full attention. "Where?"

"Out in the hall. Somebody's with her. An uncle, I think."

Leith looked at Kendall. Without a word, the two physicians turned on their heels and walked toward the double doors leading into the hall.

Nate Pontiac stayed behind to perform the procedure. Angie Bremness stayed to help him. With a disposable razor, the neurosurgery resident began to shave hair from a spot on the patient's scalp directly above his right eye. Evening visitors were beginning to arrive in Acute. Wanting to spare them the sight of a doctor going at a child with a piece of equipment that looked as if it belonged in a basement workshop, the nurse drew the curtain around the bed, then placed a white paper drape over the patient's face and wrapped his head in a towel so that only the shaven spot remained uncovered. Nate Pontiac placed a drill bit against that bare skin and began to bore a hole into Frederick Eberly's skull.

As the surgeon worked, the child's head jostled and bumped. The nurse tried to hold it still. She had yet to mark a year at Children's. Her job there fulfilled a dream she had had almost as far back as she could remember. Her youngest brother had been born with a cleft lip and palate. Surgery performed at Children's had been so successful that Angie thought someone looking at her brother now would never know he'd had a defect. People at the hospital had been very good to her family. Angie had gone into pediatric nursing hoping she could help do for others what Children's had done for the Bremnesses.

Elsewhere in Acute, the overhead lights had been dimmed a little. From across the unit Angie could hear the dull clapping sound of a child being percussed. From nearer by came the singsong voice of a nurse who was sitting in a rocker and reading to a small patient on her lap. Looking down at her own patient, wondering what kind of person he had been until this morning, Angie Bremness was suddenly struck by the thought that in the city visible through windows on every side of the hospital, most children were home eating their suppers or playing with their Christmas toys.

Freddy's mother stood against a wall out of traffic. Her purse and coat hung over one arm. She was a tall woman, Sharita Queen, and slender to the point of boniness. A scarf covered her hair. Though plainly inexpensive, her outfit had been put together with attention to neatness and style. Her eyes took in nothing. She said nothing. She might as well have been alone. Beside her, likewise silent, was Freddy's uncle, the brother of his father, in khakis, a leather jacket, and a baseball cap. She had given her son his father's last name.

The news had ended her workday an hour after she'd begun it.

Her supervisor had called. The doctors at Springfield had told Freddy's mother he was critical but had said not to worry. Only when they'd told her they were transferring him to Children's Hospital had she begun to understand how badly hurt he really was. She waited now feeling like two people. One of those people insisted that Freddy was going to be all right. The other kept saying he was going to die.

The two doctors approached her and introduced themselves. As the chief of Anesthesiology had gone home, they took Sharita Queen into his empty office. Her friend came with her. Leith was glad of that. The uncle seemed solid, a rock, and the mother was plainly overwhelmed.

The doctors spoke straightforwardly. Kendall began by telling Freddy's mother he was fairly certain that her son would live, thereby introducing the idea that he might not. The doctors gave her their assessment. The boy had sustained a major brain injury. There was a good chance that his brain would recover well. This could take weeks or months. There was a chance he would be partially paralyzed. His spinal cord seemed all right, but his legs weren't moving, or were barely moving. No one could say at this point whether the child's speech would be affected. His belly seemed to have been taken care of properly. The doctors weren't particularly worried about him on that score.

However, they expected the next few days to be marked by trouble. He would need to be in the hospital six or eight weeks or longer. After that he would need rehabilitation—perhaps months of it.

It was obvious to Leith that Freddy Eberly's mother grasped the seriousness of what had happened to her son. Yet her response was quite passive, quite trusting. She shed no tears. They encouraged her to ask questions. She had no questions. All she said was that she wanted to stay with her son.

They urged her to do just the opposite. Go home and get some rest, they said. Come back after you've slept and stay as long as you want. All right, she said, she would do that instead.

They left her in the hall where they had found her. They were still working on the boy, they told her, but she could see him as soon as he arrived back in the unit after a CAT scan.

The top of the white paper drape covering the patient's face was now stained with blood. Protruding half an inch out of the bare spot on his head was a hollow column of stainless steel little thicker than a pencil. The bolt descended through bone into the layer of cerebrospinal fluid that forms the middle covering of the brain and spinal cord. As Leith and Kendall returned to the child's bedside, Pontiac and Bremness connected the device to a transducer which would provide a continuous readout of intracranial pressure on a small screen behind the bed. A figure of 15 or under would mean the ICP was normal.

Pontiac plugged in the transducer. Four pairs of eyes riveted themselves to the screen. The numbers came up in red: 14.8. Suspense went out of the atmosphere like air from the mouth of a balloon.

"It's low," Pontiac said, as if anyone needed telling. His announcement was sober, which was the way Nate Pontiac typically expressed himself.

But Leith grinned. "Dynamite!"

"Okay," Kendall said wearily but with evident relief, "let's get him next door."

As expected, the CAT scan showed no clot. There was no depressed fracture, either—no pushing in of cracked bone against the dura, something that could have happened when the child hit the pavement. For better or worse, the problems in Freddy Eberly's head could not be solved by surgery.

The pictures did show diffuse swelling, which was anticipated, and a tremendous amount of blood in the back of the brain, which was not. The child had bled so much that Pontiac wondered if perhaps the boy had had an aneurysm before the accident, a weakening in an artery wall that had then burst as a result of the car hitting him.

The amount of blood was of serious concern. Conceivably it could block normal drainage and cause acute hydrocephalus, a buildup of cerebrospinal fluid that could itself cause pressure problems. Hydrocephalus can be alleviated by a shunt implanted surgically to divert the fluid into the abdominal cavity where it can be absorbed. This is imperfect therapy at best. Shunts have a way of developing mechanical problems. Each repair involves another trip to the OR.

Even with hydrocephalus as a possibility, however, the CAT scan films did not essentially alter the boy's prognosis. Before the accident he had been in good health. A healthy body has restorative powers unavailable to patients weakened by chronic illness or malnutrition. The likeliest course was that the boy would improve gradually, be off the respirator and free of all his tubes within two weeks, and return home within two months.

He might, however, be unable to walk.

Freddy Eberly was gone from Acute for well over an hour. During that time his mother and his uncle waited in a small lounge down the hall from the unit. They spoke little. Sharita Queen had little to say even to God. She believed that Freddy's accident had been God's will, and there was nothing much she could say to God about a plan she did not yet understand.

She did ask Him for strength. She did tell God that if Freddy was to be taken from her, she was ready to do whatever she had to do to let him go. She also said His name. The minister had taught them to do this: just to say "Jesus" over and over and over again when they could think of no other words.

She had grown up in North Carolina in a large family. Her father had always said he'd be glad when his children were old enough to leave the nest. Choosing a city where she had relatives, Sharita had come north soon after finishing high school. At twenty-one she had found a job at Springfield Hospital. She had found her spiritual home in the Baptist church. She went on Saturdays, on Sundays, on Tuesdays for prayer meeting, on summer evenings when revivals were held, and on any evening when there was a musical program. Her faith was strong. She knew she could rely on it now.

Sharita Queen opened her purse and took out her Bible. Tomorrow night Freddy was to have read the Scripture aloud at church for the first time. The One Hundredth Psalm. All week she had been going over it with him to make sure he knew it, to make sure he had memorized what he had to say afterward: "May the Lord add a blessing to the reading of His word." Turning to Psalm One Hundred, she read it now to comfort herself:

Make a joyful noise unto the Lord, all ye lands.

Serve the Lord with gladness: come before his presence with
singing.

Know ye that the Lord he is God: it is he that hath made us, and
not we ourselves; we are his people, and the sheep of his
pasture.

Enter into his gates with thanksgiving, and into his courts with
praise: be thankful unto him, and bless his name.

For the Lord is good; his mercy is everlasting; and his truth
endureth to all generations.

It was past 9:30 before a nurse touched her shoulder.

Angie Bremness had done her best to clean the child up, washing the blood off his skin so he would be as easy as possible for his
mother to look at. About the tubes and monitors she could do nothing. In the hall outside the unit, the nurse tried her best to prepare
Freddy's mom and his uncle for what they were about to see.

Leith saw them come through the door. The mother moved as if
in a trance. Her gaze was fixed on the far wall of windows. Her
companion caught sight of his nephew and stopped midstride.

Angie pointed to a sink beneath the windows. The woman
walked toward it and washed her hands carefully. She dried them
carefully with a towel that the nurse had provided. Only then did
Sharita Queen turn to behold her son.

She walked toward him very slowly. Her arms were folded across
her chest. Her purse dangled from one arm. About a yard from the
bed, she stopped and began to take the child in. Her eyes traveled
over every inch of his body. They came to rest upon his face. She
stood looking at him for fully three minutes. Her own face never
changed. She did not try to touch him.

When she was ready, she turned from Freddy and walked un-
certainly toward his uncle. He took her arm. In silence the two left
the unit.

Friday, December 28

Brandon Gregory looked much better at morning rounds than he had looked on Monday. The blood transfusion that day, a nurse had remarked the next, had made his tiny body "pink as a rose," though he did still turn dusky with handling. Apparently because his feeds had been stopped for a day and then restarted very cautiously, his abdominal distension had now disappeared, as had his lethargy. He was receiving quarter-strength breast milk at 1 cc. per hour. So far he was tolerating it well.

But his morning chest x-ray looked much worse than yesterday's. The film showed a generalized haze over the baby's lungs, a nearly complete whiteout of the lung field. The likeliest explanation was that Brandon was now developing chronic lung disease, or "concrete lung."

Bronchopulmonary dysplasia: the Catch-22 of prematurity. Babies born with lungs too immature to function properly can survive only with help from respirators. But artificial ventilation destroys lung cells. The infant's body responds with a mighty effort to replace those cells, and that very attempt to heal lung tissue renders it so tough and noncompliant that now the baby needs help breathing as a result of being on a breathing machine.

Doctors can't say exactly when this process begins. For all practical purposes, however, any child who has been on a respirator more than two weeks without making great progress can be said to have developed BPD. Brandon Gregory now fell inescapably into this category. At two weeks and six days of age, he was not nearly ready to breathe on his own. Roger Forbes made the diagnosis with reluctance. While chances were good that Brandon would eventually be weaned from the ventilator, a baby with BPD could spend months in the Intermediate Unit and might even have to go home on a respirator.

The residents learned one more piece of bad news about Brandon at morning rounds. He had a severe abrasion on the cornea or transparent covering of his left eye, and the ulcer was infected. It had been discovered by an ophthalmologist Thursday afternoon during a routine examination.

The ophthalmologist had been surprised by his findings. Lesions of this kind are unusual in very tiny babies. The only possible cause is irritation or minor trauma. In this case, the doctor had surmised, if the baby had had his eyes taped closed for surgery, perhaps a bit of tape had come in direct contact with the cornea by mistake and, when removed, had pulled up a smidgen of tissue. Or perhaps the baby's lids were so weak that he couldn't close his eyes well, so corneal tissue dried out and was torn by the lids themselves. The infection was common staphylococcus.

The ophthalmologist had consulted an infectious disease expert. Together the two men had devised a plan of treatment that involved drops, ointments, IV antibiotics, and a drug called atropine to put the patient's eye at rest temporarily. The ulcer was cause for real concern. It could eat all the way through the cornea. The baby could lose the whole eye to infection.

The ophthalmologist had given this news to the patient's mother over the phone. Before their conversation Robin Gregory had been absolutely convinced, no matter what she had been told, that the doctors were going to have to amputate her son's bruised right arm. After talking with the ophthalmologist, she had replaced the receiver in despair. So what was Brandon going to look like when he could finally come home? Was he going to have any arms or legs or eyes left?

She had been unable to stop crying.

Ø

On Friday afternoon the Welfare Department social worker who would be evaluating Jody Robinson's case paid her first visit to the Intermediate ICU at Children's. The invitation had been issued by Children's social worker Lynn Story. Gladys Wexler was to come first to Story's office, a small room without windows off the main hallway on the fourth floor.

Waiting for her there, Story typed a memo. She was a slim, pretty woman of thirty, recently engaged, with long wavy brown hair full of natural light. As a youngster growing up in suburban Detroit, Story had dreamed of one day listing herself in the phone book as "friend." She had discovered the profession of social work in high school and had been at Children's for two and a half years.

Story felt slightly apprehensive about Wexler's visit. The last social worker to come to Children's on a similar mission had left Story with a bad taste in her mouth. That woman had been from a community agency arranging foster care for another patient in Intermediate. The worker hadn't managed to get to the hospital until the day she'd come to pick up the little girl. When she finally arrived, she had spent perhaps two minutes in the unit, had had lunch in the cafeteria, and then had retrieved the child and left.

Story was not without sympathy for that worker. She suspected that the woman had been overwhelmed by Intermediate and knew that what the hospital staff had wanted of her was no small thing. In essence, the worker had been asked to separate mother from child: to actually confront the mother and say, "Look, we're taking your kid, and these are the reasons." Story had never had to do that and was glad of it. But she might have wished for someone less aloof.

Despite her apprehension about Gladys Wexler, however, she felt very glad that some action was finally being taken in the Jody Robinson situation—even gladder today than yesterday. Story had arrived at work this morning to learn that the cousins had been in to visit Jody last night. They had brought his baby sister. Considering how punky he had felt all week, the nurses had been amazed at how responsive he'd been to Sabra II. The cousins had stayed a long time with him. They had asked more questions than ever before about the kind of care he might eventually need at home.

Naturally staff members close to Jody did not like to think of him as an abandoned child. It was nice for everybody to see that he had some family who cared about him. Yet while the cousins had indicated that they *might* one day be willing to take Jody, they certainly weren't clamoring for him. *Nobody* was saying he or she badly wanted him. In a way the cousins' visit had simply underscored the absence from the child's life of anyone he could truly depend on.

"Lynn?"

The woman who stood in the open doorway was short and rather heavy. Her hair appeared to have been dyed many times. She looked to be in her late forties. Story was just beginning to feel her heart sink when Gladys Wexler extended her hand. Her grip was firm.

"Why don't you come in and sit down, and we'll talk a little bit," Story suggested, "and then we'll go on in and see Jody." Before today they had discussed the child only briefly in a phone conversation that had gone something like this:

"Does he talk?"

"No, he . . ."

"Is he walking?"

"No."

The Welfare worker had commented to the effect that if Jody was neither walking nor talking at a year and a half, he must be in pretty bad shape. Story wanted Wexler to understand that in the context of all the problems he'd had, the child was doing beautifully.

Anticipating that the Welfare worker might have allotted no more than fifteen minutes for her visit to Children's, Story summed up Jody's social history as quickly as she could. She was at pains to emphasize to Gladys Wexler how awful Jody had looked in his first weeks of life, all bloody and bloated and full of tubes and stitches, and how overwhelming he must have seemed to his young mother. Even to the social worker he had looked gross. Story could understand in those days why Sabra would come in and peer at her baby in the Infant ICU through the hall window, then take off the moment someone from staff caught a glimpse of her.

Many if not all parents are frightened at the sight of a desperately sick infant, Story told Wexler. For most that fright begins to diminish as their contact with the baby increases. Sabra had seemed to grow not more comfortable but less. Perhaps her own life had been so overwhelming to her that she had been unable to deal with Jody's too. Perhaps she had been troubled by guilt, an issue that comes up for the most devoted mothers who have never touched drugs or alcohol or cigarettes during pregnancy.

Story talked a little about the cousins. Because Gladys Wexler seemed to be in no hurry, she then told of her own frustrations with regard to Jody Robinson. An essential question about his social status remained unanswered. Was he a placement problem or wasn't he? The child's family had never been fully in the picture or fully out of it. Story had never been able to say, "Yes, he's a placement problem," and then proceed to try to solve that problem. It was in this area that she was hoping for help from Welfare. Was Jody or was he not a candidate for foster care or adoption?

As the two women made their way to the unit, Story attempted to prepare Wexler as she would a parent, assuring her that it was very normal for someone entering the unit for the first time to feel overwhelmed. Intermediate was busier than usual. For some reason there was a tautness in the atmosphere that was more characteristic of Acute. Today more than other days the unit felt like a typical ICU. Yet the floor was littered as usual with its colorful clutter of stuffed animals and plastic trucks. Story could sense the woman beside her attempting to get her bearings.

They approached Jody's bed. He was sitting up, all dressed, helping Marla to comb his hair. He was still running a fever and looked as if he weren't feeling particularly well. Story made introductions. The patient responded solemnly, waiting for the stranger to make the first move. In response to a question from Wexler, the nurse began to detail her patient's medical status. Watching Marla, Story became aware that the Welfare worker wasn't saying anything and realized that Gladys Wexler had tears in her eyes.

All told the woman stayed an hour. She asked many questions. While the three stood talking at Jody's bedside, the child's coolness disappeared. Marla wound up his monkey for him. As he always did when the monkey began playing its cymbals, Jody clapped and hugged himself and flashed his million-dollar smile. Soon he was trying to imitate the monkey. Marla got him to show how he waved hello and goodbye and how he played peekaboo with a towel. He got silly and went through all his tricks. Story was delighted. The woman from Welfare had seen the child's personality under full sail.

As Gladys Wexler was leaving, she described her plan. First she would visit the cousins and sound them out about taking Jody to live with them when he was finally discharged. Then she would try to track down Sabra and attempt to ascertain whether or not she was likely ever to function as a mother for her son. The results of these inquiries would determine the worker's next step, a plan that seemed reasonable to Lynn Story. Though she had no doubt that Wexler would reach the same conclusion about Sabra that they'd all reached, insofar as her ability to parent was concerned, Story admired the woman for starting with an open mind about Jody's mother.

Story was pleased, and Marla was especially pleased, that Gladys Wexler seemed to consider the cousins the likeliest prospect. As Marla said after the Welfare worker had gone, if Jody were with the cousins, he'd have a home with caring people, his mother could still visit him, and the hospital staff wouldn't have to turn him over to somebody who'd take him off to Timbuktu.

Ø

When a patient in coma begins to recover consciousness, the first evidence, frequently, is the person's ability to open his or her eyes.

A person in a vegetative coma may also eye-open. But the sooner the event occurs after the patient has become comatose, the likelier it is that the eye opening represents the restoration of some brain function, and the better the prognosis.

Freddy Eberly opened his eyes about 8:00 P.M. Friday evening, just thirty-six hours after a car had knocked him senseless. Smoothing Vaseline onto his lips, Angie Bremness suddenly noticed his eyelids flicker and open halfway, then all the way, then blink, then shut again. The news was announced to every nurse within earshot. Moments later, telling Freddy's mom when she reappeared in the unit what a great sign this was, Angie was still grinning.

There were other good signs. The period of greatest concern about intracranial pressure is twenty-four to seventy-two hours post-injury, because this is when the brain is most swollen. Freddy's ICP readout remained low. His gag had returned to a limited extent. He gagged and coughed a little when suctioned. He continued to react to the pain of a sharp pinch.

At 10:00 P.M., when the orthopod on duty had discharged his more pressing responsibilities, Freddy Eberly was wheeled to the Operating Room where the surgeon finally set his broken right leg. The job was done with four stainless-steel pins driven into the bone through the patient's flesh and a compact stainless-steel device which was impaled upon the pins and locked in place with screws, thus fixing the broken ends of the bones in a position that would allow them to heal together most advantageously. The nurses were asked to clean the pin sites carefully at least three times a day.

Sunday, December 30

Dr. Alan Cavanaugh stood in Radiology and read Mark's morning chest x-ray in disbelief. The film showed a pneumothorax of twenty percent.

A small air cap had reappeared on Mark's x-ray the day after Christmas. But when the remaining chest tube had been reattached to an Emerson, the patient's lung had fully reexpanded. It had remained fully expanded through last evening. The cardiothoracic surgeons had been convinced, as of yesterday, that the lung was now stable. They had left the tube in over the last day or two only to allow maximum time for the surfaces irritated by tetracycline to heal together now that they were finally in direct contact with each other at every point.

But Mark's breath sounds had been somewhat decreased this morning, and now Cavanaugh saw why. Clearly the boy still had an active air leak. On December 1 he had had a pneumothorax of twenty-five percent. Today, nearly one full month later, he had a pneumothorax of twenty percent.

Cavanaugh wondered how best to break this news. The recurrence of the air cap on the twenty-sixth had sent Mark into a terrible slump. If anything his morale had gotten worse since then. Besides being depressed about the long hospitalization and the fact that he still had a chest tube in him, he was extremely anxious about having that last tube removed. "I'm scared my lung will just collapse again," he kept saying to Cavanaugh and the nurses.

He had begun complaining of abdominal pain which he himself attributed to anxiety. He had begun to vomit several times a day. Whether the anxiety was causing the vomiting no one was sure. On Thursday he had asked if he could have something to relax him. The doctors had started him on Valium. The vomiting and depression had persisted. Though he could rally for guests or enjoy a game with the nurses, most of the time he sat hunched over in bed reading nothing, doing nothing, saying nothing.

Sipping coffee, the resident examined his patient's chest film more closely. Mark's lung disease was getting worse. Cavanaugh had been on Adolescent only thirteen days, but even in that time the shadows on x-ray had intensified and spread, indicating spaces being blocked by mucus that should have contained air. Part of the problem was that because his percussion had been stopped after the pneumothorax, and because the chest tubes had made it painful for Mark to cough up mucus, he simply had been unable to clear his lungs very well. He was now getting percussion on the right side and vibration on the left, which would help. Meantime he was still losing weight. His vomiting this week was only adding to a nutritional problem that was already severe. Even if the chest tube problem got solved, Cavanaugh thought, not much would have been gained for this youngster.

He finished his coffee rehearsing what he would say to Mark. Even in his imagination Cavanaugh had trouble meeting the boy's eyes.

Dr. Drew Cipriani came up to Adolescent and irrigated Mark's fourth chest tube for the third time. Another x-ray was taken and showed no improvement. Cipriani told the patient and his mother that the boy might need a fifth chest tube.

In tears, Ellen Price called Daniel Earnshaw at home. She told him she did not want Mark to have another chest tube. He calmed her down, finally, with a question that had only one answer she could live with. Did she intend to make this decision by herself, without consulting Mark?

Of course she didn't. If a decision had to be made, it would be Mark's to make, and there was no doubt in his mother's mind what that decision would be.

Dr. Cipriani thought the fourth chest tube might have slipped so that the tip was no longer in the apex of Mark's chest cavity. If this indeed had happened, another tube was all but inevitable.

First, however, the boy's physicians wanted to make certain that all other possible remedies had been investigated and exhausted. With this in mind, Drew Cipriani proposed to Alan Cavanaugh that he vacuum the fourth chest tube. Basically, this procedure involves hooking up to an Emerson a tube narrower and stiffer than a chest tube and threading it into the chest tube with the suction running.

Theoretically any mucus encountered is either vacuumed out through the narrower tube or pushed into the chest cavity. Vacuuming is considered unorthodox because introducing anything into a chest tube risks infection and because technically it shouldn't work. One tube doesn't necessarily slide smoothly through another.

However, the CT surgeons caring for Mark had tried this approach with some success in the intensive care units; and since the alternative in this case was a bigger procedure, more pain, and more suffering, the risk of infection seemed worth taking. At Cavanaugh's urging, Cipriani went ahead. An x-ray done afterward showed some improvement in the pneumothorax but not as much as had been hoped. Cipriani said he'd watch the lung for twenty-four hours and decide about a fifth chest tube in the morning.

At the nurses' station soon afterward, Cavanaugh fell into conversation with Julie Wixted, the nurse who had been with Mark the night of the tetracycline treatment. The two quickly realized that insofar as this patient was concerned, they were thinking along the same lines. Both had begun to wonder where medicine would take the boy from here.

Throughout Mark's hospitalization this time, everybody involved with him had been working to get his lung up and get him home. Was that still a realistic goal? Several people including the patient's mother were speculating that this might be Mark's last admission. So far as the nurses and residents had observed, Dr. Earnshaw was definitely not treating it that way. But the pneumothorax was by no means resolved, and the boy was very sick. If his doctor was optimistic, on what was he basing his optimism? Should Alan Cavanaugh and the nurses who spent the most time with Mark continue to encourage his hopes?

It seemed to the resident and Julie Wixted that a plan was needed—not just a day-to-day plan based on the morning chest x-ray but an overall plan based on the patient's progress or lack thereof. A multiservice conference was needed—a formal meeting at which questions could be asked and answered, at which everyone involved in Mark's care could formulate a plan together.

Cavanaugh offered to write a request for such a conference into Mark's chart where Daniel Earnshaw would be sure to see it. The

nurse offered to ask social worker Dick Jacoby to make the arrangements, a time-consuming task given the number of people close to
the case and the demands of their schedules.

Ellen flushed the contents of Mark's bedpan down the toilet and
was washing the pan when she heard him call to her from his bed.

"Mom!" Impatiently: "Mother!"

She put her head out the bathroom door to see him glowering at
her. "Don't do that! I don't want you to clean the bedpan. The
nurses are paid to do that."

Amazed, Ellen replied, "It's half done, Mark."

"It's not your job."

"All right," she said finally. "I'll finish this, but I won't do it
again."

He did not respond.

In part she charged herself for his depression. She had spent so
much time in the hospital before Christmas, and since Mark had
been so happy on Christmas Day, she had not come back to visit
him the day after, the day the air pocket had shown up again. He
had taken that blow alone.

She knew, too, that he was very disappointed over Dr. Earnshaw's refusal to consider transferring him to a hospital nearer
home. When Mark had made this suggestion on Christmas Eve,
Ellen had not really taken him seriously. She herself would not trust
anyone else to take care of Mark. But because he had insisted, she
had asked Dr. Earnshaw, and he had said he would not let Mark go
to another hospital as long as he had a chest tube in him.

Then the news today about the possibility of yet another chest
tube . . .

When she returned to Mark's bedside, he was leaning back
against the cranked-up mattress with his eyes closed and his face
turned away from her. She sank into the padded armchair and
closed her own eyes. She was almost asleep when she heard him say
something she didn't catch. Standing, she bent close to him. "I'm
sorry, honey, I didn't hear you."

He opened his eyes and looked straight at her. "Roll my bed
down."

She cranked the mattress down several notches. "How's that?"

"All the way down."

"What?"

"All the way down, I said."

She told herself that he wouldn't try to commit suicide with her right next to him. She remembered that he had pronounced himself willing to have another chest tube if he had to.

Watching him closely for signs of distress, she cranked his mattress down flat.

He offered no explanation. She returned in silence to her chair.

He lay silent a long time, breathing as always with difficulty. But as she herself was succumbing to sleep, he spoke again, again inaudibly.

"What did you say?"

"I wasn't talking to you. Just leave me alone."

Minutes passed, and then he said, quite clearly, "God lies."

This time Ellen Price did not respond to her son. Instead she sat staring at the Bible on his bedside table, refraining only because it was his, and only because it meant so much to him, from picking up that holy book and dashing it into the wastebasket.

His nurse on the three-to-eleven shift was Jacquie Harper. She was twenty-two and black, a June graduate of a college nursing program, tall and coordinated enough to have played basketball in high school. Off and on for several days the person assigned to Mark on evenings had been the only nurse on the floor he did not like. Since Jacquie worked permanent evenings, Ellen had asked her if she would be willing to take Mark whenever she was in so he would not have to deal with someone who bugged him.

Jacquie had said yes without even hinting that she had been avoiding Mark ever since she'd met him, because of his prognosis. Jacquie Harper had not yet come to terms with death. After three years, she was still finding the death of her great-grandmother very difficult to accept.

In her previous job Jacquie had taken care of a few oncology patients, but never when a patient was in the end stage of the disease. Except when the floor was very short-staffed, her wishes were likewise respected at Children's. She had taken care of Mark a few times, but not consistently. The fact that his favorite nurses had always fought to get him had kept the pressure off her.

But she liked Mark and knew he liked her. She could not bear to think of a child so sick being cared for by someone he didn't like. She felt honored that Mark wanted her and that Mrs. Price thought her a good enough nurse to take care of her son. So Jacquie had said yes despite her apprehensions and with a sincere but limited commitment. She knew that Mark was not expected to die on this admission. She knew that when he got worse, she could ask not to be assigned to him.

New Year's Eve

In the Children's Purchasing Department one floor below the lobby, employees reported for work as usual and then gathered in the storeroom to inventory what remained there at year's end of the items with which the Department keeps the hospital supplied— some 2,400 kinds of items in all, including lab equipment and everything else required for patient care except drugs. Those are stocked by pharmacists.

One does not look around the Children's storeroom and imagine oneself in a hospital for adults. "Ever since God invented them," according to one purchasing expert, Pampers have occupied a substantial amount of this institution's available storage space. The throwaway diapers come in five sizes, and the hospital goes through some thirty tons of them a year. Pacifiers take much less space but are bought at an average rate of more than six hundred a month. Though plain Band-Aids are used routinely at Children's, a good supply of adhesive bandages printed with Snoopy and Strawberry Shortcake is kept on hand to reward youngsters having blood drawn.

These items aside, however, the storeroom shelves at Children's are filled with articles that would be standard in any hospital, albeit many are stocked in small sizes. Chief among these are feeding tubes and suction catheters. In the past a number of the articles used at Children's had to be specially made by manufacturers in business to service adult hospitals. There are still only a few suppliers of small pajamas for hospital patients. For some reason those companies that do sell them all seem to favor shades of blue.

One shelf in the Children's storeroom is stacked neatly with cartons of Saran Wrap. It's bought "by the mile," according to a Purchasing employee. Most of the stuff is used in the wrapping of wounds. But boxes of it are sent regularly up to the Infant ICU where it is made into "blankets" for babies such as Brandon Gregory.

Ø

Making morning rounds in Acute, neurosurgical resident Nate Pontiac approached Freddy Eberly's bedside and pinched a bit of skin on Freddy's chest. So immediately did the child's eyes fly open and his limbs lift off the mattress that Pontiac was a little startled. Even the pinned leg moved slightly.

"Hey, that's not so bad!"

An anesthesiology resident who had come up beside him agreed. "Not bad at all!"

Pontiac was also encouraged by the possibility that the patient might come off the respirator sooner than expected—maybe even today. The doctors had begun to back off on his therapy this morning, decreasing the hyperventilation and letting the boy's carbon dioxide level begin to normalize. Freddy's intracranial pressure had remained low.

At the same time, Pontiac and Colin Kendall were both concerned that perhaps the boy might have more damage to his brain than had originally been apparent. Four days after his accident, he still had very little cough and not much gag. While he appeared to be making some purposeful movements with his right arm, he'd had no spontaneous or voluntary movement of his legs.

He was not obeying commands, at least not consistently enough to convince the neurosurgeons that his responses were intentional. Ability to obey commands means that the brain has resumed functioning as an integrated entity. The hemispheres eventually recover from reversible damage, as does the brain stem. But the two must hook up. When that connection gets made, the patient is able to translate signals into action and takes the giant step up from being vegetative to being conscious.

This had not yet happened to Freddy Eberly. A somewhat surprising development, given that he had started to eye-open so early. In an effort to figure out what was going on with the boy, the neurosurgeons had decided to schedule another CAT scan.

At 1:00 P.M. Freddy was taken off the respirator. Within moments he had to be put right back on again. In the rather odd terms of hospital jargon, he had "flunked extubation." Though apparently able to breathe on his own, meaning that the respiratory centers of his brain stem were functional, he couldn't keep his airway open. His tongue kept falling back and obstructing his trachea. Why this occurred the doctors were not certain, but the message was plain. The child could not breathe unassisted.

Ø

For Mark the day had brought somewhat better news. His morning chest x-ray had shown a reduction in his pneumothorax from fifteen percent to between five and ten percent. He would not need a fifth chest tube, at least not today.

Nevertheless, he had remained depressed. He had eaten little breakfast and no lunch, had vomited once—from nerves, he'd said—and had asked for Valium twice. Shortly before lunch, out of the blue, he had asked his mother to cut his hair with a bandage scissors.

"I don't want to fool around with it," he had told her. "Just hack it off." The term had saddened her. Until this admission, he had been so fastidious about his grooming.

At 2:00 Bob arrived. While Randy and Denise stayed with friends, he and Ellen would be celebrating New Year's Eve with Mark. Bob had packed his pajamas. To make the occasion as festive as possible, he had also brought in herring and other goodies they all liked and had smuggled in a can of beer apiece. But the Prices were spending one more holiday in the hospital, and they were all in odd moods—all making an effort, yet all slightly out of sorts.

About 3:00 Ellen left to take a walk in the halls and returned with news. "Lisa's back," she announced to her husband and her son, referring to a youngster just Mark's age who also had CF.

They were reading sections of the newspaper Bob had brought. Ellen was gratified when Mark expressed interest. "How is she?"

"She's not feeling very well at the moment," Ellen replied, "but she asked about you and said she'd be in to see you as soon as the antibiotics start working. Honestly, that girl has the face of an angel. She gave me a great big hug and a kiss." Ellen had been surprised at the strength of a child who looked so frail and white.

Bob closed the sports section and tossed it onto Mark's bed. "I forgot to ask," he said, reaching for another. "Is Janet still here?"

"No, Janet went home a few days ago," his wife replied.

"How was she when she left?"

Catching his eye, Ellen gave him a silent warning. The nurses were expecting Janet to go anytime. "Better, I think," she said truthfully.

When Clara Bowman arrived to give Mark a breathing treatment, he responded to her greeting without looking up. She marched to his bedside, hands on hips.

"What's all this?" Her voice was sharp enough to startle him. "If you're going to be my husband, you'd better talk to me! Don't you hold your head down reading no paper when I come up here to see you!"

He laughed.

Ellen hadn't heard him laugh since Christmas.

He was better after Clara left, brooding less, talking more. When he and Bob resumed their reading, the atmosphere in the room had lightened.

Ellen sat down, picked up the front section of the paper, and placed it on the bottom of Mark's bed. With an elbow on the edge of the mattress, she began to scan the page.

After some minutes she became aware that Mark was looking at her.

"Anything wrong?"

"No, not really . . ." He glanced away, then back at her. "Mom?"

"What is it, Mark?"

"Mom, you know I can't get up to go to the bathroom now. I have to use a bedpan right here in the room. Everybody's in and out of here all the time—nurses, doctors, technicians, students—I don't know . . . everybody. I have no privacy left. The only thing I have here, the only thing that's mine, is my bed."

Lifting her elbow, she grinned at him. "Mark, are you trying to tell me to get off your bed?"

"Would you please? It's all I have left."

"I understand completely." She drew the newspaper into her lap.

"And would you please not let anybody else . . ."

"Of course."

"Thank you."

"Oh, Mark. You're very welcome."

On his way home about 5:00, the recreation therapist stopped by with a package of two chocolate cupcakes for Mark. When Jacquie Harper came in, Mark asked her if she could get him another Coke.

She frowned. "Not when you put it like that I can't."

Her sternness made him smile. "I mean could you *please* get me another Coke."

"Now that I can do," Jacquie said, smiling back, "and I'd be glad to."

When she had gone, Mark opened his cupcakes and lectured his parents. "You know, you guys are so worried about me that you're letting me get away with stuff you never let me get away with before. Like you always made me eat my wholesome food before I could eat junk food. Now you're just happy to see me eat any old crap. That's not good. Even though I'm sick, you've got to keep me in line. You shouldn't be lenient with me. Even though I am sick, I don't want to turn rotten and spoiled."

Fifteen years with Mark had taught Ellen to expect almost anything to come out of him at any time.

"Well, Mark," she said approvingly, "I think you've made a very good point. How about wrapping those cupcakes up again and having them later. It's almost suppertime."

"You can be real cooperative, Mom."

"I try!"

Over the dinner hour, the evening fell apart.

Bob would be hard-pressed later to figure out exactly what had gone wrong. The trouble had come up almost out of nowhere, like a summer thunderstorm. Suddenly Ellen was angry at Bob, he was angry at her, and Mark was arguing with both of them. Minutes into the argument Ellen got her things together, took out her car keys, kissed Mark goodbye, and went home.

Her husband had no trouble understanding why. He had

learned that even in a happy marriage an argument can occur on perfectly pleasant days when things are going right in every direction. He and Ellen hadn't had such a day in a long time.

He called her when she got home. The storm had blown over for her as well.

But as it was far too late for her to drive back to the city, Bob and Mark saw in the new year together without her. They played cards, watched television, listened to the new radio, had herring and crackers and cheese and beer. Toward the end of the three-to-eleven shift, the nurses set out a small buffet in the playroom and invited parents and patients to help themselves. Since Mark was too weak to get up, Bob brought several sandwiches back to the room.

Just before 12:00, Jacquie and several other nurses came in to watch the Times Square festivities on Mark's TV set. They teased him about his beer, making him laugh. As the announcer counted backward—"twelve seconds . . . eleven seconds . . . ten seconds . . . nine seconds . . ."—the nurses passed out noisemakers. At precisely the instant midnight was announced, Mark and Bob set their watches to the same second so they'd be running on exactly the same time in the new year—Mark's idea—and then the youngster was inundated with nurses kissing him and wishing him well.

New Year's Day

Yesterday Jody Robinson's temperature had gone up to 105 degrees, the highest Marla Meyerle had ever known it to go. This morning lab reports showed for the first time in the nearly two weeks he'd been feverish that Jody had the pseudomonas bacterial infection so common to the children of Intermediate. He was put on antibiotics.

Marla was relieved that the problem was no worse. She'd been concerned about Jody. On the good side he had managed to be sick without exhibiting any need for increased support from the respirator. But he hadn't been his happy self recently: not as energetic, not as active. He'd been sleeping a lot. When she'd wake him, he'd be friendly but unresponsive. She'd find diarrhea in every diaper. Because of the loose stools, he was getting clear fluids instead of his usual formula, which had slowed his weight gain. The secretions coming out onto the gauze pads covering Jody's esophagostomy had continued to be heavier than usual.

He'd been refusing his green cup again. Instead of drinking the water, he'd dip his fingers in it, paddling, stalling. Marla had been worrying that he was regressing. She had mentioned the problem to the speech therapist, who'd urged her to try Jody on a little yogurt or applesauce for a change. But when she'd tried to get some yogurt down on Sunday, he'd gagged and gagged. Though he'd taken it himself when she'd offered it, though he'd obviously been interested, he hadn't been able to handle it. For some reason the thicker stuff couldn't pass through Jody's esophagus without causing him distress.

Marla was also concerned about his continuing tendency to turn blue for reasons no one had yet figured out. She wondered if he could be aspirating. Technically there should have been no way for the secretions in his esophagus to enter his windpipe if all the repairs had been as successful as the ENT specialist had observed them to be during Jody's most recent bronchoscopy. But secretions were always pooling around the trach tube in the child's throat. Maybe the tube was looser now that Jody had grown, the nurse surmised, and maybe secretions were getting in around it. Marla had started urging the doctors to insert a bigger tube. She was also pushing them to dilate his esophagostomy more frequently. It didn't have to be done in the operating room. She felt bad for Jody that he kept gagging and turning blue, and it certainly wasn't good for him.

Marla herself was recovering from disappointment. She'd been told on Monday that the assistant head nurse position in the operating room had gone to someone else.

Actually, aside from the blow to her ego, Jody's nurse had begun to feel relieved. In the past couple of weeks, several incidents had crystallized in Marla a desire to one day teach nursing. In preparation she would need certain professional experience which the job in the OR could not have provided. She had been too eager for change to realize that before. Marla knew now that she had to look not just for a different experience but for the *right* one.

Ø

Next door in Acute, Sharita Queen drew her chair close to her son's bedside and said softly, "It's Mama, Freddy. Your Mama's here. It's New Year's. Happy New Year."

He slumbered on. His tongue protruded half an inch through open lips. He was drooling. Taking a tissue from her purse, his mother dabbed his chin, his neck, the corners of his mouth.

Elsewhere in the unit dietary aides collected lunch trays. In one corner a child was crying for her mother. In another the general surgery residents conducted rounds at the bedside of an open-heart patient. At the bed next to Freddy's the father of a two-year-old who last night had swallowed half a bottle of vitamins stood rubbing his son's back. Nearby a mother and grandmother who both looked upset talked in low tones with two of the nurses. Perhaps because of the holiday the music coming from the radio behind the nurses' station was louder than usual.

Sharita Queen took her son's hand. It felt limp in her own. She sat caressing it and studying his face. Never had she dreamed that an accident could change him so completely.

She was beginning to realize that he was not dead. She was beginning to understand that he could not recover right away from the kind of accident he had had. She was beginning to believe the nurses and doctors when they told her that he was progressing.

Still, at home when the phone rang, she jumped.

She could eat nothing sweet. Since Freddy had been hurt, even the thought of cake or pie or ice cream had made her sick. Likewise bacon and eggs.

"Mama's going to read to you, Freddy, okay? I brought along some of the books you like."

Beside her on the floor she had dropped a big denim bag. She rummaged in it and chose a book. Ever since he had learned how, Freddy had always liked to read to her. Now she would have to . . .

The doctor had suggested that she make a tape for Freddy to listen to when she wasn't there. "Put his favorite music on it," the doctor had said. "Record his friends." Sharita Queen had mixed feelings about this idea. Freddy did not care about being around a whole lot of people. As an only child whose mother worked, he was used to spending time alone. So long as he had something to eat and something to play with, he was satisfied. He was not a miserable child. He knew how to make himself happy.

She opened the book and began to read to her son. At home when she read to him, he'd fall right asleep. Now she was reading because the nurses had said the stories might help wake him up.

Sharita Queen was an enigma to the nurses in Acute. They were accustomed to parents who plied them with questions and leaned heavily on them for emotional support. Freddy's mom did neither. She came in and sat quietly by her son's bedside, and after a while she left.

Yet it was obvious to the nurses that she was trying to do the right thing. Though she seemed shy about talking to him, which they urged her to do, she read to him willingly. She listened carefully when the nurses explained to her about the tubes. She had gone back to work on Monday after staying at the hospital the entire weekend but had called twice during the day, had come back to see him last night, was in again this morning. She had no car. Getting to Children's from Springfield Hospital, where she worked, took her an hour on two buses and a subway; getting home took her another hour and a half.

So the nurses knew that she cared about her son very much. They also knew that she must be terribly frightened if not overwhelmed. But because she betrayed no fear, she gave them the impression that she needed nothing from them beyond a daily update, leaving them to guess how best to help someone who was not seeking their help. They surmised that Mrs. Queen must be getting what support she needed from other sources. A Children's social worker who had talked to Freddy's mother the day after his admission had been quite impressed by the strength of her faith in God and in the power of prayer. Such composure had the woman exhibited, in fact, that the social worker had left Sharita Queen her office phone number fully expecting that her own role in the case henceforth would be minor.

In essence the nurses in Acute had drawn the same conclusion. They made it as clear as they could to Freddy's mother that they were available. They assured her that they would be glad to answer any questions or see to it that those questions got answered by somebody else. They supported Sharita Queen by according her the privacy she seemed to prefer and by looking out for her smaller comforts. For example, when Freddy's mom came into Acute to be with her son, his nurse always made sure that she had a chair.

Wednesday, January 2

Making rounds at dawn, Daniel Earnshaw stopped at the Adolescent nurses' station and scanned the notes entered in Mark's chart over the past forty-eight hours. He noted with relief that Tuesday's chest x-ray had shown no change from Monday's. The pneumothorax had remained stable with an air cap of five to ten percent.

However, according to the chart, Mark's lips and nail beds were cyanotic. He had eaten little in two days except for a couple of meals from McDonald's and one special milkshake. He was complaining of chest pain ascribed by a resident to irritation from hard coughing. He was still uncomfortable enough to be getting codeine and Tylenol once per shift. He was anxious and upset enough to have requested Valium at 3:00 this morning, telling the nurse, "I'm so nervous today that I can't get back to sleep."

The patient was sitting on his mattress bent into a circle. His breathing was more labored than usual. There was a purplish cast to his lips. He did not look up when Earnshaw approached the foot of his bed, and his greeting was a single word. In the slump of Mark's shoulders, the doctor recognized a fundamental fatigue. As little confidence as he felt in such situations, Earnshaw knew he must at least try to get through to the boy.

"You're looking very discouraged this morning," he observed gently. "Very sad."

Mark rolled and unrolled the hem of his pajama trouser against his calf. Puberty had put hair on his legs, but he was so small and thin that it looked out of place. He had lost nearly a sixth of his weight since the pneumothorax. He was down to fifty-four pounds.

"Do you want to tell me about it?"

At first the patient shook his head. Finally he said, "God lied."

"What did God lie about, Mark?"

"The surgeons lied too. And I don't think *you* know what's happening." Suddenly the boy was weeping into his hands. "I don't
think ... I can ... medically ... take another chest tube!" He
dropped his hands and drew back his pajama trousers. "Just look at
me! I'm all skin and bones."

Earnshaw sat down beside him on the bed. Passing Mark tissues
and his sputum pan, he laid his free hand over the patient's nearest
foot.

"Mark," he said softly, urgently, "I can't help but feel that you're
looking only at the negative side of all this. You're not focusing on
the fact that we've gone from four chest tubes to one chest tube,
from a lung that was twenty-five percent down to a lung that's only
five to ten percent down. We've made progress here. There really is
a possibility that your lung will stay up this time."

Nothing in the boy's eyes suggested that Mark believed this.

"I know you're skeptical, and I know you have reason to be,"
Earnshaw went on carefully. "But it's possible that we're continuing
to get air in the apex because the tetracycline hasn't had a chance to
work in that part of the chest cavity. Remember, the top part of the
lung didn't fully reexpand against the chest wall until after the
fourth tube went in. Those surfaces may not have been in contact
long enough to scar together."

"I know that already," Mark said dully.

"Well, what I wanted to say," Earnshaw continued, "was that the
tetracycline may have worked everywhere else. It's possible that the
lung *can't* collapse any more than a certain amount now. We could
reasonably assume this if the size of the air cap remains stable. If it
does, we may just decide that a five to ten percent air cap is the best
we can do and take the last chest tube out without waiting for full
reexpansion."

"What about the air that would still be in my chest cavity?"

"It would eventually be absorbed into the surrounding tissues.
The air itself is no real problem as long as we're sure the lung is
stable."

Mark said, barely audibly, "Sometimes I think I'm never going to
get out of here."

Racking his brain for a different approach, the physician remembered Norman Cousins's book *The Anatomy of an Illness* about
the author's own battle with disease. Cousins's conviction that the

patient makes an important contribution to his own treatment had impressed Earnshaw. He drew, now, on this idea.

"Mark, you've been pressing all of us to do things that will help you get better, and we've been trying to do that. But there is only so much we as doctors can do. For you to get better, we're going to need your help. There are certain things only you can do that you're not doing. For example, you've refused to do anything about that atrocious diet of yours.

"We can't make you look at things in a more positive light," the doctor continued. "You're the only one who can do that. You're going to have to say to yourself, 'Stop thinking of the negative side. Think of the positive side.' Maybe it would help you if you made a list for yourself of the things that are negative and the things that are positive. Write down how much you believe of this, how much you believe of that. Try to make some objective evaluation of what's happening."

No response. None whatever.

Earnshaw began pulling thoughts out of the air. "I interpret your sadness as a feeling that the situation is sort of hopeless. That's not true. We're not ready to give up. We haven't done everything we can do yet; there are still things we can try. . . ."

"Like what?" The boy was looking him straight in the eye.

Earnshaw went into detail about various combinations of antibiotics that could be used against the lung infection. Then he mentioned hyperalimentation, describing it as a high-calorie dietary supplement that to hospital patients is usually given intravenously. Actually Alan Cavanaugh had recently suggested this for Mark, an idea Earnshaw had discouraged. Hyperal therapy doesn't begin to show results for at least two weeks. Earnshaw was not eager to keep Mark in the hospital for two additional weeks if he could avoid it.

Furthermore, there are risks involved, including the risk of pneumothorax. With a patient as debilitated as Mark Price, the substance must usually be infused directly into a large vein leading to the heart. The surgeon placing the conduit catheter could conceivably miss the vein and puncture the lung lying right beside it. So in suggesting IV nutrition to Mark, Daniel Earnshaw did so with no serious thought of actually proceeding with it, certainly not during this hospitalization. He was trying to make a different point: that the doctors still had tricks in their bags.

But Mark showed far more interest in hyperal than in anything else the doctor had found to say to him. He plied Earnshaw with questions, and Earnshaw, somewhat startled, briefly laid out the pros and cons, glad for the upturn in the conversation and the spark of life in the patient, glad to be able to leave the boy in a more positive frame of mind.

In the hall he wondered if he should have tried to do more. "I know you're worried about dying, Mark," he could have said. "Why don't you talk to me about it?" Partly what stopped him was never really knowing when a cystic patient was going to die. In particular Patsy Loring stopped him. At ten, Patsy had gotten so sick during one admission that she'd appeared to be on her way out. Pushed by staff opinion that the child needed help confronting this truth, Earnshaw somehow had managed to go to Patsy himself and to raise and discuss with her the matter of her dying. Since that conversation two years had passed. Patsy had not been back in more than a year!

At the nurses' station Earnshaw pulled Mark's chart and found a chair, remembering the nurse who had finally come to him about Perry Smith. "It's unfair not to tell Perry he's going to die," the nurse had said to him. "Maybe he's got goodbyes he wants to say. Maybe there are things he wants to set right." Strange as it seemed to him now, Earnshaw had never thought in such terms before. He'd felt the nurse had made an excellent point.

Yet he had never acted on her suggestion. So eager had he been to keep Perry fighting that Earnshaw hadn't had it in him to say to the boy, in essence, "You haven't got a chance."

Opening the chart he held in his hands, the doctor took a pen from the breast pocket of his lab coat and wrote:

The biggest problem today is Mark's depression. He is very discouraged. This seems quite reasonable to me. The repeated insertions of chest tubes, the up-and-down optimism and discouragement accompanying the ups and downs of his pneumothorax, the prolonged hospitalization, and his severe pain are the realities which lead to worry and anxiety. Now he can see only the negatives in the picture. I am trying to help him toward better balance of the positives as well as the negatives.

Mark is basically a very strong character who has coped successfully with many difficult situations. With our help he will not give up on this one.

Soon after Jacquie Harper reported for duty at 3:00, she went into Mark's room to say hello and noticed that the fluid in his Pleurevac was no longer bubbling.

She called Alan Cavanaugh, who in turn called Dr. Cipriani, who came up and confirmed for the others what Cavanaugh had already guessed—that Mark's last chest tube had stopped functioning. There were no bubbles in the Pleur-evac because no air was coming out of the chest tube.

The CT resident made the decision to do nothing. He wanted to see whether the lung would stay up by itself without a functioning chest tube. He told Mark that if his breathing got no worse, the tube would be clamped after a while, and if the lung remained stable, the last chest tube would be pulled.

For an hour after Cipriani had gone, Mark paid very close attention to his breathing. But it proved no worse than usual.

He sat now playing solitaire trying hard not to get his hopes up. He had hit upon a plan that he thought might solve several problems at once, not just for himself but also for his family.

He knew that if the doctors got his tube out and his lung stayed up, he could be discharged. He also knew that he would be going home in terrible shape, much thinner than he had been upon admission, weaker than he had ever been in his life. If instead he stayed in the hospital and got hyperalimentation, the extra nourishment would make him stronger and better able to fight his disease. The extra weight would make him look better and feel better. The hyperal would be good for him—especially if he could get it at a hospital closer to home. Dr. Earnshaw had said he couldn't go to another hospital as long as he had the chest tube in. But what if they got the chest tube out?

"Here you go, Marcus," Jacquie said, coming in with the codeine and Tylenol he'd asked her for.

"Are you going to come back later and play Concentration with me?" Ever since he had taught her the game the kids from his woodshop had sent him, they had played it every evening she was on. So far the nurse had won every game.

"Sure. Soon as I get my other patients squared away." She turned to go.

"Could you get me some more Coke, Jacquie?"

She kept walking. "Nope."

He groaned. "Jacquie, could you *please* get me some more Coke?"

From the doorway she gave him a dazzling smile. "Of course!"

He fixed his eyes on something well above her head. "And could you please get that spider off my ceiling?"

She looked hard where he was pointing and was suddenly frightened. Was the boy hallucinating?

She was halfway to him when he burst out laughing. The intensity of her relief told her she was in much deeper than she had realized. When she spoke, it was in anger. "Mark, don't you ever do that again!"

Thursday, January 3

Freddy Eberly's second CAT scan was done at 2:00 P.M. The films yielded some good news. With his accident exactly one week behind him, the patient's brain was beginning to heal without complications.

However, the repeat scan revealed much more diffuse swelling than the first had shown. The injury had been worse than the neurosurgeons had originally thought. While the doctors remained optimistic that Freddy would make a good recovery, Colin Kendall read the scan results feeling less optimistic than he had, particularly about the return of full intellectual function.

Friday, January 4

10:15 A.M. Somewhere in the back of the Oncology Clinic, an infant was crying in fright and fury at the top of its lungs. The sound fell over the waiting room like a chill. Gina DeRose and her mother entered Clinic with sober faces, and not only because the baby's cries had accompanied them all the way down the hall. Gina had just vomited in the parking lot.

Though pale, she was matter-of-fact about this to the secretaries and, a moment later, to Sam Silver, who appeared suddenly, alerted by Charmaine, and greeted them briefly. He seemed preoccupied.

"I hear you got sick just now downstairs." He was dressed more formally than usual. He had on a white shirt and a tie with his gray corduroy trousers. His stethoscope hung around his neck.

"Yeah, I had a little cold, and I kept sniffing in mucus, and it got stuck," she told him, dropping her coat on a chair. "That's what made me throw up." She had on dungarees printed with apples, brown clogs, and a blue T-shirt showing Snoopy puckered up over the caption ALL GIRLS LOOK FORWARD TO THEIR FIRST KISS.

"For a few mornings she's been doing that," her mother told the doctor. "Mucus collects in her chest. I think it has something to do with the medications, and then maybe she was jostled in the car." Marie could contemplate this explanation without alarm.

"No fever?" Silver did not appear to be particularly worried.

"No."

"Well, I'll listen to her chest." To the child he said, "I'll have to take your blood too."

It was unlike him to state his intentions so flatly, and the content also surprised her. He had never taken her blood before. "Can't the nurses do it?"

"The nurses are all tied up with the baby."

She looked doubtful. "Do you do it like they do?"

Silver had spent the last hour talking with an eighteen-year-old who had just relapsed. In his first months at Children's, the doctor had been able to block out what bothered him in Clinic. He couldn't

do this as well now. He'd had a few days off over the holidays and
had come back feeling as if he could have used a few more. But at
Gina's insistence on knowing his credentials for a routine procedure, he finally grinned. "I hope so!"

Ordinarily she would have gone to Angie first, but Angie, too,
was tied up with a patient, and Dr. Silver had a few minutes free.
He led the way through the waiting room. For once Gina let her
mother come along. In the treatment room she boosted herself into
a sitting position on the table, and the doctor placed a clean gauze
pad against the skin above her right inner elbow. Without being
asked, she held it there. In silence he tied a tourniquet around her
arm, a tan rubber tube. He took the other things he needed from a
drawer and opened a disposable syringe. He rubbed the back of her
hand with alcohol. "Are you ready?"

"Will you do it fast?"

"Here goes."

She braced herself, knowing she would feel just a pinch, and
then it would be over.

But very little blood flowed into the syringe. He had to pull the
needle out and stick Gina a second time. Again she braced herself.
Again the flow was minimal.

At that moment Clinic head nurse Cindy Strickland put her
head in the door. Clinic policy holds that a staff member who fails
twice to draw a patient's blood must call in someone else for the
third attempt. Seeing the nurse, Silver wasted no time getting out of
his predicament.

"Cindy, will you take blood from Gina? She needs enzyme studies and a CBC." His voice was sharp with the irritation he felt with
himself.

Cindy sat down in front of Gina and caressed the hand that now
showed a small bruise. "How are you, honey?" Her manner was
very soothing.

"I'm fine," she said mournfully.

"You look a little sad right now."

The patient nodded. Silver hoisted himself onto the table beside
her and put an arm around her shoulders. "You mad at me?"

"No."

Cindy got a needle into a vein in the patient's left hand on the
first try. As Gina watched the small syringe fill steadily with her

blood, she suddenly launched into a dissertation that started out to be on Christmas.

"I got roller skates! My girlfriend Michelle has the exact same ones! Those shoe kind of skates? The others I had you just buckled, and they were metal, and you could make them any size, but see, I didn't want the other ones because these don't wear out, and they don't make you trip. My cousin, she has sneaker skates, and you know what she did? She almost fell and broke her neck!"

The adults around Gina were smiling. She scarcely stopped for breath. "I also got a fishing rod with my name on it, and so did my brother, because we go camping, and my dad is getting a license so we can get fish for breakfast instead of Mom making eggs! I caught a fish once! It flopped around on the table, and my dad had to kill it, because . . ."

Angie walked in pretending to scold. "Girl, where have you been? I've been waiting for you to get weighed!"

"Well, I've been waiting for you to give me Band-Aids!" She held out both hands for Angie to see. No sooner had Cindy and Dr. Silver left the room than the senior nurse's aide was regaled with the whole story of how the patient had had to be stuck three times because the doctor couldn't get blood the first two times!

For one reason or another, neither Cindy nor Sam Silver had remembered that Gina was supposed to have chemotherapy today. Usually the vincristine was injected through the same needle inserted to draw the child's blood for the enzyme studies, thus minimizing the number of times she had to be stuck. The patient herself did not mention chemo.

Minutes later Gina and her mother met Sam Silver in Examining Room 3. He told them that he was going to check the enzymes again and that if they were normal, he would put Gina back on a smaller dose of Methotrexate and increase it gradually. Still sounding somewhat preoccupied, Silver then began his customary questioning. The patient answered him cheerfully.

"How has school been?"

"Fine."

"Any problems?"

"No."

"How's your energy?"

"It's good!"

"Hair growing back?"

For answer she took her wig off. Her hair covered her head like a boy's. It was almost long enough to have been cut that way on purpose.

Gina could have told Silver, as she had told her mother, that she had shown her hair to her friend Christine in the girls' room at school—just lifted her wig a little because Christine had wanted to see underneath it. She had even showed a boy who wanted to see.

She could have told Silver that after weeks of running upstairs to put her wig on before going for the mail on Saturdays, she had gone out on the porch without the wig on New Year's and had talked to a neighbor—a hairdresser, as it happened. The neighbor had complimented her. "Oh, Gina, your hair looks so pretty! You should wear it short all the time." Marie DeRose could have told Dr. Silver that her daughter had been very pleased.

Marie could also have told Silver that Gina was becoming much less sensitive about the wig than she had been. The first few weeks she'd worn it to school, she had come home and taken it off immediately. Now she wore it almost all the time. Marie had even seen her taking a bath with it on. Last night during dessert the child's head had itched so much that she'd lifted the wig, scratched her scalp, and put the wig back on. Marie, Tony, and Little Tony had been hysterical. Gina had laughed with them.

Marie could have told Sam Silver further that the child talked constantly about her hair growing back in.

But Silver hadn't put any questions to Gina's mother, and Gina herself provided him with no information beyond what his eyes could see. He offered her encouragement anyway. "I suspect that next time I see you, it will be much thicker."

Turning off the overhead light, he examined her eyes with the aid of a small but powerful beam.

"Sam, where's the star?"

"There is no star in this room."

"When you put that light up to my eye, I see like little pieces of pizza, but it's my veins, right?"

"I can tell you for sure," he said, "that it's not pizza." His spirits were beginning to lift. He switched the light back on. "Okay, Gina, will you take your shirt off for me, please?"

One might have sworn that she'd been waiting for this moment. "Yeah, and watch me turn into Supergirl!" She whipped off her T-shirt and sat before her doctor in a bright blue training bra with a red S on a yellow background smack in the center of her chest. There was no indication that she needed the bra. "I have on under-pants to match, but you can't see them! I have some with Wonder Woman on, too! Underoos! My mom bought them for me when we saw a whole bunch!"

Mimicking ads she'd seen on television, Gina began to sing. "Wearing Underoos is fun, yeah! It's really something new in un-derwear, la da da da. . . ."

Silver laughed. This was the child who'd been so moody just two weeks ago that her mother had worried about relapse. He said as much to Marie, who rolled her eyes.

When he had finished his examination, Silver wrote out a couple of refill prescriptions. He had found no reason to be concerned about the vomiting. He told Gina he wanted her back in two weeks for a blood test for the enzymes. Ideally it would take only a few minutes. Could she come in after school one day?

"Dr. Silver, do you know what my reading teacher says? She goes, 'How do you always know when we have tests?'" She giggled.

But the doctor frowned. "Gina, I don't want you to miss school for this. Do you usually go back to school on the days you come here?"

Marie answered. "Sure, if we get out of here! Normally we come in at ten-thirty and get out by eleven-thirty or twelve, and then I take her right back. If we don't get out till two, by the time we get through the city there's practically none of the school day left."

This satisfied him. Handing Marie a form, he reminded Gina that her next regularly scheduled Clinic visit would be in four weeks. He was about to remind her that that's when she'd be getting her bone marrow and spinal tap when suddenly he remembered the vincristine.

"Gina, I'm really sorry. I completely forgot that you're supposed to get chemo today." He could not have been more apologetic.

She shrugged, but her face fell. She replied gamely. "Okay." Marie wondered whether the child herself had forgotten or whether, as sometimes happened with the medicines at home, Gina had simply been hoping that no one else would remember.

There is a trick to giving vincristine. Administered improperly, it can cause a bad burn. If the needle doesn't go into the vein just right, the nurse must take it out and start over. If the patient is crying, the nurse is always tempted to leave the needle in and save the child another stick. This temptation must be resisted. Severe chemo burns are very painful and can permanently disfigure the site. The child burned even mildly by vincristine or certain other agents can feel discomfort for as long as two weeks.

Back in the treatment room, Cindy broke open a sterile package and took out a fine butterfly needle. Gina offered her left hand. Cindy took it without comment. Most children let the nurse decide where to put the needle. Gina favored one particular vein in her left hand that almost always seemed to work. Occasionally, to give that hand a rest, Cindy would try a vessel in the other. If that vein failed to yield, as it sometimes did, Gina would say, "See, I told you! You should have used *this* vein!"

Cindy gripped the needle by the green plastic "wings" on either side of it and pushed the point through the skin of her patient's hand. Gina sang two lines of a song in very fast tempo. Blood appeared in the tube. The nurse asked the child to remove the tourniquet. Gina yanked the tan tube off her arm and crossed herself.

"Keep praying," Cindy said. The blood had slowed. The needle was meeting resistance. Within seconds a small rise in the flesh told the nurse that the needle had poked through the other side of the vein. She had no choice but to take the needle out.

"I'm so sorry, honey. This is really a bad day for you."

Gina made a face. "Yeah."

Yet when Cindy suggested that they walk over to a room with a sink in it and see if they could bring up a vein under warm water, the child jumped off the table eager to try. Hand submerged, she chatted on and on with her favorite nurse about needles she'd had other places where they jabbed kids, not like at Children's where they gave needles lightly.

Cindy attributed this resiliency to a change in Gina's attitude. The first few weeks in Clinic are always very stressful for kids, particularly those with acute lymphocytic leukemia, who have to go through six spinal taps in that period. Within a few months, however, the children learn that in the hands of a doctor or nurse experienced in giving chemo, the butterfly doesn't really hurt very much. Though they all fear bone marrows and spinal taps, they eventually come to understand that much of what happens to them in Clinic is far less frightening. Gina had always appeared to like the staff. Now it seemed to Cindy as if she had begun to trust them.

The nurse took the patient back to the treatment room and pierced Gina's skin with the fifth needle she'd had in less than an hour. This time the vincristine flowed into the child's bloodstream without a hitch.

In the waiting room, meanwhile, Marie DeRose talked with Ellie about a matter relating to payment. Tony had health insurance through his union. Because it fell short of what was needed for Gina's bills, the family was eligible for Supplemental Security Income, a federal program incorporating Medicaid. The DeRoses were also getting assistance from the American Cancer Society and the Leukemia Society of America. Both organizations were contributing money for Gina's medications. Even with all this assistance, Tony DeRose was still making regular payments to Children's to help cover his daughter's Clinic visits. Hard as this was on the family pocketbook, Tony could not consider it a burden. "For what I've gotten in return," he'd told his wife, "it's worth it."

As she was concluding her business with Ellie, Marie overheard two staff members say something about a child with a brain tumor who was going to have to be admitted for possible surgery. Minutes later the little girl was wheeled out through the waiting room and into the hall on a stretcher. Watching the child pass, her parents walking like zombies behind her, Marie couldn't help but think to herself that in one way coming to Clinic was good. She had never set foot in Children's Hospital without seeing somebody worse off than Gina.

Ø

Upstairs on Adolescent an hour later, with Kate, Alan Cavanaugh, and the patient's mother looking on, Dr. Drew Cipriani detached Mark's fourth and last chest tube from the Pleur-evac, folded the end of the tube over on itself twice, wrapped it in gauze, and put a rubber band around it.

"Okay, Mark," Cipriani said, smiling to allay the boy's anxiety, "we'll leave this clamped for a couple of days and see what happens. If you have any unusual trouble breathing, let somebody know right away. The residents starting their CT rotations tomorrow morning will continue to check on you just as I've been doing. We're not really expecting any problems. The lung has been fine for nearly two full days without a functioning chest tube. But as you know, we can't make any promises. If there's no change in the pneumothorax over the next forty-eight to seventy-two hours, somebody will come up and get this tube out of you." Cipriani would have the weekend off and on Monday would return to the university hospital to continue his general surgery training.

The patient's face registered both happiness and uncertainty. "I can't believe that in two days I might not have this chest tube anymore."

"*If* your lung stays up."

"Right. I know."

"Meanwhile you can get up and move around as much as you want to."

This brought a grin. "Boy, that I really don't believe! I've been sitting here looking at these same four walls for five weeks. I can't wait to get some practice on that new bumper pool table!"

Cipriani returned the grin. "Don't let us hold you up!"

"How about if I get you a wheelchair," Kate suggested, "just to get you in there. Save your strength."

He refused. He let Kate help him out of bed and walk alongside him as far as the hall. He walked slowly, obviously weak, and used his IV pole for support. But for a youngster with no muscles who had had no exercise for more than a month, he got along fine. Seeing that he did, Kate stopped at the doorway. He turned into the hall. When he looked back to wave, he was beaming.

He found the pool table in use. A big kid he had never seen before was shooting balls. A couple of younger patients Mark recognized sat at a table nearby playing chess. When the newcomer said hi, the younger boys said hi back, but the big kid said nothing, which irritated Mark.

He watched the kid's game, glad to stand still for a few minutes. He saw that the new patient wasn't very good. When the last ball had been sunk, Mark moved closer. "Could I shoot a game with you?"

The boy agreed with noticeable reluctance. Mark picked up a cue and played as badly as he could.

Beating Mark made the boy more friendly. He suggested another game.

Mark suggested that they play for a quarter this time.

The boy smiled. "How about a dollar?"

Hearing this, the youngsters at the chessboard turned in their seats. Bets are common among patients on Adolescent, but dollar bets are almost unheard of. Mark saw that the kid was trying to take advantage of him because he was small, which made him angry.

"Okay," he said, "I'll bet you a dollar."

He took a lot of pleasure in winning that dollar. A few times in the past Mark had hustled new patients on the pool table just for the fun of it—the old ones knew how good he was—but afterward had always felt bad. This time he felt happy.

"That's a lot of money to take from somebody when you don't even know what his circumstances are," his mother said to him later in a halfhearted attempt to chide him. Actually Ellen found it hard to conceal her pleasure at the thought of skinny Mark with a tube in him and an IV pole beside him wiping out a big kid who assumed he was a pushover.

Her son was unrepentant. "He's the one who upped it to a dollar, not me."

"It doesn't sound as if you showed much mercy, either!"

"Mom, my ego needed to beat him."

That she knew.

She left for home as the supper trays were being distributed. An hour or so after they'd been collected, her son had a visit from his friend Lisa Fletcher, who had been readmitted to Children's on Monday.

Lisa made her way slowly down the Adolescent hallway. She was weak, and she was having trouble breathing. Like Mark, Lisa was in and out of Children's every few months now. Her face was a heart framed in curls of palest blond. For her trip down the hall she had tied a red ribbon in her hair to match her red and green plaid bathrobe.

She and Mark had met in the Adolescent playroom when both were twelve. They had known each other well since September, when their tune-ups had overlapped for a full ten days. Because they were the same age, they shared many of the same problems. Lisa knew how it felt to be called Toothpick or Stick. She knew how it felt to have to stop going to school full-time. Because she herself had been cut from cheerleading for missing practice, Lisa understood how Mark felt about having to give up his bike. She also knew how it felt to write a letter to someone who never answered.

In September she and Mark had talked about these things and many others. They had exchanged stories about how nice their classmates in high school seemed. Mark had told Lisa about the boy who had teased him about growing tits. He had also told her about having two beers and a little whiskey on New Year's Eve and falling down in the kitchen. She had told him that she'd tried Amaretto on her birthday and had it every so often now because she liked it so much. Mark had described his reaction to his first and only cigarette. Lisa had told him that she never wanted to even try smoking because of her lungs. On the subject of marijuana, the two had agreed that they could not understand why kids with healthy bodies would take such risks with them.

Finally one day they had talked about fear. This had been a difficult conversation for Lisa. Unlike most of her conversations with Mark, it had left her feeling not less alone but more so. Lisa had been very close to Nicole, the twelve-year-old who had died of CF just three months earlier. Nicole's death had hit Lisa very hard. One day in the hall in September she had told Mark that she couldn't stop thinking about Nicole and that she was afraid to die. When she had asked Mark if he was afraid, he had said no.

"If it's going to happen," he'd said, "it'll happen." He had gone on to talk about a girl they both knew with CF who he thought was *really* afraid. Lisa had not been able to get over Mark's saying that he wasn't scared himself.

She entered his room and found him counting his money. He didn't look good to her. He was a lot thinner and paler than he had been in September.

He was glad to see her. At his invitation, she pulled a chair up close to his bed, then asked him what he was planning to do with all that money.

"Well, sixteen dollars goes to the church. Ten percent."

This surprised her. She knew Mark had faith, but she had never known he was so strong in his faith. Noticing the Bible on his bedside table, she observed to him that she didn't remember his having a Bible in the hospital before.

"I've got two besides that one," he told her, "but I keep them in a drawer so people won't think I'm an evangelist!" He explained his reading program to her and said that sometimes he compared versions.

"I never knew you read the Bible all the time."

"I didn't, until this happened." He indicated the chest tube hanging out below his pajama top. She waited to see if he would talk about his lung collapse, which she'd learned of from the nurses.

Instead he remarked that she seemed to be having a lot of trouble breathing.

She told him she was all right. But he expressed such concern for her, even offering her some of his oxygen, that she confessed the truth.

"I'm depressed about being back in here again so soon, and I'm scared. I'm just always in here. I get out, and then I have to come right back in again."

He shifted on the mattress to face her. "You have entirely the wrong attitude," he said. "You can't look at it that way. You have to look at the bright side of things. The positive side."

"I keep thinking about Nicole."

"Here," he said, surprising her, "hold my hand." Urging her to try to relax, he told her that he had done a lot of reading on CF after his lung had collapsed and had learned something that made him feel better.

"I've read," he said, "and the doctors have told me, that there are three critical periods for this disease. The first is in your first two years of life. The second is when you start school, and the third is during your adolescent years, like from eleven to fifteen. You and I are almost past that period. Nicole got too sick too soon. But with us, the damage that was going to be done during our adolescence has pretty much been done, and we're still alive. I think that once we get past this stage, we have a chance of getting stronger."

Lisa had never been able to understand how Mark could read about cystic fibrosis. Now, for the first time, she could appreciate his reasons, because what he had just said sounded right to her and made her feel better too. She told him so.

He was quiet, then, for a long time. Feeling that he was struggling with something, she also remained silent. At last he looked up at her.

"Remember the talk we had in September when I said I wasn't scared?"

"Yes. In the hall."

"Yes." He took a deep breath and then another. "I lied."

She nodded. She had known that, of course. But how it helped her to hear him say it!

"I just . . ."

"What, Mark?"

"No, I won't say it. You're too upset already."

"No, what? Please tell me."

"I was just thinking what one of us would do if something happened to the other one."

But Lisa did not want to contemplate this, and she led Mark away from the subject just as a moment ago he had led her away from her fear. "Well, I'm going to live till about eighty."

"I don't care how long I live," he answered seriously, "as long as I graduate."

"Maybe they'll come up with a cure before then," she offered. "Maybe they'll come up with something to help us. I'm not going to give up, I know that. I'm going to keep trying. At times it seems hard, and I can see why somebody would give up, but I want to keep going."

"I do too."

"We're both going to live a long time."

He told her he would take that statement as a promise.

Saturday, January 5

Shortly after noon Freddy Eberly was transferred out of Acute and into the Isolation Unit across the hall. A variety of staphylococcus bacteria growing in the heavy secretions issuing from his lungs and trachea had been discovered to be drug-resistant. Though not dangerous to him, the organisms could spread to other patients in Acute and make those children very sick. He was moved for *their* protection.

An hour later Freddy was taken off the respirator for the second time in three days. He had been weaned gradually during that period until his carbon dioxide had risen to normal levels. This time, however, instead of removing the tube from his throat, the doctors cut off the delivery of breaths to the patient by simply turning a dial. Leaving the tube in would prevent Freddy's tongue from obstructing his airway. It would also permit the ventilator to perform the limited but vital functions of providing the patient with oxygen and exerting positive pressure in his lungs to keep them slightly inflated. Nevertheless, the boy was considered to be off the respirator because it was no longer breathing for him.

Nine days after his accident, eight days after he had first opened his eyes, he remained comatose.

Sunday, January 6

Just before 7:00 A.M. the night nurse noticed that Mark's breath sounds had decreased somewhat on the left side. His chest tube had been clamped overnight because the CT surgeons had hoped to take it out this morning. But an x-ray done right after breakfast revealed that the patient's lung was down between about fifteen and twenty percent. The tube was reattached to suction.

The film strengthened Alan Cavanaugh's resolve to press for hyperalimentation for Mark. He understood and respected Daniel Earnshaw's objections. But on Saturday the chief cardiothoracic surgeon at Children's had examined Mark for the first time and had told Cavanaugh afterward that the boy ought to be on hyperal as a way of improving the healing potential of his lung. Later the resident had wondered why he hadn't thought of this angle himself. He had learned in medical school that good nutrition helps surgical patients heal fast, and obviously the same principle would apply to a burst bleb in the lung.

The resident also believed that IV therapy could contribute to Mark's overall well-being. Ellen Price had asked Cavanaugh whether he thought Mark could get hyperal at a hospital nearer home. Knowing nothing about the capabilities of the hospital she had in mind, the young doctor had nonetheless been very enthusiastic about the concept. When Ellen had offered to investigate the possibility, Cavanaugh urged her to do so.

A multiservice conference on Mark had finally been scheduled for Thursday at 4:00. At that meeting Alan Cavanaugh intended to make a compelling case for hyperal.

At the Adolescent nurses' station he noted in Mark's chart the increased pneumothorax, then added, "We have to do something more aggressive now. I think Mark feels the same way."

Ø

Early Sunday evening Colin Kendall visited Freddy Eberly for the first time in several days. The neurosurgeon had been tied up all weekend with two major emergencies. These cases had occupied the residents too, so that there had been time for only passing glances at the neurosurgical patients considered to be stable, Freddy among them. As the boy was being watched closely by the critical care specialists in Isolation, Colin Kendall was not anticipating unpleasant surprises.

Sometimes called the "bug barn," the Isolation Unit at Children's is smaller than Acute and usually quieter. Patient quarters are a row of six private rooms overlooking the courtyard. The neurosurgeon found his patient alone. The boy was propped in a semi-sitting position with pillows at his back. A rolled towel wedged under his right cheek held his head up. Beneath the sheet that covered him to his armpits, his legs had been elevated on rolled blankets. His eyes opened slowly. Kendall noted that they continued to appear downcast.

Picking up the child's left hand, the doctor attempted to close it over two of his own fingers.

"It's Dr. Kendall, Freddy. Can you squeeze my fingers?"

The hand uncurled slowly and relaxed. It was dead weight in the doctor's palm. The right hand behaved similarly. Kendall frowned. The hand seemed to have lost tone since Friday. In fact, as he went on testing the child's function, Kendall perceived that the patient was less responsive in general than he had been on Friday.

Consulting Freddy's chart, Kendall found the explanation immediately. On Friday the patient had come off the ventilator. Ever since then his carbon dioxide level had been drifting upward. On his own this boy was breathing too shallowly or too infrequently to blow off CO_2 in normal amounts.

Kendall was chagrined. Elevated carbon dioxide put the boy at risk for the intracranial pressure problems he had so far escaped and for further damage to the brain itself. The elevation was only moderate. But obviously Freddy had been less stable over the past couple of days than the neurosurgeons had realized or than the anesthesiologists, unschooled in neurosurgery, could have appreciated.

Furthermore, Kendall was dismayed by the implications. He feared that the CO_2 retention reflected damage to the patient's brain stem. This suspicion was fortified in the doctor's mind when he sat down at the nurses' station to review Freddy's chart. In the past week the patient had gone nowhere. He wasn't moving his legs. He was neither swallowing nor breathing properly. His eyes had yet to follow a physician's forefinger beyond the range right in front of his face. While his coma was less profound than on the day of the accident, the boy was not waking up. While none of these signs proved brain stem dysfunction, all were consistent with it.

There was nothing Kendall could do about damage that might already have occurred. But he could prevent further damage. Crossing the hall to Acute, he insisted to the anesthesiologists overseeing Isolation that the child go back on the respirator immediately.

Almost as soon as the machine began to pump air into the patient's lungs, the child opened his eyes and kept them open. He shifted his right arm from one spot to another on the mattress.

Rechecking the boy's reflexes minutes later, Kendall was convinced that Freddy's neurological status had improved. He concluded from the improvement that the boy still needed artificial ventilation.

Ø

Several hours later, returning to Mark's room for their nightly game of Concentration, Jacquie Harper found her patient sitting with his back to the door. At first she thought he was looking out into the court. But when he didn't answer her greeting, she walked around the bed and saw tears streaming down his face. He sobbed against her. "I'm so depressed!"

"I know. I know."

"I just want to go home!"

She couldn't answer. She was crying herself, the first time in her life that she had ever cried with a patient.

She felt he was going to die. She thought *he* felt he was dying. And instead of wanting to run from him, as she had always wanted to run from death before, Jacquie wanted to stay as close to Mark as she possibly could.

Monday, January 7

The Infant ICU nurse doing Brandon Gregory's A.M. care weighed him, subtracted the estimated weight of his tubes and the covered foam blocks that protected his arms and legs from the tape holding some of the tubes in place, and posted the baby's weight on the huge flow chart taped to the glass partition near his bed: 720 grams. As of today, he was one month old. He still weighed an ounce less than he had weighed at birth. Nevertheless, though born a whole trimester too early, he continued to defy the high odds against him.

In the ten days since an ophthalmologist had informed his mother that her baby was in danger of losing an eye, Brandon had followed a largely undramatic up-and-down course familiar to the Infant ICU staff as being fairly typical for a patient Brandon's size and known in the unit as "putzing along."

He had managed to gain only a couple of ounces. His feeding problems had been compounded by a yeast infection. In all likelihood secondary to the antibiotics Brandon had been getting for the corneal ulcer, the infection had caused the baby to retain urine, distending his abdomen enough that his feeds had had to be stopped completely for the second time in as many weeks.

They had been restarted this past Friday at a rate that engendered impatience even in Roger Forbes. But Forbes hadn't the nerve to push the baby. Any progress, he'd told the residents, was better than another defeat. Defeat had serious implications. Unless Brandon soon began to take in the number of calories needed for growth, it was possible that he would have to be given hyperalimentation through a central line which would have to be placed in the operating room. Like Mark Price but for different reasons, Brandon Gregory was a poor candidate for this procedure.

The baby's nutrition problems had been further compounded by the discovery on x-ray of too much fluid in his lungs. Without ever being definitively diagnosed, the edema had been brought under control by a reduction in the volume of fluids being given the patient intravenously. Since these were accounted for one hundred percent by hyperalimentation, however, the decrease in fluids had meant a decrease in calories for Brandon. While his weight and his fluctuations in weight were not unusual for a baby his size, they were far short of optimal.

He had run into other difficulties during his third and fourth weeks of life. For one thing, he had had episodes of excessively rapid heartbeat, secondary, perhaps, to the atropine drops in his eyes or to the drug he was getting that reminded him to breathe. He had also had periods of cyanosis. His ventilatory status had improved very little. As a result, the baby's primary diagnosis, entered each morning on the flow chart near his bed, had been changed from prematurity with respiratory distress syndrome to bronchopulmonary dysplasia: the difference between immature lungs and chronic lung disease.

The BPD, of course, had resulted from treatment. So had the corneal ulcer and thus, apparently, the yeast infection and perhaps the rapid heartbeat as well.

However, some good things had happened to Brandon Gregory in recent days. More accurately, perhaps, some bad things that could have happened had not. The abrasion and infection in his left eye had gotten progressively better. The patient's belly had remained free of even a suspicion of necrotizing enterocolitis. To the best of anyone's knowledge, his brain had not hemorrhaged. He had suffered no catastrophes. He remained a vigorous, active baby.

Brandon had also, by his fourth week in the Infant ICU at Children's, won himself two special friends among the nurses. One was Dory Hatfield, a somewhat stocky woman of twenty-seven with frizzy blond hair who loved infants and in particular loved the tiny premies. When Dory Hatfield beheld a baby born far ahead of schedule who insisted on staying alive in defiance of the odds, she saw a character full of audacity. A fighter. Her favorite patient these days was a premie now ten weeks old, Trisha, whom Hatfield had cared for since the day of the baby's admission. But she also felt close to Brandon. She was taking care of him more consistently than was any other nurse in the unit except for Lea Bowersox.

The mother of two young daughters, Bowersox was a tall woman, quiet of manner, who was a little older than Dory Hatfield and had had twice the amount of professional experience. She had liked Brandon Gregory from the beginning.

However, she had no intention of *loving* him or any other patient now. Once at Children's Bowersox had allowed herself to become very close to a tiny premie who had spent more than a year in her care. He had then gone to Intermediate. One week after he had finally been discharged, he had been readmitted to the hospital and had died. As a nurse, Lea Bowersox had experienced no death more difficult to bear. She had learned its lessons. She would not get close to Brandon Gregory.

She was glad now for the protection of her resolve. As Brandon marked his fourth week in the Infant ICU, Bowersox was beginning to wonder about the quality of life being saved in this case. She thought it quite possible that the baby would one day go home. She thought it quite unlikely that he would go home undamaged.

She had begun to worry about his future. And not just *his* future; his parents' as well.

At one time Lea Bowersox had been constitutionally opposed to aggressive treatment for tiny premies. Before having children of her own, Bowersox would say of her smallest patients, "If I had a kid that size, I wouldn't let him be treated."

Now she felt differently. Having carried and borne two children, the nurse now understood how parents could accept a child who was somehow imperfect. She could understand why, when staff wanted to turn off a baby's ventilator, parents sometimes said no. She thought now that in the same situation she might herself say no, however small the baby, however poor its chances for a normal life.

On the other hand, Bowersox had taken care of infants who had struggled along on the ventilator for six months only to die. She knew that those children suffered. Caring for a suffering child who seems likely to do badly despite the experts' best efforts is very hard on a nurse. Bowersox knew how it felt to go home at the end of a day wondering, *What am I doing and why am I doing it?*

Still, she had seen enough of the smaller babies pull through in reasonably good shape in the past few years that she was finding it increasingly difficult to say to herself or anyone else, "I think we should stop on this kid." Who was Lea Bowersox to say that Brandon Gregory was not one of the growing minority of tiny premies who would turn out perfectly all right?

So far she thought the doctors justified in continuing to treat him aggressively. But in developing bronchopulmonary dysplasia, the baby had succumbed to a serious complication of prematurity. He still had a very long way to go before he could be considered out of danger, and Lea Bowersox had begun to fear for him.

Brandon's mother was under the impression that her baby's best friend at Children's was a nurse named Phyllis. Tom and Robin Gregory had met Lea Bowersox only briefly and Dory Hatfield not at all. Phyllis had been tending Brandon on several occasions when his parents had visited. In fact, unbeknownst to the Gregorys, the nurse was about to move to another city. Already she had begun to withdraw emotionally from the Infant ICU.

But Robin thought her very good with Brandon. She had seen other nurses work with the baby as if they were merely doing a job. To her Phyllis seemed more compassionate, more sensitive, more feeling. She seemed to treat the baby with loving care. In fact, Robin Gregory had gotten the idea from someone in the unit that only with Phyllis would Brandon not go into fits of holding his breath. It made Robin feel good to know that her baby had trust in someone at Children's.

The Gregorys had paid their son three visits over the past ten days. Each had been disturbing to Brandon's parents.

During the first, they had found the baby sound asleep on his tummy, left cheek to the mattress. Robin had asked about the eye ulcer. The nurse—not Phyllis—had begun to explain, then had said suddenly, "Here, let me show you," and had actually moved to turn the baby over, tubes and all.

Horrified, the Gregorys had objected strenuously, upset that she would even have offered to bother Brandon just so his parents could see an abrasion in his eye. As it was, the baby was moved too much, in Robin's opinion. Why move him when it wasn't necessary? In her womb, where he should still be, he wouldn't have been bothered at all.

Three nights later the Gregorys had visited their son again. This time, winding up Brandon's musical bunny for him, Robin had heard a strange sound behind her and turned to face the male nurse who had urged her to hold Brandon. He stood beside a female nurse who was working on another patient. Seeing Robin's puzzlement, the young man had explained, "It's the baby crying."

"It is?"

"Yes," the man had replied, and then he'd teased her by saying, "That's the way Brandon will sound when he gets older!" The two nurses had started to laugh.

Robin had not joined in. She had found the crying terribly sad. The thought that Brandon might make such sounds when he got older had sent a chill through his mother.

Yesterday, Sunday, she and Tom had come back in once again. By this time the baby had had so many intravenous lines replaced in his arms and legs that in order to give his poor bruised limbs a rest as well as for a more technical reason, someone had inserted an IV into his scalp. A patch of his hair had been shaven, and the skin around the IV had turned bluish. Though the Gregorys had been forewarned, the sight of a catheter running into their tiny son's skull had been very distressing to them, however much Robin tried to console herself that since Brandon had tubes in him everywhere else, one more didn't really make any difference.

They had also been distressed by his scrawniness. Robin had understood in phone conversations that the baby had begun to gain a little weight toward the end of the week. Yesterday she had seen that actually he was losing weight. His ribs had been more visible than on her previous visit. He'd been down to bare bones on Sunday, and it had seemed to Robin that he was also losing some color in his skin.

The matter of how much the baby weighed had by now become a source of considerable confusion for Robin Gregory. Each day she'd call and ask about his weight, among other things; each day a nurse would answer in grams and then convert the answer for Robin to pounds and ounces; each time she called it would seem as if he'd gained; each time they visited it would seem as if he'd lost. "Well, he lost an IV board," a nurse would say.

Robin knew that when the nurses weighed Brandon, they then had to deduct all his tubing and equipment. She could appreciate that an accurate reading was probably difficult to get. But sometimes it seemed to her that different nurses gave different weights, and her confidence in what she was being told about the baby's weight had not been strengthened by the nurse who'd reported that Brandon had gone up to two and a half pounds.

"That can't be," Robin had said. The nurse had recalculated, and sure enough, the baby hadn't even weighed one and a half pounds. The Gregorys had gradually concluded that they had probably never known Brandon's true weight except on the day of his birth.

Yet Robin had expected his weight to go up and down. From everything she'd been told, she'd expected Brandon to progress in bursts: to go forward a little, then backward a little, then forward again. So the baby's mother had noted his scrawniness on Sunday without feeling alarmed. She continued to interpret the nurses' reports as good. Today, marking the end of Brandon's first month on earth, Tom and Robin Gregory remained quite optimistic about their son.

In the ten days that had passed since the ophthalmologist had informed them of the ulcer on Brandon's cornea, his parents had had virtually no communication with the hospital staff members who knew most about Brandon medically and who were managing his care: his doctors.

Hours after the ophthalmologist had telephoned Robin, the Infant ICU fellow had called her to see if the baby's parents had questions about the eye problem or about anything else related to Brandon. Later Roger Forbes would remember having talked to the parents the same day, though neither Robin nor Tom would recall a conversation with Forbes on that occasion. In the days since, they had heard several times from the ophthalmologist. But the ophthalmologist was a consultant whose role in the baby's overall management was very small.

Under optimal circumstances the doctors involved in such a case, particularly the primary physician, would proceed to educate the infant's parents in the same way Brandon's doctors approached a tiny patient's feedings. That is, they would undertake to ascertain exactly how much and what kind of information the parents could or wished to absorb and to supply that information at a rate determined by the parents' demonstrated tolerance. In this way doctors may continually deepen the family's insight into their baby's condition.

Providing such information is no easy task. Premature infants tend to be born to young women; both mothers and fathers of premies are likely to be medically unsophisticated and very frightened. Teaching these parents about their babies requires time and patience and endless emphasis on the uncertainties of treatment and prognosis, and for the doctors the job is never done. The scared young couple in the morning is followed by two in the afternoon and two more the next day and two the next. In the words of an attending physician who has worked in the Infant ICU and faced those couples, "It's the volume that kills you."

That the Gregorys did not become more knowledgeable about Brandon was due in part to limitations on the frequency with which they were able to visit the hospital. They lived an hour's drive from Children's. Subsisting on unemployment, they had little money to spare for gas, and they had two babies at home who left them little time to spare. Brandon's mother was still recovering from major surgery. Like many parents of babies in the Infant ICU, and for similar reasons, the Gregorys couldn't get into Children's every day or even every other day.

When they did visit, they came in the evening after the twins had gone to bed and could be checked easily by a neighbor. By that hour Infant ICU doctors tend to be out of the unit. Attendings work days. Unless there were emergencies, Roger Forbes usually went home at suppertime. Residents often work longer days, but they, too, go off duty in the evenings unless they are on call. The unit at night is overseen by one fellow and one resident. Technically they are available to talk to parents. In fact if all twenty beds are full, or if even one patient is in the throes of a life-threatening crisis, the doctors have little time for talk.

Furthermore, the Gregorys did not seek much attention from the medical staff. Some parents besiege their children's doctors for information. Those who press for it inevitably get more of it than those who don't. Tom and Robin Gregory were by nature passive people. They were not inclined to demand more from the experts than was freely offered. Besides, they could see every time they visited that the doctors were very busy. The parents judged the doctors on their care of Brandon. On this score, aware that she had no basis for comparison, Robin believed that the doctors were doing a good job for her baby, especially Roger Forbes.

Brandon's physicians might have kept the Gregorys apprised of their son's condition by telephone. Unfortunately, as is too often the case in pediatrics and in medicine generally, the doctors did not assume this responsibility. In the ten days that had passed since the diagnosis of the corneal ulcer, the baby's parents had not received a single phone call from an Infant ICU doctor: none from Roger Forbes, Brandon's physician of record; none from the fellow; none from the resident filling in for Logan Sadler. The resident had never even met the Gregorys. Asked why she had not tried to contact them by phone, the young doctor replied, "Negligence." She had not had time, she said, though she acknowledged initiating contact with parents able to be more closely involved with their babies.

Brandon's nurses had almost daily conversations with the Gregorys. Yet the relationship between the parents and the nurses had not become close. Had they realized that the Gregorys' understanding of their son's condition did not fully accord with reality, the nurses would almost certainly have taken steps to remedy the situation. But they never got to know the parents well enough—in part, of course, because the Gregorys were on the scene so infrequently. Nor did the nurses ever get to know Tom and Robin well enough to appreciate the problems between them.

Thus no one called in the social worker. While often she would check with the nurses and try to troubleshoot any problems they saw arising, her responsibilities covered both the Infant ICU and a larger unit, and the two together amounted to more work than one person could adequately handle.

The hospital chaplain would gladly have made himself available to the Gregorys. Robin in particular might have found his perspective helpful. Unfortunately, no one connected with the case had thought to call him.

The physicians who surrounded Brandon at morning rounds the day he turned one month old included Logan Sadler, back from sick leave, and none of the other three physicians who had been most involved in the baby's care since his admission to Children's. All had rotated out of the Infant ICU according to schedule on Sunday evening. Roger Forbes and the fellow had been replaced by counterparts in neonatology who would run the unit and make decisions about all patients for the coming month.

Late Monday morning Brandon's belly blew up a little, and his doctors decided to take the patient off feeds entirely for the third time in less than two weeks.

An hour earlier the patient's mother had gotten a call from the Children's ophthalmologist, who'd been happy to give her the news that Brandon's eye had completely healed.

Robin had hung up thanking God. She was going to bring home a whole baby.

Ø

A baby in the Intermediate Unit who would never be as whole as Brandon Gregory had always been was feeling better today than he'd felt in nearly three weeks. Jody Robinson's fever was gone. His diarrhea was nearly gone. After a week on clear fluids, he was back on his regular formula as of this morning. His secretions had become much thinner. He was bouncing around on his bed like a well child. On Sunday he had pulled himself up to a standing position in his crib without help for the first time in his life! Unfortunately, he still continued to gag, sometimes violently. Marla had decided for the time being to give him nothing by mouth but water.

Late in the afternoon Jody's social worker got a call from his social worker at the Welfare Department. Lynn Story had not heard from Gladys Wexler since Wexler's visit to Children's on December 28, and she greeted the caller with pleasure that turned quickly to dismay.

Wexler had gone to visit Sabra's cousins. She had asked them whether they would be willing to think in terms of taking Jody to live with them, assuming he one day became well enough to leave Children's. The cousins had expressed considerable doubt about their ability to handle the child. It had been Wexler's impression that the two women were already overwhelmed with the three babies they had—their own and Sabra II. The Welfare worker did not think the cousins could be counted upon as future caretakers for Jody.

Therefore Gladys Wexler thought it would be best to concentrate on the mother herself: to find Sabra, to sound her out, and to try to discover whether Jody's mother might be nearly ready to settle down and get serious as a parent.

Story listened telling herself that even if Sabra could be located, she was unlikely to agree to change her ways, and that even if she did agree, proof of her transformation would have to precede Jody's discharge. Story also told herself that there was no great hurry to settle the matter. Jody was going to be a patient at Children's for months and perhaps longer. Had he been getting ready to go next week, Lynn Story would have hung up the phone and crawled the walls.

Her impulse, which she curbed with some effort, was to wish Gladys Wexler a disdainful "Good luck."

Five hours later, at 9:00 P.M. Sabra Robinson walked into the Children's Hospital lobby and requested a visitor's pass.

Following longstanding orders, the volunteer at the reception desk called a nursing supervisor who in turn called the charge nurse in Intermediate who in turn called Jan Haver at home to ask if there was anything special the nurses should do when Sabra arrived in the unit. Haver, watching television with her mother and father, was nearly speechless with amazement.

She quickly gathered her thoughts. "Make sure Security knows they have to send somebody up with her."

The charge nurse said Security was planning to do that.

"The only other thing I can think of is tell her to call Dr. Crossin at the hospital tomorrow so he can bring her up to date on what's happening with Jody medically. You can also tell her that if she wants to call me here from the unit, I'd be very glad to tell her anything about him I can."

Sabra stayed in Intermediate about half an hour. She played with Jody, asked a lot of questions about him, and assured the nurses that while she had been in a lot of trouble, she was going to straighten out. She wondered whether her son was ready to come home. They told her he wasn't ready yet and urged her to call Peter Crossin on Tuesday.

Next morning when Haver would tell Crossin that he might be hearing from Sabra, the doctor would drop his head into his hands and groan sarcastically, "Thanks a lot."

Tuesday, January 8

After a long weekend off, nurse Dory Hatfield reported for day-shift duty in the Infant ICU and discovered that Brandon Gregory now had an IV in his head. He had also been taken off feeds again on Monday, though he'd been restarted—again—during the night.

These discoveries were upsetting to Hatfield. Because scalp IVs are upsetting to parents, staff ordinarily tries hard to avoid that site. In Hatfield's opinion, someone had not tried hard enough with Brandon Gregory. Moreover he was no further ahead nutritionally than he'd been at New Year's.

Understandably, everybody was afraid of feeding him too fast. But thinking back on his problems with feeds, Dory Hatfield wondered if they'd really merited the worry they'd aroused. It seemed to her in retrospect that nurses who hadn't taken care of Brandon regularly had tended to panic when the baby had responded to feeds in a certain way. Granted that his belly had blown up a few times, he had never once had a suspicious x-ray.

Hatfield wondered whether staff expectations of Brandon Gregory had been too low. He was going nowhere on his ventilator settings. Was that because he was already doing his best, or was it because he wasn't being pushed hard enough to improve?

The baby had reached a point in his course when some premies got lost in the shuffle, as the nurse had come to think of it. When the acute period was over, the physicians' attention turned quite naturally to newer patients and those in more immediate danger. The infant who had been through a lot and looked it, yet to whom nothing very dramatic was happening medically or developmentally was sometimes less attractive to nurses than he or she had been at first.

Of course the baby continued to get good care. But if no one undertook to champion his or her cause, to be diligent about pushing the patient to his or her limits, that baby would continue to putz along more slowly than might actually be necessary.

Dory Hatfield did not want this to happen to Brandon Gregory. Convinced that he was good protoplasm, she wanted to help him as much as she could.

From Brandon's bedside Hatfield walked out to the nurses' station where Logan Sadler was talking to the new Infant ICU fellow, another woman. The nurse shared with the two doctors her concerns about their tiny patient. The fellow had spent three months in the unit on another rotation. She and Sadler both agreed with Dory Hatfield that Brandon Gregory might be able to tolerate being pushed a little more than he had been.

The three devised a plan. They would increase the baby's feeds to half-strength breast milk at 5 cc. an hour. Unless he did something awful, they would build him up as quickly as possible over the next three days and get him to a level of nourishment at which he could begin to gain weight. Unless he did something awful, only the nurses who knew him would be permitted to stop the feeds. If he could not tolerate the feedings and did not gain weight, Sadler and the fellow, in consultation with Brandon's new attending physician, would seriously consider sending the baby to the OR for placement of a central line through which he could receive maximum infusions of hyperalimentation.

Hatfield would henceforward refer to this plan as "The Conspiracy to Help Brandon."

Ø

11:00 A.M. Mark and Julie Wixted sipped sodas together on the bench in the sixth-floor hallway. He could leave his room because his chest tube had been reclamped this morning. The CT resident strongly suspected that the chest tube had somehow slipped out of communication with the air cap and was doing the patient no good. So now the resident had clamped the tube again to test this theory.

"We'll take an x-ray now and another one tomorrow morning," he had told Mark at breakfast time. "If there's still no change by tomorrow, we'll take the tube out. If the pneumothorax gets worse between now and then, we'll have to go with a fifth chest tube."

Suspense over the behavior of his lung had become so agonizing for Mark that the prospect of something definite being done within twenty-four hours, even if it had to be another chest tube, had lifted his spirits. He was telling Julie of his willingness to have a fifth chest tube when his mother appeared in the hall from the elevator and caught sight of them.

The nurse would have expected Ellen Price to be more pleased at seeing her son up and out of bed with his tube clamped. She realized that Ellen was angry.

"Well, Mark," said his mother tightly, dropping her purse and overnight bag on the bench and unbuttoning her coat, "if they're not going to give you hyperalimentation here, they're willing to do it up at St. Michael's."

Warning signals went off in Julie's brain. "Let's call Dr. Earnshaw and find out *why* he doesn't seem to want Mark to have hyperal," she suggested, "or even if the decision is definite."

To Earnshaw she said from a phone at the nurses' station, "You'd better get up here."

Earnshaw came. He sat with Mark and his mother in the hall and listened to their thoughts, then told them his. He began by laying out possible courses. Mark's chest tube could come out in the next few days, and he could go home. The tube could come out and a surgeon could insert a catheter for hyperal in a large vein near Mark's heart, and if St. Michael's was equipped to take care of a patient with a central line, Mark could be transferred up there as soon as he was stable. Or the pneumothorax might increase over the next few days, and Mark would have to have another chest tube. If this happened, the pediatrician said, he would consider putting Mark on hyperal as a means to heal the air leak in the lung.

Yet if the lung healed on its own, Earnshaw continued, he had real reservations about putting Mark on hyperal. The surgery would be hard on him. His lungs would not tolerate general anesthesia, and he was very debilitated. There were risks involved: of infection, clots, a punctured lung during surgery, liver damage, bruising, discomfort. The last thing Mark needed was to encounter new difficulties after having endured so many already.

Earnshaw did not discuss with the Prices the delicate matter of what good the therapy would ultimately do. Its use in cystic fibrosis was relatively recent. While some CF patients had gained weight on hyperal, there was no proof that weight gain altered the child's course in any way. But the pediatrician did wonder aloud whether St. Michael's could offer a patient on hyperalimentation the kind of support that was available to Mark at Children's.

Ironically, all the while he sat attempting to lead the Prices away from hyperalimentation, Earnshaw himself was being drawn toward it by his observations of the patient. In bed in his small room, Mark's emaciation was less dramatic than it was in the big hallway among many healthy people of normal size. He looked to his doctor like a survivor of Buchenwald. He was so run-down nutritionally that Earnshaw found himself thinking of hyperal as an attractive possibility even if Mark did not need it to heal his lung.

The patient's enthusiasm for the therapy was almost as remarkable as his appearance. The subject made the boy's eyes positively dance. Mark seemed to have his fight back. He was ready and willing to commit himself to one more painful procedure, one more tube, and several more weeks of hospitalization on the grounds that that commitment might improve his general condition and his ability to handle his disease.

The pediatrician was not yet aware that at 7:00 this morning Neil Martinson had presented the case of Mark Price to a weekly conference of chest specialists from all over the county who had ultimately concurred that the best way to proceed would be to put the patient on hyperalimentation.

But Earnshaw did know what he saw in Mark's eyes. Mark's en-

thusiasm alone would not have swayed Earnshaw, any more than
Alan Cavanaugh's enthusiasm had swayed him. Rather he was finally persuaded by a combination of factors. Mark wanted therapy
that would very likely be good for him and most likely do him no
harm. The staff at Children's had a way of giving it to him. Therefore, Earnshaw told Mark on the hall bench that if he could convince himself that St. Michael's could take proper care of his
patient, he saw no reason not to go ahead with hyperal. *If.*

After lunch Mark initiated with his parents a conversation unlike
any he had ever had with either of them before. It was a conversation unlike any he had ever had with his doctors, his nurses, his
social worker, or his recreation or respiratory therapists; and it was
a conversation he had never had with the psychiatrist called in by
Bruce Griffin to help Mark grapple with his fears. He talked to his
parents about his dying.

Bob Price had taken the afternoon off to be at Children's. No
sooner had he arrived on Adolescent than Mark asked his mother
and father both to sit down.

"We have something serious we need to talk about," he explained. He sat cross-legged on the mattress using no support from
pillows. He seemed nervous. Bob and Ellen exchanged glances.

"I want to ask you a question," Mark said, looking from one
parent to the other, "and I want you to answer honestly." Behind
his glasses his blue eyes were enormous.

Bob had a sense of scrambling for bearings on unfamiliar
ground. "I can't promise that, Mark, until I hear the question," he
said, "but I'll try."

Ellen nodded, preparing.

He looked directly at her. "Mom, how long do you think I'm
going to live?"

The question shook the earth beneath her and catapulted her
back to Dr. Earnshaw's office in late October. Fragments of their
conversation flashed in her mind: ". . . final stages of the disease . . .
a month . . . years . . . no way to know." He wanted an honest answer. How could she be honest? He wanted to live. She did not want
to take that away from him.

She shifted in her chair. "Well, Mark, I used to think you could
live a long time. To forty, maybe. But you've been sick so much

lately that several times in recent weeks I would have told you a few days. Today I feel optimistic. I would say maybe early twenties. Twenty-five."

He turned to Bob. "How long do *you* think I'm going to live?"

The man saw that the boy had set them on a course from which they could not turn back. He had never admired Mark more.

"Well, when you're feeling well, you look so good I think you could last forever. Sometimes when you come in here you look so sick that I think you could die any week."

Mark noticed that his father had given no specific age.

"I don't think you guys realize how sick I am," he told them earnestly. "You come in here day after day acting like everything is okay."

Ellen looked at Bob and laughed in astonishment. "When do I get my Oscar, now or later?" She found it difficult to believe that Mark couldn't see that his mother knew what his condition was. His comment would puzzle her for months.

"Put yourself in our shoes," Bob suggested. "If we could reverse roles, with me in the bed and you sitting where I am, would you come in with a long face and exhibit all sorts of distress and worry?"

"No, I'd probably come in looking just like you look!"

"Mark," Ellen said, "how long do *you* think you are going to live?"

There was nothing she had ever wanted more to know about her son than how he saw his future, and no question she had felt less able to ask him. Now he had paved the way. Waiting for his answer, she literally held her breath.

"I think I'll live to be at least twenty-two or twenty-three," he said simply. "One of my goals is to at least graduate from high school. I don't know if I will, but that's what I want. Mom, up until a year ago, you talked about me going to college and maybe becoming a psychologist or psychiatrist. A college education would be wasted on me. Not wasted, but I'm not going to live long enough. You know what I mean."

She nodded, wordless.

He began to cough. As he dropped his head, heaving and hacking in his effort to bring up mucus, Ellen pushed his sputum cup into one hand and some tissues into the other. After many seconds he deposited a large tannish blob into the shiny stainless cup and covered it over with used tissues. He set the cup aside and sipped some cola. He cleared his throat. A minute or two passed before he got enough breath back to talk.

"I want you both to know," he continued finally, meeting their eyes once more, "that when I go back to school, I'm going to be a different person. When we moved up there, I hated it." He grinned. "Now I just dislike it! No, seriously, the cards from the kids and the computer game from my woodshop have given me confidence. Before, I was quiet. I didn't really try to make friends. Instead I concentrated on my grades. I did pretty well at that. But I've decided I'm not going to worry about grades anymore.

"Now that doesn't mean," he added quickly, "that I want anyone to think I'm stupid. I want to be able to talk intelligently to people. But I'm not going to worry about bringing home A's anymore. I want to have some fun. There are things I want to do before I die. I want to learn to drive! I don't have the strength to be a good student and have a social life too."

Bob nodded. "Mark, we understand completely. If you bring home nothing but C's, that's perfectly fine with us. Your life has been shitty, and . . ."

"No!" He sat up straighter, eyes blazing. "I have a good life!"

His mother could not believe her ears. "You can say that after all you've been through these last six weeks?"

"Yes," he insisted, "my life is good. There have been moments in this hospitalization when I thought I might want to die, but I knew that if I said I wanted to die, I would. I'm not ready to die yet. When I am ready"—here he smiled, but he continued slowly and with great emphasis—"I'll tell you, and I'll mean it!"

He took another sip of cola and dropped his head. As Ellen reached for the sputum cup, he looked up again, and his eyes were filled with tears.

"Now here's where I get emotional," he said. He cleared his throat several times. "When I do die . . . not to say I'm going to die first. You guys could die before me! But I'm pretty sure I'm going to die before you. When I do die, I don't want you guys to miss me so much that you'll ruin your lives."

He explained. "I've read about situations where the wife loses her husband and misses him so much she kills herself, or the family loses a child and the family falls apart. This scares me. When I die, I know you're going to be sorry, I know you'll miss me, but I just hope you can live normal lives afterwards. I don't want your lives to be shattered so you have to go to a psychiatrist . . ."

He was having trouble talking. "I want you to go on and be happy. Just try to have happy memories of me."

Bob spoke over a huge lump in his throat. "Mark, there's no way that we're not going to grieve. We'll miss you terribly. I'll feel sorry for myself, for your mother, for all of us left behind. But . . ." He shook his head. Unable to look at the boy, he examined his palms instead. "But I'll be happy for you, because as a Christian, I know you'll be happy after you leave us."

Now he did look at Mark, eager to reassure his son. "Your going will hurt, but time will make the pain easier."

Ellen, too, wanted Mark to know that she was ready for whatever happened.

"As long as we are being completely open," she said, "I'll tell you straight out that there have been times when I've asked God to take you. I wanted your suffering, mental and physical, to come to an end. I'll tell you something else. I've even thought about your funeral. If you have any thoughts about that, I'd like to know them. Bob knows I want to be cremated."

Mark was surprised and somewhat taken aback by these comments. He hadn't thought the discussion pertained to his funeral.

But he had an answer. "I think I want to be buried. Nothing fancy! And I want an autopsy done."

"An autopsy!" Once again Ellen was taken off guard. "It's a good thing you told me, because if the doctors asked me, I think I would have said no."

He grew solemn. "Mom, how else can the doctors learn about this terrible disease? I think CF is one of the worst diseases there is. If I could stop one person from getting it by donating my body to research, that would make me feel good."

"Then that will be done."

He said he had told them everything he'd had on his mind to tell them. Dazed, his mother went to him and kissed him. "I love you, honey."

"I love you too."

They embraced. Then Mark and Bob embraced. Ellen observed this show of love between her son and her husband feeling utterly overwhelmed. Though she had always known that Mark was special, she realized now that she had never fully appreciated how special he really was. She felt deeply privileged to have been part of the conversation through which he had just guided them. For that conversation above all other reasons, Mark was, and to her would always be, a hero.

In the evening he played bumper pool in the playroom with his father and his friend Lisa. He was in high spirits. The x-ray taken after the chest tube was clamped this morning had shown no worsening of his pneumothorax, and it had begun to seem to Mark that everything he wanted for his immediate future was about to come true. Though he continued on Tylenol, he had needed no codeine for three days.

"Hey, Bobby, I'm going to take this hyperal, and it's going to make me fat!"

"That's right," said Kate, who was working three-to-eleven, "and nobody'll even know you!" She, too, sensed that a huge weight was being lifted from all of them and that nothing else could go wrong.

"Right, I'll be so fat that nobody will be able to recognize me!"

Bob said, "You'll have to wear a name tag!"

"Right! I'm going to get so much meat on me that all the girls will fall in love with me!"

"And," said Kate, "they won't worry about crushing you when they hug you!"

"Are you playing," Bob asked his son, "or shall Lisa and I just do this one by ourselves?"

"I'm playing! How about thirty cents, double or nothing?"

"Thirty cents? Naw, that's too much for me. I want to play for a dime. Lisa wants to play for a dime too, don't you, Lisa."

Mark looked scandalized. "A dime? Ten cents? How can you be so cheap?"

"So I'm cheap!"

"*Ten cents?*"

"Hey, Mark," Kate put in, "how are you on this new table, anyway? Won any games?"

"He's won every time," Lisa said mournfully. "He always wins. He was always the best."

Wednesday, January 9

After a poor night's sleep, Mark awoke feeling great anxiety about what the day held for him. But the morning chest film again revealed that the air cap in his pleural cavity had not increased. At noon, thirty-nine days after Mark's original lung collapse, his fourth and final chest tube was removed. A follow-up x-ray showed that the pneumothorax had improved slightly.

His long siege of pain had come to an end.

Ø

Downstairs in Isolation, nurse Frannie Lambert placed a red rubber ball in Freddy Eberly's left palm and tried to close his fingers around it. She was in her mid-twenties, the girl next door grown up but with the same bangs and barrettes.

"Squeeze the ball, Freddy."

His eyes seemed to study the ceiling. A crescent of tongue lay on the ledge of his lower lip, provoking associations with mental defectiveness. He was drooling. He wore a pale blue hospital gown, white socks striped in red and blue, and ankle-high white sneakers to prevent foot drop. The shoes and socks were brand new, bought for Freddy by his mother.

His left hand reverted slowly to recumbency. The red ball tipped onto the mattress. But Freddy could squeeze a little now with his right hand. As of this morning he was also feeling his tubes with that hand, holding onto the side rail of his bed, and pulling at the suction catheter whenever Frannie used it on him. He was alert enough now to feel discomfort when suctioned.

He was also beginning to communicate, Frannie thought. Sometimes he seemed to be looking straight at her. The nurses had been urging him to blink once for yes, twice for no. This morning it seemed to Frannie that Freddy was beginning to make those connections, to reengage with the universe he had left the morning the car had hit him.

He was improving in other ways. The bolt had been removed from his head, the drainage tube from his abdomen, the bandages from his broken right leg. He no longer needed an IV or a bladder catheter. The large incision in his abdomen was healing nicely. The pin sites in his leg were free of swelling or infection. The bruise and swelling over his left eye were diminishing. The tube draining his stomach contents out through one nostril had been replaced by a feeding tube into his small intestine. He was now being fed canned formula.

But he was still very far from being well. He swallowed poorly. He drooled and needed suctioning almost constantly. He needed percussion every twenty or thirty minutes to keep his lungs clear of fluid. He had to be put through range-of-motion exercises every four hours to minimize loss of muscle tone. He needed pin care on his broken leg once per shift or oftener. He required mouth and ear care. His position on the mattress had to be changed frequently to prevent bedsores. He had yet to regain control of his bowels.

Furthermore, Freddy's breathing difficulties had persisted. Thirteen days post-injury, the child still needed the respirator. While this of course raised questions about his future, it had also become a cause for immediate concern. Ever since his accident, the patient had been ventilated through a tube which entered his throat through his nose. Inevitably the tube rubbed against the vocal cords. Inevitably it would soon begin to erode that tissue. The only way to prevent this breakdown was to ventilate the patient through a tracheostomy, a hole cut into his windpipe below the vocal cords.

Doctors try hard to avoid taking this step. A surgical opening is a potential site for infection, and the patient will be left with a scar. But a trach tube can stay in for months without endangering vocal function. In cases such as Freddy's, a hole in the neck is the lesser of two evils. Unless the boy's own respiratory competency improved, he would have to be trached within the next couple of days.

Ø

Christmas was now more than two weeks gone. Most of the decorations had disappeared from the units, and the hospital chaplain noticed as he walked the halls and talked to staff and families that the load which had lightened somewhat toward the end of December had grown heavy again.

Scarcely a bed stood empty. Some of the sicker children who had been able to spend Christmas at home were being readmitted. Those whose deaths had been staved off for the biggest holidays of the year were now just marking time. It was the chaplain's impression that the incidence of meningitis and a viral infection called Reye's syndrome decreased in December, as if disease itself took a vacation. In recent days such admissions had started to increase. The chaplain had begun to gear up for January.

He was thirty-eight, a tall, slender blond man with the face of a boy and the short bangs of a storybook prince. Like most other professionals at Children's, he went about his business dressed informally. His business was to give pastoral support to parents and children in crisis and to the staff as needed. A Baptist minister and the stepfather of a seven-year-old, he had once studied nursing and had been brought to Children's originally because the oncologists wanted to make spiritual help available for their patients. The chaplain continued to devote nearly half his time to children with cancer and their families. The rest of his time went to anyone showing a desire for it. Many of his referrals came from nurses. Mostly, though, he walked the halls with his antennae out.

In his work with parents who acknowledged a religious force in their lives, the chaplain was sometimes asked to explain why God would permit the illness or death of a child. That mystery, he had observed, was nearly intolerable for many parents. Some reacted by interpreting the illness as God's punishment for their own sins. Punishment, genes, air pollution, bad luck, God's wish to test parental faith—some mothers and fathers could accept almost any explanation more easily than they could accept that the reason was unknown. How could God possibly not heal their child?

The chaplain did not get involved in defending God. His own philosophy held that sickness is part of life, and that God's involvement is to bear some of the suffering. He believed that parents who insisted on knowing the unknowable could become mired in despair. The chaplain attempted to lead parents away from that abyss. He attempted to help them toward an understanding that God's way was not necessarily their way or God's thoughts theirs.

Once a father had punched him for his efforts. The man's son had died after open-heart surgery. For a day or so the chaplain had wondered whether he wished to continue in a job that taxed his resources at every turn if he was going to be socked by the very people he was trying to help. But seeing that father again, he'd realized how badly the man had needed a punching bag.

For the same reasons parents got angry, the chaplain encountered anger in himself from time to time. He walked the halls of Children's Hospital feeling daily doubts about God. Hurting with parents, watching children lose their battles, the chaplain occasionally wondered why God was not more forthcoming about His purposes, or even more in evidence. He accepted these doubts as the essential ingredient of his faith. Doubts, as he saw it, were the difference between believing and knowing. Without them faith could not exist.

At times the demands of his job at Children's made the chaplain feel like a dried prune. He had learned that certain children had the power to restore his energy. He had learned this first from a little girl in Acute with a beautiful smile. She had eventually died. But whenever the chaplain had gone to see her, had held her hand, he had come away feeling that *she* had been ministering to *him*.

There were others. The children wrung the chaplain out, but they also kept him going.

Thursday, January 10

Late in the afternoon, Daniel Earnshaw having established to his complete satisfaction that St. Michael's Hospital was indeed equipped to care for a young patient receiving intravenous nutrition, the Children's staff members present at the multiservice conference called to review the management of the case agreed unanimously to start Mark Price on hyperalimentation and to transfer him to St. Michael's for the duration of the therapy.

Friday, January 11

On the third morning into The Conspiracy to Help Brandon, the patient woke up weighing 760 grams. While this was only a fraction above his birth weight, it was the heaviest he had been in nearly five weeks of life. Not only was he tolerating his feedings; he was also producing the little white worms of feces that are typical of early feeding stools. Furthermore, though needing a fair amount of oxygen support, he was down to only four breaths a minute now from the ventilator. The rest he was taking on his own.

He looked better than he had in some time. The bruises on his limbs had all but disappeared. His skin color was good. The outline of his rib cage had softened. He kicked vigorously but amiably under his blanket of Saran Wrap. In the pale blue stocking cap that Dory Hatfield had put on him for warmth, he looked positively elfin. He appeared to listen to every word she said to him.

She did his A.M. care feeling delighted about his progress and worried about his parents. Hatfield had never met the Gregorys. She had talked to them by phone just three times, the third time late yesterday afternoon. Brandon's mother had told the nurse during that conversation that she and her husband were fighting. The nurse had had the impression that Robin would have liked to visit her baby much more frequently than was possible to arrange.

Hatfield felt sorry for Brandon's mother. She felt sorry for his father. She'd heard that Tom Gregory had had a premie by his first wife and that the baby had died. If Brandon's father was protecting himself by keeping his distance, Hatfield could understand why. Yet she could also understand that his standing back must be hard on his wife.

Wanting Robin to know that she wasn't alone, Dory Hatfield had assured her that many parents in their situation had fights. She had encouraged Robin to look at things from her husband's point of view. Maybe because he wasn't working, he was feeling inadequate. Were the Gregorys able to talk with each other about how they were feeling?

Robin had said that they were, and that this had helped a little. The nurse had been glad to hear it. Now, however, reconstructing the conversation in her mind, Dory Hatfield made a mental note to call Brandon's parents more often and also to ask the social worker to give Brandon's mom and dad a call.

Ø

Freddy Eberly was scheduled for surgery at 1:00. Last evening for the second time since his accident, the doctors had attempted to free him from the ventilator by removing the nasotracheal tube to which he and the machine were both connected; and for the second time Freddy had flunked extubation. He had had trouble maintaining his airway and had blown off too little carbon dioxide. Obviously he still needed help from the machine, yet he could no longer be ventilated through an NT tube without endangering his vocal cords. The doctors had no choice but to send the patient for a tracheostomy.

Freddy's case had turned into a major puzzle for Colin Kendall. The boy was clearly conscious now. He was obeying commands, he was moving, he was keeping his eyes open at least half the time and making eye contact, he was apparently blinking now for yes. Aided by a physical therapist, his movement had progressed rapidly over the last two days. With his right limbs he could apparently do anything he wanted. This morning when a nurse had lifted Freddy's gown to bathe him, he had slid his right hand down his abdomen and covered his penis!

So he was definitely awake, and he looked awake enough to breathe on his own. Yet here they were two weeks out having to do a tracheostomy. Despite never having looked all that bad, the patient still wasn't looking all that good, in Kendall's opinion, and he had a hell of a long way to go. His legs continued to be of major concern.

The neurosurgeon was convinced that Freddy's problem resulted at least in part from brain stem injury, but he could not figure out exactly how such injury could have occurred. The boy had suffered diffuse brain trauma: not a direct blow to one spot but generalized trauma resulting from the snapping back and forth of his head on the pivot of his spine. As a rule in such cases, motor function tends to be preserved better than anything else because the brain stem, buried deep in the cranium like the core of a cabbage, is so well protected. The brunt of the insult is borne by the more vulnerable hemispheres, the centers of intelligence and awareness. Usually after diffuse head injury which does not inflict irretrievable damage, the most basic functions—breathing and movement—come back first.

With Freddy it was just the reverse. His consciousness appeared to be recovering better than the motor function below it.

The likeliest explanation, Kendall surmised, was a blood vessel spasm or stroke occurring as a result of the accident. An arteriogram might have shed light on this matter, but the test is an invasive procedure with known hazards. For now, at least, Kendall did not think the information gained would be worth the risk to the child. If spasm and cell death had occurred, there was nothing anyone could do about it. Injured cells that had survived would heal in their own time.

While the exact nature of Freddy's condition remained a mystery, however, his immediate future had been laid out for him. He would have to remain at Children's at least until he was breathing on his own. From Children's the boy would go to Leverett House for two to six months of intensive physiotherapy. Leverett House is a pediatric rehabilitation center with facilities at two sites. One is in a rural setting some ninety miles from the city. The other, the Annex, is located in leased space on the fifth floor of Children's Hospital. Freddy would go first to the Annex, where Kendall could keep an eye on him a while longer, and then would be transferred to the country when a bed there became available.

Meanwhile, now that the boy was conscious, Kendall wanted him out of Isolation as soon as his tracheostomy was stable. Freddy would be emerging from his coma with no idea of what had happened to him over the past two weeks. Being in a room that was void of activity could only delay his progress. Kendall wanted the patient up on a floor where he could be with other children. The doctor also wanted to get rehab specialists involved as soon as possible. The most important thing to be done for Freddy Eberly right now was to help him reenter the world.

Ø

While Freddy was in the Operating Room, Mark waited anxiously for his surgeon to visit him. Dr. Abe Weinberg was due up sometime this afternoon. Supposedly the surgery was scheduled for Monday. No one had told Mark that for certain. The uncertainty was making him nervous. So was the prospect of one more new experience. He had a lot of questions that nobody had answered yet. A little while ago he had asked for Valium because he was so anxious. Now he had a stomach ache, also because of nerves, he thought, and had asked for some Maalox.

He sipped some cola from the can on his bedside table. Next to the can lay the get-well card that Lisa had brought in to him yesterday just before she was discharged. He reread the note she had written. It said:

Mark,

I just want to say I think you're a really great person. Thank you for our talk. It helped me. I know in my heart it's going to work out for both of us, so just hang in there. Even if we have to come in again, I know it's going to be a good year for both of us. Take care,

Love always,
Lisa

Inside the card she had put a five-dollar bill. Her giving him money had upset him. He told himself now that when he got out of the hospital, he would buy her something nice with the five dollars and send it to her.

Shortly after 3:00, Mark had a visitor—not the visitor he was waiting for, but someone he was glad to see: Pastor Arthur Stroud, his minister from home. Mark welcomed him warmly, telling him how much he appreciated the cards and letters from his new friends in the congregation.

The pastor had visited Mark once before at Children's, in December. They had talked that day about the nurses, the doctors, the food, the care, the boy in the next bed, the game room, the hospital itself. Today Stroud could hardly believe the change in Mark. The child looked very ill. His feelings also seemed closer to the surface than they had in December. When describing his joy over being transferred to St. Michael's, Mark also expressed concern for his parents' fatigue and said how glad he was that now they wouldn't have to travel so far. He gave Stroud the impression that he felt himself to be a burden to his family. As they talked, the pastor realized that while in December he had been visiting a boy, he was now in the presence of a mature individual.

At one point in the conversation Mark pulled open the drawer of his bedside table and took out his Beck Bible. People being visited by a minister are often moved to bring out a Bible. However, Stroud was surprised to hear Mark talk at some length about his habit of reading chapters nightly, and the pastor was not expecting specific questions. Mark said he had quite a few. However, since he was tired, he said, he would like only one answered now, if Pastor Stroud wouldn't mind. Would the pastor talk a little bit about Jesus saying He had come to raise swords and divide families? He showed Stroud Matthew 10, verses 34 and 35:

> Don't think that I am come to bring peace on earth. I didn't come to bring peace but a sword. I came to set a man against his father, a daughter against her mother, a daughter-in-law against her mother-in-law.

The pastor assured the boy that the passage was simply a historical statement referring to the fact that when Jews joined the Christian faith, their families had declared them dead.

The boy seemed much relieved by this interpretation. After a moment he said to his pastor, "If something happened to me, what would it do to my parents?"

The question was unique in Stroud's experience. He replied, with a firmness he truly felt, "They will be capable of taking it."

They talked a little longer. Death was not mentioned. But it was obvious to Stroud by the time he left that Mark had made peace with his conflicts and had reached the point of being able to let go.

As the pastor was leaving, his young parishioner reached out to shake his hand. "Thank you so much for coming," he said. "I really appreciate your driving all the way down here."

"Next time I see you," Stroud said, "you'll be up at St. Michael's. When you get there, I'll be glad to have communion for you and your parents at the hospital, if you'd like."

The patient said he would like that very much.

He waited the rest of the afternoon for the surgeon growing more and more upset. By evening he was depressed enough to refuse dinner. It was Friday. Except for emergencies, the surgeons would not be working over the weekend. Could the surgery still take place on Monday? If not, that meant three days' delay for him in getting up to St. Michael's.

About 7:00 P.M. he was started on a dilute dose of hyperal through a vein in his arm. Kate's efforts to cheer him up were totally unsuccessful.

"In poor spirits today," she wrote in his chart at midnight. "Wanting to sleep the day away."

Sunday, January 13

In the wee hours of the morning, Dory Hatfield dreamed that one of the babies in the Infant ICU was going to do badly.

Once in a great while she had dreams about what certain patients might be like at four or five. Otherwise the hospital left the nurse alone when she slept except for occasional dreams that something was about to go wrong.

This had not happened for more than a year. The last time the subject had been an older baby Hatfield had taken care of in the Infant ICU who had gotten well enough to go upstairs to the Stepdown Unit. The night after her dream the baby had arrested and died.

Almost any nurse has the ability to come in at the beginning of a shift and say, "There's something wrong with this baby." Predicting, Hatfield believed, was another matter.

Nurses sometimes have a feeling about how a given patient is likely to turn out. Hatfield thought her roommate very good at being able to say right at the beginning whether a baby was or was not going to do well without ever having had any exposure to the patient. When she felt someone was not going to do well, she never took care of that baby. She had guessed wrong on occasion. So had Dory Hatfield. They had both been right often enough, however, that they had learned to pay attention to these inner voices, even though Hatfield found them scary. Wondering if these feelings were in any sense supernatural, she rarely talked about them to anyone.

But whenever she dreamed that a baby did badly, she always called in before going to work. Once she got to the unit, she was always extra careful to go over her patients with the greatest attentiveness.

The patient in her dream early Sunday morning was the little girl Hatfield had taken care of for the whole two and a half months of the baby's life.

But on the phone a few hours later, the nurse learned that Trisha was just fine, and so was everybody else in the unit except those patients who'd already been doing badly or who had been expected to do badly.

At 10:00 when Robin Gregory called the Infant ICU to find out how Brandon was, she was told he was doing well. A bladder infection he had developed on Friday was responding to treatment. His respiratory function had greatly improved over the past few days. His ventilator settings had been decreased to almost nothing. After nearly a week of successful feeds, he was still digesting without difficulty. In fact his doctors had begun to anticipate that the baby's transfer to the Stepdown Unit was not too far off.

Robin was thrilled. "We'll be in this evening," she told the nurse who answered. Low on money, low on gas, the Gregorys had not been to Children's for eight days. Robin couldn't wait to get there.

But within a very short time after his mother's phone call, Brandon's rosiness began to fade. He began to look poor and then very poor. The doctors ordered tests and x-rays. None of the studies yielded any hard information to suggest what might be going on.

Hours later, at approximately 9:15 P.M., Brandon Gregory's parents arrived in the Infant ICU to find a baby who seemed to them to have lost all his color.

Shocked, Robin said to the nurse who was suctioning Brandon, "What's wrong?"

The nurse drew the suction catheter out of her patient's throat. For some reason she stalled answering. "He doesn't look so well right now because of what I'm doing to him. He usually turns a little blue when I'm taking the mucus out."

But when she had finished, the baby looked no better.

"He looks really sick," Robin said. "He looks like he's dying."

The nurse replied quietly, "He hasn't looked good all day."

"Well, are they doing anything about it?"

"They're running some tests, but so far they can't find anything wrong with him. They'll be doing some more tests and really keeping an eye on him through the night."

"Will they let us know as soon as they find something out?"

"Of course."

Alone with her baby, Robin slipped her hand under the Saran Wrap covering Brandon and began to stroke his hand. She saw immediately that this bothered him.

So instead of touching him, she wound up his bunny and played the bunny for him over and over again. When he first heard the music, he opened his eyes and looked all around. He even moved his head toward the bunny. He seemed to be lying there listening. After a while he dropped off to sleep.

But it was obvious to Robin that something was wrong with him. Taking off her gown in the anteroom some minutes later, she said to her husband, "It's like every time you go in there and think he's doing well and get a little bit of hope, the next time there's something to take that hope away from you."

Monday, January 14

On the morning of his thirty-seventh day of life outside his mother's womb, nine weeks and five days before the date upon which he should have been born, Brandon Gregory crashed. His deterioration was so swift and so decisive that by the time the doctors understood what was wrong with the baby, they were virtually powerless to help him.

The first solid sign of trouble appeared in the results of a blood gas study which reached the Infant ICU about 2:45 A.M. Read by the second-year resident covering the unit overnight, the study showed an acid imbalance in the patient's system.

The resident was concerned but not alarmed. While acidosis can reflect the beginnings of necrotizing enterocolitis, NEC is not the likeliest explanation. Acidosis is rather common in tiny premies. Their immature kidneys cannot metabolize acids very well.

All the same, the resident ordered an abdominal x-ray. She also ordered a dose of bicarbonate for Brandon. He received it about 3:00 A.M. and responded to it well. The x-ray done about the same time confirmed the absence of even a hint of NEC. Had there been a hint, the resident would have stopped the patient's tube feedings imediately so as not to exacerbate the problem. A second x-ray, done at 6:00 A.M., was likewise innocent. Feeds were continued.

At 7:00 A.M. Dory Hatfield came on duty. As usual she checked on her patients before going into the nurses' lounge for report. Brandon didn't look bad to Hatfield, but something about him didn't look quite right either. Hatfield discussed this with the night nurse, who agreed and who mentioned the acidosis. Two words came into Hatfield's mind: necrotizing enterocolitis.

When report was over about 7:30, she went to Brandon's bedside, slipped a narrow tape measure under his back, and measured his abdomen. His girth was no bigger than it had been on Saturday or Sunday. Next the nurse tested a little of the baby's stool for occult blood. Negative. With a syringe she drew back on the patient's feeding tube, checking to see whether he had residual feeding in his stomach. No. He was absorbing the feeds. He was not cyanotic.

At 8:00 Logan Sadler reported for duty. So did the fellow who was the third member of The Conspiracy to Help Brandon. Motioning the doctors to his bedside, Dory Hatfield told them she had a funny feeling about the baby.

"It's nothing I can put my finger on," she said to the others. "He's not doing anything specific. But he's just not up to snuff."

The three agreed that they would watch the patient extra carefully over the next few hours. When at 8:30 Logan Sadler was called out on transport to pick up a newborn at another hospital, she asked the resident covering the unit to please walk by the baby's bedside a little more often than she otherwise might while Sadler was gone.

At 9:00 the residents came through on rounds with the neonatologist replacing Roger Forbes as this month's attending physician in the unit. The doctors took note of the patient's acidosis. They talked about his need for sodium supplements. As they stood watching him, the baby was kicking and active. The attending commented that Brandon didn't look too bad. When he added, "Maybe it's his belly," he was speaking facetiously. NEC occurs most often in babies about two weeks of age. This patient was really too old for it. The doctors continued on their way.

At about 9:15 Dory Hatfield left Brandon to work with a patient at the other end of the unit. Fifteen minutes later she happened to pass Brandon's warmer bed on an errand. Glancing down at him, she stopped short. He was cyanotic. His heart and respiratory rates were way up. His belly was distended. He looked ghastly. Hatfield took her measuring tape from her pocket. The baby's girth was three centimeters larger than it had been at 7:30.

Just then the head nurse walked by. Before even noticing the baby, she caught sight of the stricken face of her colleague.

"Get the guys back here," Hatfield said heavily, "and call a STAT x-ray."

The doctors returned in a group. Seconds later the grim-faced attending physician said aloud what Dory Hatfield already knew beyond a doubt and what everyone else could plainly see. The baby had full-blown necrotizing enterocolitis. The x-ray done a few minutes later showed bubbles of air in the walls of Brandon Gregory's gut from stem to stern.

The only hope was surgery. If the affected bowel were removed, if enough good bowel were left to provide Brandon with a functioning digestive tract, the baby might pull through—if he survived the operation itself.

A call was placed to the surgeons. While the stunned pediatricians began instituting treatments to attack the acidosis and counteract the dangerous fluid loss which accompanies NEC, Brandon's abdomen grew so distended that it began to interfere severely with his breathing. Within no time he required maximum respiratory support from the ventilator. The baby could no longer breathe at all on his own.

Roger Forbes walked into the unit about 10:00. He had arranged to meet a mother there to discuss the possibility of transferring her baby to a hospital in a city closer to where the parents lived. While not in charge of the unit this month, Forbes was also paying daily visits to a couple of the patients he'd felt most concerned about last month, one being Brandon Gregory.

Standing with the mother near the unit clerk's desk, Forbes was aware of a general sense of commotion around him which he took to mean that things had suddenly gotten very busy. He and the mother completed their business in fairly short order. A moment later Forbes fell into conversation with an English physician who happened to be visiting the Infant ICU. As the two stood chatting, a resident came over to take a phone call, saw Forbes, and handed him the x-ray she was holding.

"Take a look at this," she said, picking up the receiver, "and tell me if you've ever seen necrotizing enterocolitis as bad."

Forbes and the Englishman looked at the film long enough to see that it showed a terrible case of NEC. Having no idea where it had come from, Forbes read the film as any doctor might read any interesting x-ray. Moments later he handed it back to the resident with a comment or two and resumed his conversation with the visitor never dreaming that the x-ray belonged to a patient he knew.

The truth hit him when he started toward Brandon's bedside. Suddenly Forbes became aware that several people were working over his former patient, and one of them was the fellow in general surgery.

The baby's appearance shocked Roger Forbes. Brandon was still active and alert, was still looking at the people around him, but he was gray all over, his belly was extremely tense and ugly-looking, and the abdominal blood vessels were distended like bad varicose veins, a sign of liver involvement. The belly got bigger and grayer as Forbes stood watching.

He could hardly believe his eyes. The doctors tending Brandon were having the same problem.

"He was fine at rounds an hour ago," they kept saying to each other in disbelief.

In all his years at Children's Hospital, Roger Forbes had never seen a case of NEC progress so fast.

The news was conveyed to Robin Gregory over the phone by a resident she had never met. Wanting to give the baby's parents time to adjust, the resident did not tell Robin that the surgeons had already been called. She simply said that Brandon would have to go to surgery if he didn't improve within an hour.

Robin had called the unit at daybreak. Exceedingly concerned about the way Brandon had looked to her on Sunday, she had questioned the night nurse closely. The nurse had reported to her that while the baby still looked a little off, the doctors had been unable to find anything wrong with him, and he seemed to be doing okay. Or so Robin had interpreted the nurse's answer. Now she was being told that in the space of two hours the baby's belly had blown up, and they had discovered something so wrong with him that he would probably need another operation.

The mother responded in shock, fear, and indignation. "Couldn't they have found this last night?"

The person she was talking to told her they had x-rayed Brandon last night, and the x-ray had shown no sign of trouble. In fact they'd seen no sign of trouble on a second x-ray done at 6:00 this morning.

Robin Gregory found this statement very hard to believe.

A surgeon called her back an hour later. He needed the parents' permission for surgery.

Tom Gregory gave his permission over the phone. He told the surgeon that he and Robin would be in as soon as possible.

The surgeon told the Gregorys that their baby was not likely to survive.

The surgery could not take place immediately. For one thing, Brandon would have to wait until a table opened up in the OR and a general surgeon was free to work on him. For another, the Infant ICU staff wanted to build the baby up for the operation as much as possible by giving him blood products and everything else they could think of that might help him come out of the surgery alive.

At 11:15 Logan Sadler and the other members of the transport team entered the unit with their new patient. As they wheeled the incubator toward an empty warmer bed, a nurse stopped the resident with a hand on her arm and said simply, "Brandon's in bad shape."

Sadler went immediately to the baby's bedside. Dory Hatfield watched with sympathy as the young doctor's chin hit the floor.

Ø

The morning had been little kinder to Mark Price. His surgery had finally been scheduled for Tuesday, but at approximately the same time as Logan Sadler had gone out on transport, Mark had been told that because Tuesday was Martin Luther King's birthday and a holiday for some hospital staff members, his operation would have to be postponed until Wednesday. This news had brought him close to tears.

Besides having ragged nerves, he had a headache, his stomach hurt so much from coughing that he'd had to ask for a heating pad, and at breakfast time the hyperal needle had infiltrated his vein and had had to be replaced. The day so far had been so lousy for him that he had asked his mother not to leave his room unless she had to, telling her he didn't want to die.

Yet amazingly, he could still see a bright side. He actually thought he could feel the hyperal beginning to work a little bit. He was surprised at how much energy he had. When he walked around, he didn't get out of breath as quickly as he would have expected himself to after six weeks in bed. When the social worker came in to see how he felt, Mark was able to reply that aside from the nerves and the headache and the fever and the stomach ache, he felt pretty good.

When the social worker had gone, Mark showed his mother a Valium tablet taped to the inside of his right knee. Her amazement made him grin. "I asked them for one when I didn't really need it so I can have it handy in case I really need it in a hurry!"

Around 2:00 Dr. Griffin visited Mark, and when he left, Ellen followed him out of the unit and handed him a three-page synopsis of the talk Mark had had with her and Bob about his future. Profoundly touched by that event, she had later reconstructed as much of it as she remembered, and Bob had had her summary typed and photocopied at his office. She had titled it simply "A Conversation with Mark."

Reading the document back in his lab, Bruce Griffin was impressed by the openness evident between the boy and his parents. After a long time on separate wavelengths, they appeared to have gotten together very fast. Griffin was further impressed by Mark's realistic grasp of his situation. On the day he'd demanded admission so many weeks ago, he had seemed controlled by his fears. Now, Griffin thought, he seemed in charge of them.

Upstairs Ellen Price was showing the Conversation to the head nurse on Adolescent, who, upon reading Mark's innermost thoughts about his life and death, wept in his mother's arms.

Ø

At 3:00 Lea Bowersox reported for duty in the Infant ICU and, along with all the other three-to-eleven nurses coming on at that hour, was dumbfounded by the news of what had happened to Brandon.

By this time the baby's eyes were half shut and very glazed. Bowersox was convinced he was in pain.

There was still a lot to be done for him before surgery, and there was a lot of paperwork. Lea Bowersox was assigned to Brandon at her own request. One of the first things she did for him was to administer baptismal rites. After that, unable to speak, she tended him in utter silence.

He was Bowersox's patient now, but Dory Hatfield could not bring herself to go home.

He was wheeled out of the unit at 5:30. Shortly thereafter his parents arrived. Lea Bowersox went out to talk to them. To prepare the Gregorys, the nurse told them how poor Brandon looked, how blue he was, how little like himself he would appear when they saw him after surgery if he survived the surgery. The Gregorys asked few questions. Because they seemed to need nothing from her, because she was having almost as much trouble talking as they were, Bowersox soon left Brandon's parents and went back into the ICU.

Ø

Meanwhile Dr. Abe Weinberg had left his office and started for the Adolescent Unit. A short, balding man in his mid-thirties, Weinberg had sleepy eyes and baggy cheeks that made him appear perpetually fatigued. His sensitivity to children and concern for all aspects of their well-being had given him a reputation as "the most un-surgeon-like surgeon" at Children's.

Asked to name the operations he most liked doing, Abe Weinberg would not have mentioned the insertion of hyperalimentation lines. In children this surgery tends to be highly frustrating for the surgeon because a child's veins are so small. Mark Price posed additional challenges. At the patient's bedside, this fact bore in upon Abe Weinberg within minutes. He was reminded immediately by the dressing on Mark's chest that this boy had had one pneumothorax already which had taken weeks to stabilize. To avoid puncturing the other lung by mistake, Weinberg would have to proceed with extreme caution.

While they talked, the doctor noted the respiratory distress Mark was having just sitting in bed. Hearing from the boy that he was unable to lie down any longer, that he breathed while eating by gulping air between bites of food, and seeing this patient in what should have been the prime of his life suffering literally for every breath made a very painful impression upon Weinberg. He saw a boy in no condition to tolerate the usual approach to the kind of surgery he was about to have.

This approach, similar in principle to the placement of a chest tube, requires the patient to be lying down. Since Mark could not tolerate that position, he would have to have a cut-down. Instead of inserting the catheter blindly into the selected vessel, Weinberg would have to make an incision in the skin to actually visualize the vein. Ordinarily a cut-down is also done with the patient lying down. However, the supine position is not vital for this operation.

Weinberg explained the procedure. Mark then asked him questions which told the surgeon that somebody had taken a lot of time with this boy. He also saw a youngster articulate in expressing his needs. Without at all complaining, Mark made it very clear to the doctor that he did not care to suffer during the operation.

Weinberg left his new patient pondering the ethics of the situation. He thought just looking at Mark that it would be surprising if the boy lived a year. The use of hyperal in CF was recent and controversial. Weinberg knew there was some evidence that the therapy made those patients better for short periods. Improved nourishment greatly affects any patient's sense of well-being. Mark's doctors had agreed that the boy would benefit from hyperal. Presuming that they had not drawn this conclusion lightly, Weinberg felt he could perform the operation with a clear conscience.

But he would perform it with reservations. If hyperal made the boy temporarily stronger, wasn't that just prolonging his agony? He was in such dire straits that Weinberg wondered whether nutrition could possibly make a difference. What the therapy offered Mark at this point, the surgeon feared, was too little too late.

Ø

Two floors down in the Operating Room, a colleague of Weinberg's had made his incision into Brandon Gregory's massively distended abdomen with precisely the same fear.

Now, drawing forth loop after loop of gangrenous bowel into the stern light of the operating field, the surgeon saw that the situation was hopeless.

He did the only thing he could do. He replaced all of the bowel except one small portion which he cut and anchored to a small hole he made in the baby's abdomen. As a vent for noxious gases, this would provide a measure of comfort for the patient in his final hours. Then the surgeon sewed up his original incision, and at 7:20 P.M. Brandon Gregory was returned to the Infant ICU to die.

The surgeon talked with the parents in the unit waiting room. Lea Bowersox sat with them. When the doctor had gone, Robin Gregory began to cry.

Dory Hatfield came in and introduced herself. She, too, was crying. She told the Gregorys that she had come to love Brandon very much.

In her own anguish Robin heard this and was glad. At least someone else had loved him.

The Gregorys were told that their baby would probably die before morning. Robin wanted to stay with Brandon. Tom Gregory wanted to take his wife home. He thought that would be best for both of them. While Robin did not think so, she saw that she was not going to change her husband's mind.

But when Lea Bowersox asked them if they wanted to see Brandon before they left, Robin told Tom that she did not intend to leave the hospital without saying goodbye to her son.

Bowersox tried again to prepare them, but the sight of the baby made his parents stop walking a few feet short of his bedside.

Robin Gregory went a little closer. Tears streamed down her cheeks. Though his eyes were shielded by his sunglasses, Tom Gregory, too, had tears on his cheeks. Neither touched the baby.

Lea Bowersox stood wishing the Gregorys were different people. There was so much she could be doing to support them if only they would give her the opportunity, if only they would say what they were thinking, if only they would express a need.

Dory Hatfield stood nearby wishing that Lea Bowersox would offer the parents a chance to hold the baby. Hatfield did not make the suggestion herself because to do so might be taken as an invasion of the other nurse's domain.

Brandon's mother stood looking at the huge bandage covering her son's belly and wished with all her heart that she had not let the doctors cut him again.

Ø

As the Gregorys made their sad way home, Mark received a visit from anesthesiology resident Susan Carlson, the same doctor who had assisted with Candy Rudolph's operation.

She found him eating raw onions from a plate. As they talked, he moved on to a dish of vanilla pudding and then to a couple of cupcakes. Making mental notes, Carlson examined him. The instant she placed a stethoscope to his chest, she knew that general anesthesia was out of the question for this patient. Aided only by a little sedation, she would have to talk him through surgery.

He began to question her about the procedure. Though he never said so specifically, most of his questions related to his fears about feeling suffocated. Never in her brief career had Carlson been so thoroughly questioned by any patient, adult or child.

Nor had she ever encountered a child who so fully understood the gravity of his illness or so badly wanted to live. In the course of their conversation, Carlson was struck again and again by the boy's incredible drive to stay alive. In fact she thought his will had to be keeping him alive, because his body was a wreck.

As they talked, the role she would play in his surgery assumed rough shape in her thoughts. Her goal would be to get his mind off what the surgeon was doing. She would talk to him about junk food, for example, and the books he had been reading. Through the power of suggestion, she would encourage Mark's thoughts in a positive direction, saying not "Does it hurt?" but rather "You're looking pretty good." Without presuming to minimize his situation, she would try to have an intelligent, adult conversation with the boy on aspects of life other than the surgery.

Talking someone through an entire operation, particularly a youngster, is fairly rare. Children ordinarily aren't very amenable to such techniques, which is one reason local anesthesia isn't used much in children. Nevertheless, Carlson felt reasonably confident about meeting this challenge. She had been trained in the techniques she would use with Mark. To some extent anesthesiologists use these techniques with all patients, adults or children. Basically, Carlson would be providing distraction.

The greater challenge with this patient, she felt, was medical—to give this boy enough narcotic to keep him comfortable without suppressing his respirations. She left his room never dreaming that the intellectual struggle she faced in the operating room on Wednesday morning would score her soul.

When she had gone, Mark sat alone shuffling cards and feeling grateful for the concern shown him by both the anesthesiologist and the surgeon. He had liked them and been happy to finally see them. From the way they had described the operation, it seemed it wasn't going to be as bad as having chest tubes put in, and they were going to knock him out more. They'd said if all went well, it would only take about thirty minutes.

He hoped he wouldn't do anything dumb or make stupid comments or say anything really obscene.

He told himself that whatever he might say, they'd have probably heard worse.

He hoped he wouldn't be naked.

He dealt the cards out for solitaire. His mother had gone home tonight but would be returning tomorrow to stay overnight so she could be with him before he went to the operating room.

He couldn't wait till she got back. He thought she probably realized that he was being a little overanxious about the operation and would comfort him and relieve his overanxiety.

Ø

Robin Gregory tossed and turned most of the night. She awoke Tuesday morning about 6:00 surprised that she had slept at all. The phone rang at 6:30.

Tuesday, January 15

Roger Forbes arrived at Children's at 7:30 A.M. Leaving his coat in his office, he went up to the Infant ICU to check on Brandon Gregory and saw that the baby's bed was empty.

He found the staff very downcast. Those feeling worst were the three women who'd launched The Conspiracy to Help Brandon: the fellow, who yesterday had been near tears; Logan Sadler, who in losing Brandon had experienced the first death among the babies she had taken care of regularly in the unit; and Dory Hatfield. All kept thinking they had somehow failed their tiny patient.

Feeling rotten himself, Forbes sat down with the women at the nurses' station and discussed with them what might have been done differently. How could they have saved the baby?

They went over events with a fine-tooth comb. The first hard sign of trouble had been the acidosis at 3:00 Monday morning. Had the resident covering overnight missed something? Reviewing the facts, Forbes saw nothing the young doctor should have pursued that she hadn't.

If feeds had been stopped right then, might that have changed the ultimate course of the disease? Extremely unlikely, Forbes's experience told him. Had they pushed the baby too fast on feeds that first weekend after Logan Sadler had been hospitalized? Had his caregivers, feeling high because Brandon had come through PDA surgery so beautifully, become cavalier about what the baby could tolerate?

But the only result, Forbes pointed out, had been a little distension which had gone away. Meantime three weeks had elapsed. Over the week just past, the baby had been absorbing his feedings without difficulty. Except for the acidosis, which could have indicated a variety of other problems, the usual hints that the patient was developing necrotizing enterocolitis had been absent in Brandon Gregory right up until he suddenly exhibited all the signs at once.

Would he have gotten NEC, Sadler wondered, if he had received no feeds, if he had gotten only hyperalimentation through a central line? But the baby might very well have died on the operating table while the line was being placed, Forbes reminded her. Babies on long courses of hyperal develop a liver condition much like cirrhosis which can be fatal. Eventually a baby has to eat. If they'd waited any longer to feed Brandon, he might have died of malnutrition.

No, Forbes said to the women, if we had it to do all over again, there really isn't a thing we'd do differently. There was no way we could have prevented what happened to Brandon Gregory on Monday. In essence the baby had been dead within an hour. All the rest, Forbes said, was just scrambling around.

The three women nodded looking unconvinced. Two of them stood on the threshold of careers in medicine. Roger Forbes gave the three a pep talk.

He could have used one himself.

Tom and Robin Gregory arrived at Children's at about 10:30. Logan Sadler went into the parents' lounge to talk with them. Robin had not known until now that the Dr. Sadler she'd heard about was a woman.

The resident attempted to convey to the family her own distress about Brandon and the distress of the entire ICU staff. Wishing to neutralize any guilt the parents might be feeling about any aspect of the baby's life or death, Sadler assured them that he could have gotten no better care than he had received in the Infant ICU at Children's Hospital. If the Gregorys ever needed to talk to someone about Brandon, the young doctor told them, or if they ever wanted moral support, staff was available a day from now, a year from now, anytime.

Robin sat weeping. Tom stared into space. He did mention to Sadler that he'd had a premature infant by his first wife and that that baby, too, had died. He also told the resident that he had never expected Brandon to live. It seemed to Sadler that the Gregorys wanted only to be alone. To be elsewhere. To sign the autopsy papers, to see the baby, and to be gone.

The doctor did not blame them.

They had been asked to consider an autopsy by the person who'd called to tell them that Brandon had died. They'd said yes over the phone. Tom hoped an autopsy would reveal something helpful to other kids. Robin wanted it done because last night when she'd seen Brandon looking so sick, she'd felt he was being neglected. Reluctant though she was to put the baby through it, his mother wanted an autopsy for her own satisfaction.

Dory Hatfield brought the infant into the parents' lounge and laid him in his mother's arms.

When the nurse had asked them upon their arrival whether they wanted to hold the baby, Tom had said no for them both. He did not want to hold Brandon himself, and he did not want his wife to hold him. She was too upset already, in Tom's opinion. He didn't like seeing her so upset.

But Robin had told her husband that if she didn't hold her baby one more time, she'd regret it for the rest of her life.

He was swathed in blankets. Just his head and one little hand were showing.

Crying, Robin took his hand. She was struck by how peaceful he looked. Realizing that all his tubes were gone, his mother also realized that for the first and last time, Brandon Gregory was just a baby in a blanket.

Ø

Evening. The volume on Freddy Eberly's TV set was turned up high. The program was a rerun of *I Love Lucy*. Freddy's dark eyes gazed steadily at the screen. So he could look straight at it by merely opening his eyes, the back of his bed had been cranked up and his head propped with rolled towels. The child was now connected to the respirator through a small opening at the base of his neck. On his head was a brand-new red baseball cap. On one shoulder was a towel put there to catch the secretions drooling from his open mouth.

The action on the screen turned frenzied. The studio audience laughed uproariously. The boy's expression did not change.

His mother had brought in some photographs. Several of the pictures had been taped inside the rails of his bed, others to the big window between his room in Isolation and the room next door— photographs to remind Freddy Eberly who he was and to whom he belonged: a studio picture of Freddy with his mom when he was six and wore an Afro; a photo of his maternal grandmother in a green dress smiling at the camera from a green field; snapshots of Grandma Baker all dressed up and holding a birthday cake; a group of happy kids, one holding a doll; Freddy and a male cousin in suits, hamming for the camera; a girl and a boy playing with toy soldiers in front of a fireplace.

And the patient's last school picture: the head and shoulders of a boy in a blue-gray suit. On his serious face was the hint of a small, stiff smile. Undoubtedly in response to instructions, the subject had fixed his eyes on a point somewhere to the right of the camera. The result was a faraway gaze that made Frederick Patterson Eberly appear to be a child with his future on his mind.

His nurse had gone on her break telling Freddy that his mother was on her way in. Was he waiting for her? Had he understood that she might be late because a heavy sleet was falling? Now that he had regained consciousness, did it frighten him to be alone? What did he know? think? feel? perceive? remember?

Of the two weeks he had spent unconscious, he would remember nothing. Coma looks like sleep but is actually much closer to the state induced by anesthesia. Though the brain still responds to such stimuli as flashing lights, intellectual functions cease. Awareness is suspended. Events go unrecorded. The person awakes with no appreciation even that time has elapsed.

Freddy Eberly could hear what was said to him and could carry out an assigned task. But what did he understand about himself? Severe head injuries may obliterate memory. The worse the trauma, the more history is lost, which inevitably affects a person's sense of identity.

One patient referred to Colin Kendall had fallen headfirst through a stairwell onto a concrete floor. The boy had been ten at the time. When he had awakened after a month in coma, his own name had meant nothing to him. His mother and father were strangers—nice strangers, but people he did not recognize. He did not recognize photographs of himself in family albums. The first few times his parents had taken him home from Leverett House for weekend visits, he had thought he was being kidnapped.

The boy had recovered beautifully. Now thirteen, he was back in private school and doing well, though with some adjustment problems. But his fall had erased most of what he'd known about his life until that moment. In a humorous mood, he would fix his date of birth at the moment of regaining consciousness. "Remember, now, I'm only three years old!" As for the strangers who had finally brought him home to stay, they had become his family the day he had realized that only parents would have done so much for him. If they cared that much, he must be their son. That they had conceived him and raised him he had decided to take on faith.

Freddy Eberly had been almost as badly hurt. Waking up now to find his body unusable and his life in the hands of strangers, he had to be suffering deep confusions. Months or even years might pass before he could sort them out. Though he might soon become conscious enough to talk—providing his injury had left him able to talk—he would be mute until he came off the ventilator and his tracheostomy was closed. Until he found a way to ask them, his questions would go unanswered. Until he found a way to express them, any fears he had would go ignored—unless a nurse looking into his eyes or his mother imagining his thoughts divined his need and stroked his cheek at just the right moment.

Otherwise he was alone.

His mother stood in line at McDonald's and shivered. Melting sleet dripped from her raincoat, the umbrella she carried in one hand, the plastic shopping bag she carried along with her large denim bag in the other. She was glad for the light, the piped-in music, the presence of strangers she did not have to talk to. The trip in tonight had been especially long and cold. Once or twice Freddy's father had brought her in. Other people had also offered. She preferred to set her own time, to come early instead of after supper, because by then the staff had been working on him all day, she reasoned, and her attempts to make him respond were very tiring for him.

She purchased a container of black coffee, found herself a small table in a corner, and sipped her coffee slowly, planning how she would spend her time with her son. She had a surprise in her shopping bag: a new baseball glove. She tried to have something special for him each time she came. She had brought in the photographs, some bright pictures clipped from magazines, his wallet, his radio, the times table chart he had made with the answers behind little flaps. He loved doing times tables. In fact he'd been teaching them to her.

Maybe tonight she'd say, "Freddy, do the Robot." The kids didn't do that dance much anymore, but he still liked it. If he wasn't responding very well, she would read the book about a daughter learning to set the table. Freddy liked to set the table, and his mother wanted to give him a memory.

It was Sharita Queen's understanding that wherever Freddy's mind was these days, he was probably someplace he wanted to be. Believing this, she also believed that he could bring himself through whenever he was ready. He and the Lord were going to have to work that out. The doctors did everything they could, but they didn't know what was on Freddy's mind any more than his mother did. The child had always liked to try to help himself. This was the time for him to show her that he could take care of himself. She only wanted to be able to say that she had done everything she could for him.

The nurses and doctors had told her she could help him by talking to him. In fact, they'd told her that the more people talked to him, the better off he'd be. Sharita Queen believed this too, believed that to help Freddy come out of himself, it would take more than his mother. This was why she had brought in his cousin Justine on Sunday. Justine was ten. Ordinarily a child that age would not have been allowed to visit, but the nurses had said to bring her because Freddy needed the company.

There were others whose help Freddy's mother would have liked to enlist, had she had that power. His grandparents lived in the city but were waiting for him to come home. They had their fears, she knew that. But Freddy needed company now, in her opinion, not when people got ready to see him.

His father. His father had never had much contact with Freddy, but he had gone to pieces when he'd heard about the accident. He had started to visit his son at Children's. About this Sharita Queen had at first felt very pleased. Ever since the child's birth she had been trying to get his father to be closer to the boy and take more of an interest in him. Now she had stopped trying. Urging Freddy's father to spend time with him at the hospital, she would suddenly realize that she was pushing him more than he wanted to come. Or she'd be talking to Freddy about his father and suddenly think: *Well, he might not want to be bothered with his father right now.*

The truth was that all Freddy had ever cared about was her. Whenever she went out, he always wanted to know what time she was coming back and who was going to take care of him until she got home. His concern was all for her and for what she was doing. So she was not going to push anybody else, and she was not going to worry about anybody else. She was going to concentrate on him and her. The others could do as they wished.

Nonetheless, her son's father was a sustaining presence for Sharita Queen, as was her godmother, Grandma Baker, who had been with her when Freddy was born. Beyond these two people, she needed no one. She believed she could concentrate better just keeping to herself. She wanted nobody to pity her. This situation was in the doctors' care and the Lord's.

It was teaching her to be a strong person. Sharita Queen felt proud of the way she was handling Freddy's accident. Not being a nurse, she would not have thought she could accept what had happened to her son.

But she had had to accept it, and she had been able to carry on. She did not moan and groan when she came in to see Freddy. She did not feel she was putting a lot of pressure on the nurses. In fact most of the time the nurses asked *her* to help *them*! Each day she prayed that she would get stronger, that she would be able to accept whatever lay in store for him. Each day she did feel stronger. It strengthened her to see him responding more and more. The worst time had been that first week, when he'd seemed to be at a complete standstill. She just thanked God that she had held up and had come far enough now to begin to relax.

Minutes later she entered his room, greeted the nurse, greeted her son. His head turned slowly toward her.

"You watching TV?"

He held up one finger.

"I see you've got your ball." He held it snugly in his left hand.

"He's really been working at it," the nurse said, smiling.

He watched his mother set her bags down, take her coat and shoes off, put on a pair of soft pale green bedroom slippers from her denim bag. She was wearing a black skirt and an emerald terry-cloth top.

Next she took from the bag a large pink plastic comb. Going to the sink, she washed it carefully, then returned to the bedside and began to pull the comb very gently through her son's thick nap. His hair had grown since he'd been at Children's. Hair was even beginning to grow in the bald spot where the bolt had been.

"I realize I can't do much for him right now, but I have a tendency of just combing his hair," Sharita Queen explained shyly to the nurse. "Sometimes if I'm close to him, I feel more secure. I concentrate so he won't feel he's not cared for by his mama."

A moment later she spoke again. "You got on some pretty sweat socks, Freddy. You like the sweat socks Mama got you?"

The child held up one finger. Then, looking up at her, mouth open, tongue protruding, he gave his mother the first smile anyone had seen on his sweet, solemn, nine-year-old face since the car had knocked him flying.

Wednesday, January 16

Noon. Sitting propped against pillows on a wheeled stretcher in the big square Operating Room holding area, Mark began to cough into his sputum cup. The sound brought concern to the faces of a small boy on a litter next to Mark's and several OR nurses chatting outside the glassed-in nurses' station at one end of the room. One came to him, lifted a small black oxygen mask from the wall source behind him, and held it just in front of his face.

This irritated him. "I don't think I need this right now."

She replied soothingly, stroking his hair very lightly, "It's not good for you to get too worked up before surgery."

"I don't want any more oxygen," he said a moment later, pushing the mask away. "My doctor doesn't want me to have it because having it increases the need for it."

"Well," she said, "you seem more relaxed. You're not having those coughing spells now."

"I'm not having them because the mucus hasn't had a chance to collect." Didn't *anybody* down here understand CF?

An aide had brought him down about 11:00. Half an hour later someone had told him that his surgery would be delayed because Dr. Weinberg was tied up with a newborn heart emergency. In view of the delay, and because Mark could not be premedicated, his mother had been invited into the holding area to wait with him, for which she was very glad. Her son was in a state. He hadn't spoken ten words to her last night. She was terrified that he was too frail to survive the surgery.

His head had been hurting him since he'd awakened. Knowing it was probably nerves, he had had Valium at 8:00 but nothing since because he wasn't supposed to drink anything. He'd had no breakfast, either, because of the surgery. Waiting and noise had made his headache worse. The holding area was busy. People came in and out, nurses called to each other, kids cried. In the play corner a little boy in pajamas kept dialing a play telephone. Another little boy kept winding up a musical Ferris wheel. Real phones rang in the office. Mark had asked if he could have Valium intravenously and was waiting for an answer.

At 12:30 anesthesiology resident Susan Carlson came through the double doors leading from the operating rooms to tell Mark that while she wanted to give him something to calm him if she could, she would first have to determine the amount of oxygen in his blood so that she wouldn't endanger him with too large a dose. Dismayed, he asked her bluntly whether she had ever drawn arterial blood before, then said, less irritably, "I mean, I know you've done it, but . . . why don't you lower this railing to make it easier?"

She disappeared with the sample and was soon back saying she could give him enough Valium to last about forty-five minutes. She injected a small amount of the drug in its liquid form into his IV line. Grateful now, he told her, pleading, that his mouth was very dry.

"I don't know if you know about CF—you probably do—but I had my last drink at eight o'clock, and my mucus is getting really thick. They told me I couldn't drink because of the surgery."

This made her angry. He couldn't have had any fluids before general anesthesia, but he wasn't having a general.

She got him a cup of ice chips. "There's no reason why you can't have these as long as you promise to swallow very little."

"I will." Taking some into his mouth, he rinsed the insides of his cheeks with the first few drops that melted, gargled, and spit into the sputum cup. "Gee, I never thought water would taste so good!"

He took another gulp of chips, tipped his head back so they would sit in the back of his throat, and signaled elaborately to Carlson that he wouldn't let it go down any further. He returned her smile.

At 1:00 Ellen asked her son if he was beginning to feel the Valium.

"Well, it's not a wonder drug," he replied, "but I'm not getting as mad."

At 2:00 he persuaded a nurse to get him some more ice chips by swearing to her that he wouldn't swallow any water.

His headache was getting worse.

Ø

Jody Robinson was as happy at this moment as Mark Price was apprehensive, the reason being that Jody was attending a birthday party.

The honoree was Scotty, the little boy with chronic lung disease whose crib stood opposite Jody's. Today was his second birthday and the second anniversary of his arrival at Children's Hospital. His parents were in, his bed was piled high with presents and surrounded by streamers hung from the ceiling, and the Intermediate nurses had spread out a buffet on a long counter nearby.

They had turned Jody's bed slightly so he had an unobstructed view of Scotty. Dressed in a diaper and a yellow terry-cloth shirt, Jody sat with bare feet dangling out between the crib rails and flirted with every partygoer who looked his way. He was in his element. A nurse squeezed his bare foot. He loved it. Another bent to kiss his toes. He loved that. Scotty's new engine chugged under his bed with bells clanging. Jody was thrilled. When Jan Haver brought her full plate to his bedside to stand with him while she ate, he basked in his own happiness.

When she dabbed a smidgen of white icing onto the baby's lower lip, however, he frowned.

The nurses laughed. "Put it in your mouth, Jody! Taste it!"

He touched it to the tip of his nose, leaving most of it there.

"Not your nose! Your mouth!"

He laughed at her outrage, kicking at air.

"Ta-daaa!" The phony trumpet was sounded by a nurse. The play therapist entered the unit half-carrying, half-dragging a gigantic tawny teddy bear with a big green bow around its neck—a gift to the birthday boy from the whole Play Therapy Department. On impulse, two nurses grabbed the bear by his front paws, and as the three women danced the animal through the crowd toward Scotty's bed, the nurses watching burst into a rousing chorus of the Intermediate theme song. "Oh, when the saints go marching in . . ."

Jody joined in on the clapping, so beside himself with excitement now that his heartbeat quickened suddenly and set off an alarm. Reaching calmly to turn it off—high spirits were no cause for worry—a nurse teased the patient. "Listen, Jody, let's not get tachycardic just because of a bear!" He laughed, the life of a party that might as well have been staged entirely for his benefit. All vestiges of his most recent pseudomonas infection had disappeared.

Ø

At 2:30 a hyperal nurse came to see Mark in the OR holding area and was asked by his mother whether she would feel comfortable asking someone for something to make Mark calmer.

"He had Valium at twelve-thirty," Ellen explained. "The anesthesiologist said it would last him forty-five minutes, and two hours have passed."

The hyperal nurse went through the double doors and reported back that Room 5 was being cleaned and would be ready for Mark in ten minutes.

At 2:45 a doctor finally came for the little boy who had been so captivated by the musical Ferris wheel. The boy burst into tears. An OR aide put her arms around him. "Come on, Georgie, go see Dr. Raney. He'll cry if he doesn't see you."

"*I want my mommy!*"

The surgeon picked up the screaming child and took him through the double doors.

At 2:55 several doctors came out through those doors laughing and talking. The operating day was over for them, almost over for the nurses on the day shift. An air of relaxation began to drift into the holding area. Nearing tears, Mark dropped his head into his hands. "I just want to get this over with."

In the play corner the Ferris wheel turned on its axis, repeating its single tune for the umpteenth time. Suddenly Ellen leaped to her feet and seized the toy in both hands. After several unsuccesful attempts to wind the key backward, she frantically buried the plaything under a pile of stuffed animals.

A nurse asked sympathetically, "Is that thing driving you crazy?"

"No!" Ellen cried laughing, her voice pitched high. "I always do this to toys!"

After a wait of more than four hours, he was rolled into Operating Room 5 at 3:20 P.M. Eight or nine people surrounded him, all dressed and masked in green. A tall, thin anesthesiologist who would be supervising Dr. Carlson during the surgery lifted Mark onto the table. Two nurses slipped his gown off. One covered him with the blanket from the stretcher. Just as the other nurse moved to crank up the ends of the table slightly, he went into a spasm of coughing and brought up into his sputum cup some foul green stuff that looked to Abe Weinberg as if it had come out of a sewer.

The moment was upsetting for Weinberg. It resurrected a nagging question in his mind. Were they really doing something worthwhile here?

The boy was breathing fast. "We'll give you something to help you relax," Weinberg told him, "and wash the area really well, then we'll give you some freezing medicine and get the catheter in. I'm sorry that I can't let you sit up. We'll put you at about a forty-five-degree angle. If you absolutely have to sit up, you can, but I have to know that in advance, okay?"

Mark nodded watching the nurses drape his lower body. "Okay," he said thinly.

They put a blood pressure cuff on him and told him he would feel his BP being taken every minute. They asked him to adjust the nasal prongs for oxygen to his own comfort, then they taped the prongs to his face. As soon as he began to inhale the oxygen, they adjusted the ends of the table and asked him to lie back.

He did so very, very tentatively. "I'm not used to breathing this way," he explained.

"Don't talk," one of the nurses advised kindly, "because that will use energy you'll need for breathing. Get as comfortable as possible. Want something under your knees?"

"No, but can I have my toes uncovered?"

"Sure."

The boy lay as if on broken glass, afraid to move, unable to surrender his body to full repose.

"How are you feeling in that position?" Dr. Weinberg asked.

"What do you want me to do?"

"Nothing. Maybe turn your head to the left a little. Fine. Is that okay?"

"Um-hm. Will I be able to have pain medication?"

"I'm doing that right now," Dr. Carlson said. She injected 2.5 cc. of liquid Valium into his IV line.

"Feeling better?" she asked moments later.

"No." For the first time since arriving in the operating room he made no effort to please.

A nurse swabbed his right chest from neck to nipple with yellow liquid soap, then painted his skin with Betadine solution. He kept clearing his throat but began to seem calmer.

Next the surgeon and a nurse opened up a sterile sheet of clear plastic, removed the backing, and laid the plastic on Mark's chest, sticky side down, to seal in the skin bacteria and maintain a sterile field. A precut hole was positioned over the spot where Dr. Weinberg would cut. As an added caution, the nurses slipped what looked like a large croquet wicket into brackets on either side of the table so it crossed the patient's body above his neck, then draped the frame with towels which hung to his chest. This barrier between the boy's head and the rest of his body would prevent him from breathing germs into his own incision.

"I can't see anything," Mark said. His view was the anesthesiologist's face upside down above him.

"This keeps a clean field down here," Weinberg explained. "But you're breathing okay, right?"

"It feels tight around my throat."

"That may be the sticky stuff."

Weinberg prepared a syringe containing Xylocaine to deaden

the area and relax the blood vessels. "Okay, now you're going to feel a prick . . ."

"Wait, wait, wait!" The boy's voice was panicky.

"Listen. That was the prick. Now you'll feel some burning. It won't be any more than you feel now."

"I thought I was going to feel real woozy."

"Mark, if you feel any pain, tell us." Weinberg put his hand out for a scalpel, grasped it, and made a half-inch cut into the boy's skin just above the collarbone.

"I feel a little . . ."

"Pressure," Weinberg finished.

"It hurts. Can you give me a little more stuff to relax me?"

From behind him Susan Carlson leaned over him and stroked his hair. "That was that burny stuff I gave you. I want to make sure your breathing is okay before I give you any more. Let's just wait another minute or two."

She was finding it extremely difficult to monitor his breathing. His lungs sounded as if they were barely hanging on. So while attempting to make conversation and count every breath he took, she was trying to ensure that the amount of narcotic she was giving him wasn't depressing his respirations too much, and she was also watching his blood pressure and his heart rate, which was twice the normal rate for a person his age, partly because she could not give him as much drug as it would have taken to calm him.

"Okay, Mark, I just gave you a little more narcotic for pain relief," she said. She had given him a quarter of a cc. "You just keep breathing. You're doing fine."

Weinberg was probing, seeking the vein that had appeared most obvious under Mark's skin. But as soon as he had isolated and cut into it, he saw that he was going to have trouble. The vein was occluded, a complication of the intravenous antibiotic therapy Mark had been getting all his life. The boy's veins were shot. Certainly this one appeared to be. Though it was four to six times the diameter of the catheter, Weinberg could not make the cath go in.

He picked up a narrow metal dilator and began to try to open up the passageway in the vein.

"Your mother's a nice lady," Dr. Carlson said to Mark. "I'm glad she came down so I had a chance to meet her. Did she stay here last night?"

"Yes." He sounded alert in every cell.

"You okay?"

"Yeah." But he was frowning, wincing, pulling for air.

"Your breathing sounds fine."

She was unable to lead him into a single discussion of any depth. When only half an hour had passed, she was totally without resources. She felt that Mark's eyes were looking straight through her. He seemed to be all eye, and his eyes held knowledge that she could scarcely bear to behold. In other circumstances she would not have had to behold it. But Mark's being awake forced Carlson to think about her profession, about life, and about death in ways that made her exceedingly uncomfortable.

He looked up at her thinking how nice it was to see a face. "Is everything going okay?"

"Just fine, Mark," Weinberg replied, wondering whether the veins going down into the boy's heart were also occluded. The surgeon rolled his shoulders and glanced at the clock. He had been in the OR nearly eight hours. This was his last scheduled operation today. A smooth procedure would have been just about over.

"Is something wrong?"

"Everything's just fine," Weinberg repeated. "Now, Mark, you're going to feel another prick, and then some burning again." He injected more Xylocaine, hoping to relax the blood vessels enough to open them up a little more. "You're doing just fine. Mark, this should be the third and last prick, a little lower, and then some more burning."

"Ow, ow, ow!" There was fear in his voice. "I thought you said the worst part was over!"

"Okay, you're going to feel quite a lot of pushing now, Mark," said Weinberg.

"Okay. No hurt, though, right?"

"You feel pushing?"

"Yeah."

"No hurt, though, right?"

"No. I'm sweating up a storm back here."

"Because of the curtains," Dr. Carlson suggested.

The surgeon was sweating himself, struggling to advance the catheter in the vein and getting nowhere fast.

"You must be tired, Dr. Weinberg," the patient said.

"Well, we probably should have done you first," Weinberg said, impressed by the boy's perceptivity, "and then we wouldn't be tired."

"I thought that baby probably tired you out."

"That baby did tire me out, but we have a fine health care team here, Mark. . . ." He glanced around the table acknowledging the smiles behind the masks.

"I thought you'd be too tired to do me."

"Oh, no."

"I didn't think this would take so long."

"There are several different ways to do this," Dr. Carlson said. "We want to do it the best way."

Silence followed and lasted several moments. Reading the silence as trouble, Mark again asked, "Is something wrong?"

The surgeon sighed. "Everything's going very well, Mark, but I think we might have to use a different vein, because this one has been inflamed in the past and has closed up. Let me try just one more time, and if it doesn't . . ." Attempting to concentrate on what he was doing, the surgeon let the sentence trail off.

"Have you ever run into this kind of problem before?"

"Yes, unfortunately. We've run into all these problems before."

The surgery took three hours.

Eventually Weinberg managed to get the catheter into a third branch of Mark's subclavian vein. The placement was imperfect but acceptable, and the patient had reached the limit of his tolerance. After two hours Mark's nerves had been completely frazzled. By the end of the third hour he was crying.

He was returned to Adolescent at 6:45 P.M. The thick yellow solution that had been dripping into his wrist was now flowing steadily into a vein in his chest. Weinberg had told Mark's mother that he expected the line to last about a month, to which Ellen Price had responded, "That's all we need."

The patient requested a cola. When he had drunk his fill, he slept soundly for two hours and awoke around 9:00 saying he was starving. Jacquie ordered his dinner tray. After eating everything on it, he sent his mother downstairs for a hamburger and two candy bars. He ate every crumb. Later in the evening he played a game of

Concentration with Jacquie and lost to her for the third night in a row.

But when he settled down to sleep again, using oxygen, Mark Price was as happy a person as could be found that night at Children's Hospital. He was scheduled for discharge to St. Michael's on Friday morning.

Thursday, January 17

When Daniel Earnshaw walked into his room on rounds, Mark interrupted his breakfast to give his doctor a big grin.

Earnshaw smiled back. "You look pretty chipper for this hour of the morning!" He was glad to see the boy getting a decent meal for a change.

"Oh, yeah! I feel like I'm going home tomorrow!"

Earnshaw nodded. "I have to be away for a few days," he said. "But all the arrangements have been made for your transfer." After listing them, he added, "You'll be on the service of Dr. John Asher at St. Michael's. I gather you know him?"

"He's been our family doctor since we moved. I've met him a few times."

"This should be a good change for you," Earnshaw continued. "You'll be close to home. Your family can visit you. We're hopeful that the hyperal is going to be a big help. I think we're thinking in terms of about three weeks."

The boy looked shocked. *"Three weeks?"*

"At least," the doctor said, unable to believe that he was giving news.

But Mark showed relief. "Oh, *at least*. I was thinking more of like six weeks. I want to gain some weight. I don't want to do anything halfhearted."

He asked about his lung. Reminding him that the pneumothorax had remained basically unchanged for ten days, Earnshaw said he expected that either the air would resorb slowly or the space would fill with fluid and scar in. Mark had now started per-

cussion again on the left side. His doctor told him that the frequency could be increased slowly. Earnshaw examined the incision
site of the last chest tube. He listened to Mark's chest. The boy's
lungs were quite congested. Recent sputum cultures had shown that
his mucus was now ninety percent pseudomonas bacteria.

In his heart of hearts, Daniel Earnshaw did not want Mark to go
to St. Michael's. The boy was his patient. When his patients were
sick, Earnshaw wanted to take care of them. Mark had been
through a very rough period—the longest hospitalization an older
cystic had ever had at Children's. His doctor wanted to see him out
of it. But his reasons for wanting to keep Mark were purely emotional, and therefore, in his own opinion, not good enough.

He finished examining his patient and wished the boy well.

"This has been a long haul," Earnshaw said. "I hope you have a
good trip tomorrow, and I hope everything goes as you want it to at
St. Michael's. I'd like to see you about two weeks after you're discharged from there just to check on how you're doing."

Mark nodded. "Meanwhile I know my mother won't hesitate to
call if there's a problem."

"I'm sure. Okay, then, anything else?"

"Not that I can think of."

"Take care."

"I will."

Giving his patient's toe a squeeze, Daniel Earnshaw left to finish
his rounds.

Ø

Shortly before 2:00, Candy Rudolph and her parents got off the
elevator on the third floor. They had driven in from Long Island to
see Dr. Rolfe Lorimer for the first time since Candy's operation. It
was Lorimer's practice to see all his craniofacial patients six weeks
after their surgery. The swelling had usually disappeared by then,
and most of the changes that were going to occur in the patient's
appearance as a result of surgery had already taken place. The
Rudolphs stopped first in Neurosurgery, where the patient surprised Guillermo Perez by walking toward him shyly, letting herself
be taken onto his lap, and giving him a big smile.

"We-ell! Such a pretty girl, and you came all this way to see an
ugly guy like me!"

Pleased, Candy nodded. She was wearing the same pink dress and white tights and black patent sandals she had worn on her last visit to Children's two days after discharge. Today, though, she was also wearing a wig: a little-girl hairdo of shiny brown wave and curl so cute and natural and becoming to Candy that a stranger would never have guessed it had been purchased. The hair transformed her. The doctors had yet to finish their work on her face—her eyelids looked a bit tired, a bit odd, somehow—but the hair bestowed a softness that restored the child to Planet Earth.

"How are you feeling now—okay?"

"Fine." Shyly, but without uncertainty.

"Would you take your wig off for me?"

She lifted it from her head. Her own hair was now half an inch long.

Perez scrutinized her crown. "The forehead looks good. Perfect! My part is perfect! You remember," he said across Candy to her parents, "how the eyes protruded? That was the worst part of the whole thing, and now we don't have that anymore."

There remained little to discuss. When he had answered their questions and written Candy a new prescription for phenobarbital against her occasional seizures, the physician bade the Rudolphs farewell.

"You won't have to see me specifically again," he said, standing to offer his hand to Candy's parents, "but when you come back to see Dr. Lorimer, stop over and say hello."

"Yes," Yvonne said, slow to grasp that the neurosurgeon was bowing out of their lives, "but when do you want to see her again?"

Perez said, chuckling, "Only socially!" He looked down at the child looking up at him and gave her a wink. "Right, Candy? From here on only socially!"

They were seen by Rolfe Lorimer in an examining room near his office. He was dressed in a suit and tie. He looked, as he always looked during office hours, elegant.

"Hello, Miss Candace." His manner was friendly, but Lorimer was a more measured personality than Guillermo Perez, and Candy responded to him, though willingly, more bashfully.

"Hello."

She was sitting on the examining table. So as not to tower over her, he pulled up a stool. "How are you feeling?"

"Fine."

"What have you been doing?"

"Playing."

"Playing what?"

Embarrassed: "Everything."

"How's your chest?"

"Fine."

"Will you take your dress up for me? I always ask the girls to do that."

When he had checked the rib graft incision, Lorimer stood. He asked Candy to take her wig off. Turning on a bright light over her head, he examined the incision in her scalp, then sat back down on the stool facing the child and began to assess the results of his work on her face.

Lorimer almost always felt disappointment when he saw a patient back for the first checkup. While the face was no longer distorted by swelling, the features he had deliberately overcorrected in the operating room were still somewhat exaggerated. Months of healing still lay ahead. Lorimer was as eager as the parents to see the final outcome. The surgeon as perfectionist always saw things he wished he had done better. In this child the asymmetry of bone structure had yielded that slight bump on her left temple. The left socket was a mite shallower than the right.

Thinking rationally, however, Lorimer knew he had done what he'd set out to do with Candy Rudolph. Her forehead looked great. He had expected more irregularity. The plane was smooth. Running a finger along her brow, he could feel a bony prominence that was also plainly visible. The child's nose was more assertive than it had been. Her eyes no longer bulged. The tilt of the lids looked good for this stage. So did the bone grafts below her eyes, which had filled her cheeks out nicely.

Lorimer made note of these improvements to Candy's parents. He reiterated with the Rudolphs that the forces of healing are unpredictable and that when anatomy is abnormal to begin with, the likelihood of perfect results is remote. The new architecture of Candy's upper face would probably require minor adjustments. These could be done easily during the second phase of surgery, the operation on the child's midface.

But Lorimer's caution could not conceal his pleasure. "Eighty-five to ninety percent of what's going to happen as a result of the operation last month has already happened," he told the Rudolphs. "Ten to fifteen percent will continue to occur over the next six months, and then there'll be a subtle change over a period of years. In general, at the moment, in view of what we've done, I think she looks super."

The Rudolphs' response was enthusiastic. "It goes without saying," said Candy's father to Lorimer, "that you've done a fantastic job."

Yvonne did retain some concerns about Candy. Mainly she continued to worry about the slanty look of the child's eyes. The week after the family had finally returned to Long Island, Yvonne had taken her eldest to a shoe store where a clerk had asked about Candy's scar. Told simply that the child had had neurosurgery, the woman had brightened, as if suddenly understanding, and said, "Oh, was it Down's syndrome?"

Candy hadn't heard the comment. Whether she would have understood it Yvonne didn't know. Yvonne herself had been badly shaken by the incident. She knew the healing would take time, she told Lorimer. But it bothered her greatly that after all Candy had gone through, they were still getting questions about Down's syndrome.

"Oh, but it's so soon," Lorimer said reassuringly. "If people were to say that a year from now, then we'd be a little disappointed. But we do overcorrect on purpose, and that area around the eyes is the last to settle. It will adjust. If it doesn't, we can fix it up when we do the second surgery. You've just got to be patient."

Part of the problem now, he pointed out to the Rudolphs, was that with the most dominant defect corrected in the upper third of Candy's face, the middle third looked even flatter than before. Until the upper jaw surgery was done, the child would still have a very obvious deformity.

There remained in Yvonne's mind the matter of school. Candy had already missed a month of kindergarten. Her eyes still looked somewhat odd. Yvonne hated to put her on the school bus looking as she did, hated to send her back to Mean Brian and others in her class who had teased Candy about her appearance before surgery and would certainly tease her now.

Yvonne had once taught elementary school. Using materials obtained from Candy's teacher, she was giving Candy individual in-

struction every day so she wouldn't fall any further behind. The
mother wondered what the doctor would think of Candy continuing
this way until summer and then starting first grade with her classmates in the fall.

Lorimer had no objection. Candy's defect had been moderate.
The surgeon had operated on a number of other people born with
moderate Crouzon's syndrome in whom deformity was no longer
visibly discernible. If all went well, this child could one day be
among them. By September she would look quite improved over
the way she looked now. A kindergartner did not have to compete
academically. The year was about half over anyway. If the Rudolphs
had wanted to get Candy back to school right away, Lorimer would
have said fine. Their wanting to keep her out was just as fine, and
he told them so.

Parents and surgeon discussed dates for the second procedure.
Lorimer preferred to wait at least five or six years. Changes made
surgically in the upper face responded well to growth processes, he
said, and very rarely needed to be redone. This was less true of the
midface. Lorimer did not want to subject Candy to the same operation twice if he could help it. Though impatient to have all the surgery behind them, the Rudolphs felt the same way. Until the
surgery was scheduled, the child would return to Children's for
periodic checkups.

Ø

As the Rudolphs were saying goodbye to Rolfe Lorimer, Kate
McDevitt was saying goodbye to Mark Price. Not knowing exactly
when Mark would be leaving, Kate had made plans to spend a long
weekend visiting her boyfriend in another city. She would have
loved to accompany Mark in the ambulance but knew that because
several of his favorite nurses would be working Friday, he would
definitely be leaving in the company of somebody he liked.

For Kate as for the other nurses in Adolescent, it was hard to see
Mark go off to a "foreign" hospital, as they termed it, where he
wasn't known and which had no pediatrics department. How effectively could the people at St. Michael's treat a youngster who had
had CF all his life? Yet the nurses knew Mark badly wanted to be
nearer his family, and they supported that wish.

On Wednesday the x-ray therapist who had taken so many of Mark's chest films had confided to Kate that she didn't think the boy would live a week at St. Michael's. Kate felt nothing of the sort. To her it seemed that Mark was over the hump, at least this hump. Of course he'd be back in Adolescent sooner or later. But Kate was optimistic. She kissed him goodbye convinced that he would now be free of worry about his lungs for a while, and feeling glad for him.

"Behave yourself up there, you rotten teenager. Don't give the nurses too much trouble."

He hugged her back. "I won't!"

Late in the afternoon Alan Cavanaugh wrote Mark's transfer summary feeling better about the case than at any other point in his involvement with Mark. While the boy was well in no sense of the word, his chest tubes were out, his lung was apparently stable, and he was getting hyperal, which held out the promise of making him stronger and able to enjoy his life at home awhile longer. The resident had also been very gratified to learn from Ellen Price what Mark was thinking about his life and death. The boy seemed to have his situation well in hand.

Cavanaugh thought him an incredible kid. A very wise kid. Though glad that Mark's wish was coming true, Cavanaugh knew he would miss him.

Jacquie Harper took care of Mark that evening with very mixed feelings. As usual, he and she played Concentration after dinner. This time, after a losing streak of four nights and with no help at all from her, Mark beat her fair and square.

Friday, January 18

Mark's bed had been stripped to the mattress. The wall that had held his cards was now bare. Packed and set to go, the patient himself sat in an armchair next to the bed wearing slippers and a pair of his own pajamas, wishing the ambulance driver would hurry up and come for him. He was jittery—nervous about the trip, nervous about the new hospital, nervous about leaving Children's. People had been in and out of his room all morning to say goodbye and to make a host of final preparations for the transfer. Julie Wixted would accompany him in the ambulance. His mother would meet him at St. Michael's.

"Hey, Marcus!" A nurse from the IV team hailed him from the doorway and walked in. "So are you glad you're going back home?"

"Yeah. I've missed my family. It's been a long stay this time." Again he looked at his watch. "Seven weeks and one day."

"You going to miss people?"

"I just hope the nurses are nice up there and not mean."

Julie came in. "The man has arrived and is on his way up," she said. "Are you ready? Shall we take a bottle of Coke?"

"No, I've got a can in this bag. Got a can of beer too! I was going to drink it yesterday, but I didn't feel like it."

"You'd better not let them catch you with beer at St. Michael's!"

There were delays. Certain things had to be done with his hyperal hookups, certain equipment found. Mark had several coughing spells. As he grew edgier, his breathing grew faster, and he asked for Valium and aspirin. For several minutes Allyson couldn't find the keys to the cabinet in which the Valium was kept. Someone suggested that since it was nearing noon, he should probably have his 12:00 meds. He asked to use the urinal once more. It was 12:05 before he was finally settled, sitting, on the stretcher. A swag of clear tubing connected his central line to the IV pole that would go with him in the ambulance. At his feet were his Bible and the dress shoes he had worn the day he was admitted. In one shoe was the photograph of Daniel Earnshaw's future son-in-law.

They rolled him out to the nurses' station where a small crowd gathered to say goodbye. "Where's he going?" a technician asked one of the nurses, who replied, "To St. Michael's, where they'll give him better care!"

"Next time you see me," Mark said to the nurses and to Alan Cavanaugh, who had joined them, "I'll be fat!"

"Don't be insulted if I say I hope we don't see you very soon," a nurse said, and the others chimed in their agreement. They wished him well. With Julie in a blue ski jacket pushing the IV pole and carrying Mark's bag, the ambulance driver rolled the patient out of the Adolescent Unit and down the hall to the elevator. It was there that Clara Bowman caught up with them. She had gone to Adolescent thinking he would not be leaving till 1:00 and had run frantically down the hall to say goodbye to him because she did not expect to see him alive again, did not think he would be able, in his condition, to manage much more than a week.

But she joked with him and kissed him as if this thought had never occurred to her.

The day was gray and damp. In the chill January air, Mark shivered. "Whew! I'm not used to this!" The white van was parked outside the Emergency Room. Within five minutes the stretcher, the IV pole, the patient, and the nurse were in their places. The driver shut the rear door and took his seat in front. As they felt the motor turn over, Mark and Julie looked at each other.

"This is exciting!" said the nurse.

"Yeah," the patient agreed, "something out of the ordinary!"

Easing the vehicle out of the driveway and onto the boulevard, the driver hit the accelerator heading north.

Ø

In her office down the hall and around the corner from Adolescent, Children's social worker Lynn Story picked up her ringing telephone and heard the voice of the social worker from the Welfare Department who was assigned to Jody Robinson. In their last phone conversation, on January 7, Gladys Wexler had indicated that she thought Jody's best hope for a permanent guardian might finally lie with his mother. Today Wexler had called to let Story know that the Department itself was going to file for custody of the child.

Wexler's change of heart had come about for two reasons, she explained to Story. First, she had discovered that Sabra Robinson had been released from prison to an inpatient drug rehabilitation program where she had stayed one night. In skipping out, Jody's mother had not only violated the terms of her probation but had also shown herself uninterested in taking the hard steps that would be necessary if she were truly to get her life in hand.

Then, after announcing to her cousins that she had beaten up a couple of people in the drug center, Sabra had begged the women to let her move in with them. When they'd refused, she had threatened them. "Okay," she'd said angrily, "then I'm going to come back and get you and take my daughter, and we're leaving. You can't keep her here." The cousins had thought she looked ill. Drugs? They didn't know. Frightened, they had phoned Wexler wondering what they should do if Sabra did return and try to take her child. The worker had given them the Welfare Department's emergency number. The cousins by their own admission had been scared to death.

Given those two events plus Sabra's history, Wexler had decided that it was in Jody's best interests to be in Welfare custody. Furthermore, she intended to seek permission for the cousins to be given formal custody of Sabra II so they had some legal backing for keeping the child out of her mother's hands.

Hearing this plan, the Children's social worker felt relieved but not surprised. In the face of all that she herself had learned about Jody's family situation over the past year, Story had always believed that for Gladys Wexler to reach the same conclusions she had was just a matter of time. Still, the news was the best thing that had happened to Lynn Story all week. Finally something concrete was being done toward getting a permanent caretaker for Jody. Slowly, slowly the wheels were beginning to grind forward.

Or so Story thought till the end of the conversation. At that point Gladys Wexler informed her that she was leaving in the morning for a three-week vacation in Europe—three weeks during which the wheels would not grind forward at all for Jody Robinson.

Ø

At St. Michael's Ellen Price led the way to Mark's new room on the third floor. Julie noted that the hospital was very clean and pleasant-looking, and she was delighted with the room—a single, fairly good-sized, with a big window overlooking beautiful hilly scenery. On the bed table was a telephone.

Mark was thrilled. "I can talk to anybody I want whenever I want!" At Children's the phones are in the hall.

While Ellen helped her son get settled, Julie found the head nurse and talked with her and several other nurses about Mark's care, stressing the role he liked to play himself. It pleased her to see how receptive the nurses were to the information she gave them. She left them with the phone number for Children's, the extension for Adolescent, and her own home phone number.

By this time the ambulance driver was paging Julie. She returned to Mark's room to find him in bed with a grin on his face. "Look, Julie, electric beds!"

His mother seemed to be adjusting with more difficulty. "Do you really have to go right now?" she said as Julie hugged and kissed her and her son. "Can't you stay at my place tonight?"

Julie explained that she'd have to stop at Children's to write in Mark's chart, and then her husband would be expecting her home. But embracing Ellen one final time, she herself was struck by what a milestone this day was for Mark and for all of them, and when the two women parted, the nurse, too, had tears in her eyes.

Ø

Back in the city, Gina DeRose arrived at the Children's Oncology Clinic carrying a heavy red schoolbag which banged against her leg when she walked. Her mother was with her, and so was her brother. Little Tony had just turned three on Sunday. He bore a strong physical resemblance to Gina but was, like his father, a person of few words. Whenever the Clinic secretaries made a fuss over him, he hid behind his mother.

Gina started telling Charmaine and Ellie about her brother's birthday party before she'd even gotten her coat off. "Wanna know what I gave him? I gave him a catcher's mitt and a ball, and I made him a truck out of paper and bought him a hat, a baseball hat, and . . ."

Charmaine interrupted. "Where'd you get all that money, lady?"

She giggled. "Well, my dad bought everything, but I put my name on it! I gave it to him in a bag! And my mom made spaghettis and lasagne and mashed potatoes and . . . What else, Mom? Oh, yeah, a roast and salad, and then she made this kind of sponge cake that you can put chocolate or vanilla pudding in, and my brother had chocolate, because you get the dessert you want on your birthday! You know what? He eats peanut butter, but he doesn't like jelly!"

Head nurse Cindy Strickland ran a finger down Gina's spine.

The child spun around to face her. "I just came to get a blood test! Oooh, I love your necklace! What is it?"

"It's amber. Thank you. Shall I draw it now and get it over with?"

"Let Dr. Silver do it," Marie said, deadpan. "He's pretty good."

For one second Gina thought she was serious. "No, Mom, he couldn't even get any blood after he stuck two needles in me last time!"

Cindy suggested that they find an empty room and said she'd be right with them.

Little Tony was digging into a toy box near Ellie's desk. Leaving him where he was, Marie and her daughter headed back toward the examining rooms. Gina hurried. Room 4 was her favorite, because it had pictures of Little Bo-Peep and Humpty Dumpty and Jack Be Nimble and Mary Had a Little Lamb. The door to Room 4 was closed. All the others were open. Giddy with choices, deliberating aloud—"This one's better! No, maybe I should take this one!"—she darted from room to room until her mother said finally, with warning in her voice, "Gina, this is a hospital!"

She might as well have tried to plug a spring. The child picked a room and bubbled on, hardly stopping for breath when the nurse came in. "I want *you* to do this!"

"Dr. Silver's coming right in," Cindy teased. "He said if I'd let him do it, he'd be nice to me all year, and I want him to be nice to me, because sometimes he gives me a hard time."

"Don't listen to the doctor! Listen to your patient!"

Cindy began to slap Gina's left hand lightly to bring up the vein that almost always worked. Marie stood in the doorway thinking of Little Tony's birthday party. Sunday was the first day since Gina had gotten sick that her mother had felt somewhat peppy while entertaining company. Thanksgiving had been a disaster. Christmas had been a little better. But on Sunday Marie had found herself humming as she cooked. She had really enjoyed her guests. For the first time since September, she had felt there was nothing wrong. She knew the leukemia could start up again, but she'd been able to push it into the back of her mind and to relax.

It was getting easier to handle, thank God. They were even beginning to think forward a little. For the past several years they had rented a campsite from Memorial Day to Labor Day and had

camped every weekend all summer. It was the cheapest way she and
Tony knew of to have a good vacation. The kids loved it. When
Gina had gotten sick, Marie had expected no more camping. But
now that the child was well again, there was no reason in the world
not to plan to go.

Cindy had gotten the needle in without difficulty. As the syringe
filled slowly with blood, the nurse asked the child how school was
going.

"Good. I got my report card!"

"Really! How did you do?"

"I got second honors!"

"Congratulations! What does that mean?"

"It means I didn't get first honors, but I got second honors! No,
I'm just kidding. It means you did good. Not great, but good. Usually I get first honors, but see, this was for the first quarter, and I
was sick then, and I missed a lot of work, but then I did it and
worked hard and all, and I got second honors! Miss Kelly was very
proud of me!"

"I'll bet she was! I'm proud of you too!"

She withdrew the needle from Gina's hand. "Okay, would you
like a sticker with your Band-Aid, or do you want your sticker separate?"

"Separate! Ohhh, do you have a strawberry? I wanted to get a
strawberry the last time, but there weren't any, so I got a watermelon instead!"

"I'll check." Cindy tore open a Band-Aid, and Marie asked, "Will
Dr. Silver call me with the results?"

"Yes, I'll be sure and tell him to." She applied the Band-Aid. "Is
she on Methotrexate now?"

The patient answered for herself. "Yeah, he called up and put
me back on two last week!"

Cindy found a strawberry sticker. Gina put it on the collar of her
blouse while telling her mother she wanted to go upstairs and see
the nurses in the Oncology Unit where she had been a patient.
Marie said maybe next time. Going to the Unit brought back too
many memories for her, and today she had a good excuse. She and
her husband were returning to Children's at 7:30. Every few
months a Clinic social worker runs a series of evening meetings for
parents whose children have been recently diagnosed. Tonight the

group in which Marie and Tony had been involved was to gather for the last time. Marie wanted to get home and organize herself so she could put dinner on the table, get the kids squared away for the evening, and be on time for the meeting.

"Maybe you can do it on your next visit," Cindy suggested.

"Next visit I'm getting the needles in my back," Gina replied.

This comment astonished her mother. At home the child would not permit the subject to be mentioned.

"Will you be here when I get the needles in my back?" The tone of her voice had changed ever so slightly.

Cindy bent to kiss her cheek. When the nurse spoke, it was to make a promise. "I sure will."

A child with cancer poses brand-new problems in most households. Discussing those problems with friends and family members who have never gone through such experiences, parents frequently feel isolated or even crazy. The evening meetings arranged by the Clinic staff are set up specifically to reassure parents on this score: to give them the chance to express any and all feelings triggered by what has happened in their lives in an atmosphere of understanding and acceptance.

The meetings are also intended to be social events. They provide parents with an opportunity to get away from the problems at home without feeling guilty. They encourage parents to have an evening out as a couple. The sessions are held in a lounge full of comfortable chairs. Refreshments are served. The social worker leading the group makes every attempt to keep the conversation informal.

While format varies slightly depending on the needs and desires of those present, the first session usually focuses on the discovery of the child's illness and the family's initial response. Themes identified in this discussion become the subjects of future meetings: guilt, changes in parental expectations, discipline problems, the tendency to baby a child with cancer, differing reactions in husband and wife, the importance for parents of continuing to tend their marriage, the hope for cure, the fear of relapse, the family's relationships with the doctors. Most groups meet every other week for six sessions. Experience has shown that when more than six sessions occur, topics begin to repeat themselves.

Gina DeRose's father had attended five of the scheduled meetings without enjoyment. He thought the social worker and the other parents were nice people. He could see that group was a good place in which to express and compare feelings. He knew that the meetings had helped his wife. He could even acknowledge that they might have helped him. Nevertheless, Tony had not appreciated the conversations. He did not like discussing the fact that Gina had cancer.

He did not like discussing the fact that any child had cancer. Before ever hearing about the group, he had known that other parents were in the same boat he was in and had the same feelings he had. Knowing this had been of no help whatsoever to Tony DeRose. If the decision had been up to him, he and Marie would not have attended even one of the meetings at Children's.

His wife knew this without his having to tell her. Tony had never liked to talk about what bothered him deeply. They had lost their firstborn daughter to crib death. The baby had been five months old. Afterward Tony had maintained a silence about it that for years had caused Marie to walk on eggs, to hold in her own hurt, believing that if she brought up the subject herself, she'd only make him feel worse.

To some extent he had reacted the same way to Gina's illness. When he'd grow quiet, and she'd say, "What's wrong?" he'd say, "Oh, nothing." In Marie's mind there was no point in pursuing it, if he didn't want to talk about it. She'd let it go.

So she was neither surprised nor dismayed that he kept quiet in group most evenings. He'd been this way all the years that she'd known him. Marie did not imagine that she was going to change him now. In fact she wasn't trying to change Tony, any more than he tried to change her. They had a good marriage, thank God. They never had bad arguments. If Marie did occasionally flare up and say, "The hell with you," Tony was the type of person who'd forgotten it in five minutes. She did not believe he owed her her dreams. He made no demands on her that she did not gladly meet. They respected each other in every way. As for the group meetings, Tony went because she wanted him to go. He never put up a fuss. He went for her, and that was perfectly fine with his wife.

Marie did find the meetings helpful. She liked to talk, and when something was bothering her, she needed to talk. Holding in her feelings so as not to hurt Tony had sometimes made her feel alone.

In the group she had been able to get many things off her chest. Once or twice she had even cried in a meeting. It had happened the first time because another parent had said something that had brought back very fresh memories for Marie. The man had been so apologetic about upsetting her. But she had replied that they were there to unburden. Seeing the same people session after session had made Marie feel comfortable among them. She had gained much from their understanding. They had made her see that she and Tony were not alone.

She had also learned in group how to handle the words "leukemia" and "cancer" without getting the creeps.

Unlike her husband, Marie DeRose felt sorry that the sessions were ending. She would miss the other parents. Already they had all exchanged phone numbers. Marie looked forward to keeping in touch with them.

But she knew it wouldn't be quite the same. And she thought maybe that was as it should be. The children were all doing well now. It was time for their parents, too, to move on to the next phase of their lives.

Saturday, January 19

The parents of Robin Gregory's father had died when her dad was a child. They had been buried in a Catholic cemetery a short drive from the trailer park where the Gregorys lived. On Saturday morning at 11:00, Brandon Gregory was interred beside his great-grandparents. Prayers were spoken by the assistant pastor of a Lutheran church which Robin attended on occasion. The coffin and burial services had been donated by the director of the funeral home. Robin's father had paid for the digging: twenty-five dollars.

The funeral director had called on Thursday wondering if the family wanted their son buried in special dress. Robin had not thought about this. The twins' baby clothes were much too big for a baby Brandon's size. But she had told the funeral director she would bring in a blanket. She had also given the man a tiny cross to put around Brandon's neck and a little teddy bear of Tommy's to lie next to him. Standing miserably now at her baby's grave, Robin took comfort in thinking of Brandon lying cozy in his blanket with his cross and his bear.

Her husband stood watching Robin's father. Imagining that his father-in-law was thinking about his own parents' burial in this same plot of ground, Tom Gregory had an idea that Robin's father was hoping, as he himself was hoping, that Brandon and his grandparents would meet somewhere and would find pleasure in each other's company. In Tom's fantasy those three would then meet up with his own father, who had loved children, and with his father's parents, and maybe even with the premature baby born to Tom's first wife.

Tom believed that heaven was wherever a person wanted it to be. As a teenager he had run away from home and hitchhiked to his grandmother's place in Altoona, Pennsylvania. There he had often lain on his back in his grandmother's front yard, chewing on a weed and looking up at the sky. He'd been content there. Had Brandon been formed enough to have thought, to have dreamed of somewhere he wanted to be? If not, Tom Gregory just hoped that the baby would go to a place as peaceful as he himself had found his grandmother's yard in Altoona.

Robin's thoughts during the brief graveside service were far more troubled. She was wondering what kind of God would allow a baby to be born only to die.

Robin had done a lot of praying about Brandon. When the baby had made it through heart surgery, and when his eye had gotten better, she had truly felt that her prayers were being answered. At the end she had realized that only a miracle could save him. If there was a God, and if He was able to perform miracles, why hadn't He done it then?

She wondered if He had withheld His miracles to punish her. Robin felt that she did have much to account for—not only the two abortions she'd had before the twins were born, but also certain things she'd said to Tom during some nasty fights they'd had while she was pregnant with Brandon. Confused about what the future held, wanting to hurt the person causing the confusion, Robin had told Tom in a rage on several occasions that she wished she'd lose the baby.

She could scarcely believe that God would put Brandon through so much pain and suffering just because of what his mother had said in a fit of rage. Yet what other explanation could there be for Brandon Gregory's life and death?

Robin still believed in a hereafter and believed that wherever it was, her tiny son was there. But she was not sure now that there was a God. If there was, He was not, in Robin's opinion, the God everyone liked to think He was. He was not all-forgiving or all-powerful or ready to perform miracles. If he existed, Robin Gregory was not at all sure that He was someone she wanted to know.

Many people, she knew, had lost loved ones and had remained faithful. Remembering the Biblical story of Job, Robin recalled that Job had remained faithful although he'd lost everything.

Her own faith was not that strong. All Robin could think of, watching the pastor throw a handful of dirt on her tiny son's casket, was that if this had been a test, she had flunked it badly.

Monday, January 21

At 10:00 A.M. Kate McDevitt was called to a phone at the Adolescent nurses' station and heard a familiar voice say cheerfully, "Hiya, Kate!"

"Mark! What a surprise!"

He laughed. "I have my own phone up here, so I thought I'd say hello."

"I'm so glad! How are things going? Julie said you have a really nice room."

"Yeah, I like it. The only problem is that the nurses don't talk."

"That's because of the note I wrote them about this obnoxious fifteen-year-old brat they were getting!"

Saddened by his disappointment, she nonetheless assumed that when the nurses got to know Mark better, they would talk to him more. She said this to him.

Their conversation continued for perhaps ten minutes. Mark told Kate that he was using continuous oxygen. He said he was upset with the respiratory therapist who was supposed to give him percussion and couldn't seem to understand that he needed it before meals. But he also reported that he had gained a little weight. He sounded good to Kate. She was not especially concerned about his respiratory distress. She thought it probably related to his anxiety about being in a new setting, which was more or less the conclusion Mark's mother had drawn.

The floor to which he had been admitted at St. Michael's was a general medical-surgical unit specializing in oncology. All the nurses there had seen adults in the final stages of cancer. Few had seen a child in the end stages of cystic fibrosis. It was rare for them to have a teenager in their care at all, let alone a youngster who was so sick, so obviously bright, and so obviously dying. It amazed them that he was never heard to complain. Forty-eight hours after his arrival Mark had become the key patient on the floor. Every nurse on all three shifts either knew him or knew of him.

Inexperienced in pediatrics, they were nevertheless attempting to give Mark what they thought he needed. He had been assigned at her request to a nurse with four grown children, one of whom had had a friend with CF in elementary school. Unfortunately, weekend staffing had prevented her from spending much time with Mark. Yet it was obvious to this nurse and to her colleagues that the boy's mother did a lot of his care, that Mark seemed to want her to, and that his mother anticipated and met his needs without his having to say anything. The St. Michael's nurses tried to respect this special relationship by interrupting the family's privacy only when necessary.

Ø

Toward the end of the afternoon on Monday a group of doctors gathered at the nurses' station in the Isolation Unit at Children's to review the puzzling case of Freddy Eberly. Those present included neurosurgeon Colin Kendall, anesthesiologist Stuart Leith, the chiefs of Anesthesiology and Nephrology, several residents and fellows, and Spencer Dunleavy, the anesthesiologist in charge of all three ICUs at Children's for patients over three months old.

The meeting had been called by Dunleavy. On Monday morning

he had begun a four-day rotation in Acute and Isolation and had emerged from rounds determined to orchestrate a plan for Freddy's management that would get the boy out of intensive care as soon as was feasible, both for the patient's sake—because being in the ICU was holding up his rehabilitation—and to free up his bed for a sicker child.

At issue was the question of when the patient could come off the ventilator. The neurosurgeons were not ready to withdraw respiratory support. They wanted the patient's carbon dioxide level kept low for the sake of the healing brain. The anesthesiologists, while conceding that the needs of the brain were paramount, were concerned about a strange acid imbalance that had hung on in Freddy's system for nearly two weeks. These doctors felt that hyperventilation prevented the patient's body from correcting the imbalance as it ordinarily would.

After some twenty minutes of discussion, the doctors were able to agree upon a plan. They would leave Freddy on the respirator and continue to hyperventilate him, but they would wean him gradually over the next few days, letting his CO_2 rise slowly. If all went well, the wean would continue until the boy was ready to come off the respirator entirely. But he would not be taken off entirely unless and until Colin Kendall gave the word.

An hour or two before this meeting took place, the patient who was its subject sat on the edge of his bed for the first time since his accident.

He did not sit without help. A physical therapist sat beside Freddy supporting his back, his left shoulder, and his chin. A tall, redheaded nurse named Paula Hewitt held a rolled towel around the back of his neck to support his head.

Nor did the boy appear to sit comfortably. Being upright caused him to cough hard and to wheeze hard. Without the mattress at his back, his body jerked like a rag doll's when he coughed. Strain showed all over his face.

But he was not dead weight by any means. He held the edge of the bed with both hands, and Paula could feel him helping himself to stay erect. His back seemed strong. The nurse was delighted.

"Pro! You look better than you ever did!"

A stranger on the scene might have been taken aback by this

burst of enthusiasm. The child had a feeding tube in his nose, a breathing tube in his throat, and a brace affixed to four stainless-steel pins anchored in the bone of his right thigh. His heart and respiratory rates were being monitored by a machine at his bedside. He was sitting with difficulty, staring straight ahead out the window overlooking the hospital atrium as if he couldn't spare the energy to even look around him. Saliva washed his chin. He swallowed when told to but infrequently otherwise. So long had Freddy's jaw hung slack that his front teeth had made a shallow indentation on the surface of his tongue. Though he was obviously alert, though his eyes were bright, his poor mouth control continued to make him appear deficient mentally. Without support, his head tended to tip to the left. On his left forehead was a small fresh pink scar.

"I didn't think he was this bad," the minister of Freddy's church had said to Paula in the hall on Sunday after delivering some four dozen get-well cards made that morning by the children in Sunday school.

"This is good," the nurse had told him. "You should have seen him two weeks ago."

In recent days the child had become a real person, a real personality, in Paula's opinion. He would smile now whenever the nurses told him to. In fact he'd now do anything they told him to if he could. When he smiled he looked so cute and sweet that every smile delighted Paula. She loved the way he held on to his ventilator tubes as if they were a security blanket, loved the expression he got on his face when she was about to suction him, as if to say, "I'm going to get you for this!" Yet he always cooperated.

He also had a sense of humor. Yesterday she had returned to the room to find that he'd put a towel over his face. When she'd taken it off, he'd laughed! He'd done it for a joke! He was such a rewarding child. Paula felt he had almost become more a friend than a patient.

Hearing her congratulations as he fought for balance at the edge of his bed, Freddy raised his eyes to her for an instant and managed a brief smile.

The physical therapist watched him closely. As his body seemed to need it, she shifted her support. "How're you doing, buddy? Do you think you can stay up another few minutes?"

When he didn't respond to the question, Paula encouraged him.

"Are you all right, Fred? If you think you can sit a little longer, raise your hand."

His right hand came eighteen inches off the bed. At that moment a transport nurse who had taken care of the child on several occasions bounced into the room.

"Fred-o! You look wonderful!"

Paula beamed. "Doesn't he? And you should have seen what he did yesterday morning! First of all, he's helping me brush his teeth now, aren't you, Pro? When I put the brush in, he can move it back and forth. Then yesterday I squirted some Cepacol in to clean his mouth out, and he started swishing the stuff around! Didn't you, Freddy!"

He seemed to be trying to concentrate on what she was saying. But he was also clearly laboring to meet the demands on his body of an unaccustomed position.

Paula continued. "I thought that was amazing! I said, 'You want to do it again?' He said yes. So I put some more in, and he swished that around, and then he opened his mouth so I could suction it out! I went out and told everybody, didn't I, Pro! That was so great. I couldn't believe you were doing that! You're a riot!"

He seemed preoccupied. Paula sensed that he was feeling tired. She began to massage the child's upper back. "You want to lie down, Pro? Raise your hand if you've had enough sitting up for one day."

His right hand left the mattress forefinger first.

"Are you tired?"

He raised the hand like a man taking an oath.

At the foot of the bed, the transport nurse exploded. "He's so good!"

Paula could have passed for a mother at graduation. "He's the most cooperative child in the world," she said as she helped the therapist ease Freddy back up into bed. "He never, never refuses to do anything. Even if fifteen people come in and tell him to squeeze a hand fifteen times in a row, he'll do it. You know the rotten looks you get from some kids? Not Fred. He's so cute and so sweet, aren't you, Pro?"

He did not respond. Though his eyes remained watchful, looking from one to another of the adults around him, he lay back on his pillows as if very glad to be there.

The physical therapist pulled a sheet up to the child's nipples. On command he lifted his right arm to make way for it. His left arm had not been responding well to commands and did not now. But when the therapist raised it off the bed herself, the arm left her hands, and the patient laid it across his waist.

Paula drew breath. So far as she knew, Freddy had not moved that arm as much since the accident. "Hey! I hope I wasn't the only one that saw that!"

She was not. Both the therapist and the transport nurse were grinning.

"Hey, buddy, good for you! That was good, Freddy! Excellent!"

"Pro, that was great! Your mom's going to be so happy!"

When the other two had gone, Paula began to clean the child's pin sites. She'd noticed a little bleeding start when they'd sat him up. Dabbing away, she happened to catch his eye.

"Are you all right, Pro?"

His eyes rested on her soberly.

"If you're uncomfortable, shake your head."

He didn't.

"If something hurts, tell me and I'll figure it out."

No response. He looked perfectly comfortable.

She smiled. "Can you put your tongue in for me, Freddy?"

His tongue receded slightly. She nudged it the rest of the way with a knuckle. "Now button your mouth."

His lips closed as if over a jawbreaker.

"Now smile, Pro. Can you?"

Lips together, Freddy gave her one of the sweetest smiles she had ever seen. She thought it the cutest thing in the whole world!

But it was more than cute. In that moment, for the first time in the more than two weeks Paula had been taking care of him and, so far as she knew, for the first time since his accident, something happened with that smile that might never have occurred had the car been going slightly faster, had the nearest hospital been in another county, had the medical team at Children's been a little less skilled, had the child been born a few years earlier, had luck gone against him. For the first time since an event which under other circumstances might have taken his life or destroyed his brain, Freddy Eberly looked normal.

Ø

Mark could not get comfortable. Propped nearly upright by pillows, he shifted from side to side to his back and onto his side again, taking oxygen but pulling for air. Though his night light was on, the room was nearly dark—darker than his room at Children's had ever gotten. He checked his watch. It was nearly midnight.

He began to cough. Reaching for his sputum cup, he bent over it seized by coughing. After a minute or so of effort that made him weak, he felt some mucus come up, and he spit it into the cup. For some reason the mucus tasted strange to him. He turned on his lamp to inspect it.

The stuff in the cup was bright red.

The phone rang in a dark house. Bob was away on an overnight business trip. At first Ellen thought the ringing of the phone was a dream. When she finally answered, Mark was crying.

"Mom, please come. I'm coughing up blood. I'm really scared."

He had coughed up blood before, of course. But he had never before called her to come to the hospital.

Dressing quickly, delaying only long enough to alert Denise and Randy, Ellen jumped in the car and drove to St. Michael's. The hemorrhaging had stopped by the time she arrived. A nurse took her into Mark's bathroom and showed her what was in the sputum cup. The blood did not alarm Ellen greatly. Though it was more than he had coughed up in the past, it was not a lot of blood—perhaps a tablespoonful or two. She knew that hemoptysis is not usually serious in itself and that it usually stops of its own accord. When Dr. Asher made rounds in the morning, she would tell him then what had happened.

She was less upset about the bleeding than about its effect on Mark. She didn't see how he could possibly have much time left. Why, why, why was he being put through hell every step of the way?

He was calmed by her assurances that she wouldn't leave him. Eventually, after a dose of chloral hydrate, he dropped off to sleep.

Tuesday, January 22

Ellen Price spent a restless night dozing off and on in the armchair beside her son's bed. But Mark slept fairly well and woke at 7:00 A.M. saying he felt pretty good, although Ellen thought him rather subdued. Dr. Asher came in about 7:30. He looked at the blood in Mark's sputum cup and responded as Ellen had expected him to: he was not particularly worried.

Even so, she would not have left Mark alone. But as it happened, his natural father had promised to spend the whole day with him. For this reason Ellen felt free to leave, and she wanted to leave, because in anticipation that Mark's father would be with the boy, she had invited her good friend Sandy to spend the day with her— the first fun Ellen had planned for herself in weeks. Mark urged her to go on home.

The two women were laughing over coffee at the Prices' kitchen table at 10:30 when the phone rang. Mark was in tears. He had brought up more blood. Would Ellen please come to the hospital?

Her first reaction was to cry out, "No, damn it, I'm not just a mother, I'm *me*, I'm a person! When am I going to get some time to myself?"

This impulse was immediately replaced by worry. "Of course, honey. Aunt Sandy and I will be right there."

Again the hemorrhaging had stopped by the time she arrived. Again her presence calmed him. The amount of blood was no greater than it had been last night. Ellen felt Mark out: did he want her to stay? When he pointed out that her favorite soap opera was coming on soon, Sandy left and Mark's father left, and Ellen stayed with her son for the rest of the day.

Ø

Daniel Earnshaw was working at his desk about 2:00 when his secretary called to say that Janet's mother was on the phone. The doctor thought this odd. The seventeen-year-old who was so determined to drive to Florida this spring had just been discharged on Saturday after a brief stay for treatment of a serious complication involving strain on her heart. Bruce Griffin had thought she'd looked much better when she went home.

"How are you?" he asked Janet's mother.

She told him she had found her daughter dead in bed this morning with her sputum cup in her hand.

He expressed his sympathy and asked what he could do. Janet's mother wondered if he could arrange for a death certificate. When he had done so and called her back, Earnshaw returned to the work on his desk. He did not expect to grieve Janet. He hadn't been that close to her. Though her death was a sad event, he had known it was coming and felt a lot of relief.

Several minutes later, Daniel Earnshaw's secretary heard him slap his office wall.

Wednesday, January 23

Jody Robinson began his day by taking one more small step toward freedom from the respirator. Since mid-December the machine had been breathing for him once per minute. As he had encountered no real difficulty at that level of support, he was started this morning on one breath every other minute. Of course the machine still supplied him oxygen along with the continuous positive pressure that kept his lungs slightly inflated. Nonetheless, when Jody became able to take all of his breaths unassisted, he would be considered by his caregivers to be, in essence, off the respirator.

The residents had lobbied for taking him off today. Though willing to entertain this idea, Peter Crossin had sensed that an interim step might be preferable. To check his hunch, he had spent an hour on Tuesday reviewing the entries of the past week or two in Jody's chart. The chart had told him that the child was awfully close to being able to breathe on his own. But Jody's respiratory rates were a shade high, suggesting that the patient was having to work to breathe, and his secretions were consistently described as moderate, thick, and yellow, which suggested a recurrence of bacterial infection.

Peter Crossin had seen many children come off respirators who had been on a long time. He knew that when weans near their conclusion, people get excited and anxious, and there is a tendency to sprint a little. Yet the slow process of developing respiratory capability does not accelerate in the last two weeks. If Jody Robinson were pushed and then got a serious infection, there could be a big-league setback. Crossin was determined not to make a mistake with this child. So he had agreed to one breath every two minutes on the understanding that if the patient did well, they would take him off the machine entirely sometime next week. Jody had been at Children's for nearly twenty months. There was no reason to rush.

Ø

Heading out of the Adolescent Unit on her way to lunch, Kate McDevitt saw that the head nurse's office was empty and, on impulse, dashed in and dialed Mark at St. Michael's. As soon as he answered she signaled several other nurses, and they took turns talking to the boy for nearly half an hour. At his bedside his mother sat feeling grateful to his friends for making him so animated and happy.

Early in the conversation he told Kate about the hemoptysis. "This time I'm really scared," he said, sounding scared. "There's gobs of blood coming up."

His choice of words made Kate nervous. Mark knew the difference between streaks and gobs.

In deference to the lunch schedule, Kate finally went off to eat leaving Julie on the line with Mark's mother. Julie gathered that Ellen was not particularly upset about the bleeding. Later all the nurses who had talked to Mark kept commenting on how good he had sounded. This had been Kate's impression as well. Though hearing concern in his voice, she had noted nothing unusual about his breathing.

What had upset and hurt them all was Mark's saying that none of the St. Michael's nurses would come in and talk to him.

But what stayed uppermost in Kate's mind that afternoon was the term "gobs." She found herself saying little prayers for Mark.

His breathing grew increasingly labored throughout the day, and at 7:30 in the evening, he coughed up more blood. This time his adoptive father was with him. Bob was unnerved by his son's fear. In the five years they had known each other, he had never before seen Mark frightened.

As had happened before, the bleeding soon stopped. Nonetheless, Mark remained extremely agitated and upset. He called his mother at home. On the phone she said the things that had calmed him down on Monday night and Tuesday. This time there was no comforting him.

"Would you feel better," she asked finally, "if you could talk to Dr. Earnshaw?"

"Yes, I want to talk to him."

"Do you remember that Dr. Asher was going to have a lung specialist come in and see you tomorrow?"

"Tomorrow is going to be too late," her son replied. "I'm going to die tomorrow."

Ellen took this comment not as literal truth but as a gauge of Mark's distress.

She dialed Daniel Earnshaw's home number. She told him about the bleeding and described the amounts. "And just to give you an idea what Mark's mental state is," she added, "he feels he's going to die tomorrow."

Hearing in this statement the overreaction of a boy to a mother who sometimes tended to overreact, Earnshaw replied without thinking, with an edge of impatience in his voice, "Mrs. Price. Let's not overdramatize this thing." His regret was instantaneous.

"I'm not overdramatizing," Ellen said simply. "I'm merely quoting to you what Mark said."

But the notion that bleeding had brought the boy to death's door was contrary to everything Earnshaw and his colleagues had experienced with CF patients who developed hemoptysis. The overwhelming experience at Children's and elsewhere had been that if the patient were kept quiet and the Mucomyst treatments and percussion were held, the bleeding would cease.

Earnshaw first called John Asher, in part as a courtesy: Mark was Asher's patient now. But the pediatrician also wanted a physician's assessment of the boy's status.

Asher was optimistic. Mark had gained a couple of pounds. His pneumothorax had decreased, bearing out Earnshaw's theory that the residual air would eventually be absorbed. Yes, Mark was having hemoptysis, but the amount of blood loss had been unremarkable. Asher was doing everything for it that Earnshaw would have done.

The St. Michael's doctor did mention that he thought the boy was having some adjustment problems. Earnshaw was not surprised. At Children's Mark knew the system and knew how to get what he wanted in the system. Probably there was no way he could have anticipated how strange surroundings would affect him. However, Dr. Asher seemed to feel that these problems were lessening for Mark.

His own sense of the patient's condition fortified by this conversation, Daniel Earnshaw phoned Mark. At the doctor's request, the boy described the bleeding. When he had finished, Earnshaw said, "Remember the patient you heard about at the hemoptysis conference who coughed up so much blood? That man was successfully treated. If he could be, you certainly can be."

"That was a bigger patient," Mark replied. "He had a lot more reserve than I have."

"Yes, but he coughed up a lot more blood than you did. You only coughed up a couple of tablespoons."

"I know I'm going to die. I'm not going to live through the night."

"Mark, that's not true," Earnshaw said very earnestly. "This thing stops. It always stops. It's going to stop for you. I always level with you, don't I? Haven't I always told you the truth?"

"Yes."

"Believe me, this is going to stop." The doctor had no reason to think that this boy was the exception to the rule.

Yet when he had given all the encouragement he could and both had said goodbye, Daniel Earnshaw hung up feeling he had not gotten through to Mark.

John Asher, meanwhile, called the St. Michael's respiratory specialist who had agreed to see Mark on Thursday and asked whether under the circumstances he could possibly visit him within the next few hours. As the specialist was still at the hospital, he said he would see the patient right away.

The man was rather young. When he began by asking Mark whether he knew anything about his disease, Bob Price settled back anticipating with pleasure a scene he had witnessed on any number of occasions—young doctor up against a kid knowing so damned much about cystic fibrosis that he could probably have written a book about it.

This time, however, Bob soon realized that the specialist had something to give the boy as well as something to learn from him. The doctor began explaining to Mark the difference between efficient coughing and wasted coughing, showing the boy how to lie on his side to get the best benefit from his effort to bring up mucus. Mark picked up on every suggestion. Bob found himself wishing this man had talked to his son years ago.

By the time the specialist left, it was 8:30. Visiting hours at St. Michael's were over at 8:00. Standing at the bedside, Bob told Mark he'd have to go now but would be back tomorrow after work.

Mark was lying on his side in the position the specialist had recommended to him. He was breathing with great difficulty. He had been breathing with great difficulty all evening. For a long time, he didn't acknowledge his father's comment. At last he said, his voice hoarse and very weak, "Bobby, I don't know how to explain it, but I feel so crappy."

In all the time they had known each other, Mark had never, not once, brought Bob any of his troubles.

At that moment the father happened to look down at his son's feet. He saw that Mark's feet were quivering, as if a tremendous nervousness had come upon them.

"I promise you this, Mark," Bob said, deeply moved. "I will be back tomorrow morning. I'll take my lunch hour early, and I'll come in here and eat my lunch with you. How would that be?"

"That would be fine." The words were barely audible.

Bob crossed the parking lot revising his prayers. For weeks he had been asking God to get Mark out of his pain and make him feel better. Now it came to Bob that he really had no right to pray that way. The course of Mark's life had been decided a long time ago. Whatever they were, the Lord had His reasons. Maybe He had a reason for not delivering the boy from his suffering. Maybe Mark wasn't quite ready.

Driving home, Bob Price made a new request for his son. "Dear God," he prayed, "please strengthen Mark's faith as much as You absolutely can, help *us* to strengthen his faith, give him tremendous faith, and once You've done that, take him quickly."

Ninety minutes later a nurse did what she could to make Mark comfortable for sleep. She left him lying on one side on pillows against the raised mattress, breathing hard. In the dim glow cast by the night light over his bed, his face was exceedingly pale.

Shortly after 11:00, as the unit clerk and another nurse were leaving for home, they passed Mark's room and saw that he was sitting bowed low over pillows in his lap, a dark form silhouetted against the blackness out his window. The two women went in to say good night. Seeing that he was in great physical distress and very anxious, the nurse urged him gently to try to lie back and get some rest.

He shook his head. "I don't want to lie down," he answered, heaving for air. "I'm afraid I'll fall asleep and never wake up."

The women reported this comment to the charge nurse on the night shift. Soon thereafter the resident covering the floor received the results of blood studies ordered earlier by the respiratory specialist. The studies were worse than had been expected, showing a very low level of oxygenation. Reached by the resident at home, the specialist ordered that the patient be made to lie in a certain way and be kept calm.

The resident then called the respiratory therapist on duty and asked her to assess the patient, to ascertain whether he was short of breath because he was apprehensive or the other way around. After a few minutes with Mark, the therapist concluded that both things were true. The boy asked her to percuss him. She did so very lightly. He got rid of some mucus and told her he felt better.

When the therapist left, a nurse came in to stay with Mark. "I'll just be here," she said. "You don't have to say anything." Leaving just the night light on, she pulled up a chair and sat down close to the bed. Within a short time, though his breathing remained extremely labored, he appeared to grow calmer.

Suddenly he grabbed her hand. "Please don't leave me alone," he said. "I'm not going to make it through the night."

The woman was young, a June graduate. She had never cared for so sick a child. It occurred to her that he was going to die—not somewhere in the future, but soon.

"Do you want me to call your mother?"

"No. She would be too upset."

"Mark, there's a chaplain who stays at the hospital. A priest. Would you like to see Father Carroll?"

He shook his head. No. He asked her what it was like to die.

The question shook her to the core. She had no idea how to answer him. To an older person, she might have said, "You probably just close your eyes and go to sleep." This boy was in so much distress that for him it might not be that simple.

"I don't know, Mark," she said, feeling for words, "but I was knocked unconscious once when I fell roller-skating, and when I woke up, it was like I had been somewhere else in the universe without even knowing or experiencing it. I just knew that wherever I'd been was not a frightening place."

He nodded. "I know I'm dying," he said hoarsely. "I just don't want to die tonight."

She gripped his hand in both of hers, for both their sakes. "Mark, are you afraid?"

"I'm not afraid, but I don't want to be alone."

"I won't leave you."

He was awake all night and alone not even for a moment. When one nurse had to leave for some reason, another took her place. The resident and the respiratory therapist were in and out. Every staff member on the floor kept trying to think of things to do for Mark to make him more comfortable. He refused every offer. He wanted nothing to eat, nothing to drink, though they kept a chilled can of soda at his bedside; he did not want to be suctioned; he would not, until early morning, accept oxygen.

He did ask several other nurses what it was like to die. The only thing he seemed to want was information they couldn't give him.

Finally around 5:00 A.M. the nursing supervisor placed a call to the chaplain.

"I'm sorry to awaken you, Father, but we have a fifteen-year-old boy with cystic fibrosis down here who seems to be dying and very much afraid," the supervisor told the chaplain. Actually Mark had expressed fear to no one. "Could you come down and see him?"

Thursday, January 24

The priest dressed and made his way to the third floor. He was a man of forty-two years, clean-cut and slim. He had lived at the hospital half a decade. At the door of the patient's room, Father Carroll paused momentarily to adjust his eyes to the near-darkness inside. He could see the figure of a boy who looked much younger than fifteen sitting cross-legged on the bed, clutching a pillow to his abdomen, using oxygen prongs, and gasping for breath. As the priest entered the room, a nurse who had been sitting at the bedside excused herself and slipped out into the hall.

Father Carroll approached the patient slowly and with awe. He sensed himself in the company of someone about to enter into the presence of God. He touched the youngster's scrawny shoulder.

"Mark, I'm the hospital chaplain, Father Carroll. I just want to say hello to you. I know you're not able to talk too much right now. I just want to be here with you."

The boy nodded. Very gently the priest began rubbing Mark's arms and his heaving, bony back. Out the window he could see the black forms of trees and hills under a clear sky scattered with stars.

"Is this all right?" he asked after a moment.

Again the boy nodded. "Yes," he whispered. "Thank you."

While having no notion of the patient's background, the priest had gotten a feeling from the supervisor that Mark might be needful of religious succor. He attempted to address this need.

"God loves you very much, Mark," the chaplain said softly. "God is close to you." Because the boy seemed so alone, he added, "And your parents are going to be in in a little while."

"Father?"

"Yes?" The man bent over him to hear.

"Could . . . you open the . . . soda . . . that's on my bedside table?"

"Of course." Father Carroll picked up the cola can, turned away from the bed, snapped the tab, and held the can to the boy's lips. Even with only the tiny night light burning, he could see that the lips were tinged blue.

"Thank you, Father," Mark whispered after swallowing several sips.

The priest thought it extraordinary that this boy would use the little bit of breath he had left to express gratitude.

For at least the next hour, Father Carroll was more a nurse to the boy than a chaplain, rubbing the patient's back and arms, giving him soda, handing him tissues, trying to ease his distress and help him get more comfortable. Few words were spoken. Each kept his own counsel, the child suffering, the priest wrapped in thoughts about the child's suffering and the redemptive agony of Christ on the cross. When the stars began to fade and the sky to become less intensely dark, Father Carroll, feeling slightly stiff from standing so long in one position, went around the bed, took the chair the nurse had vacated, and resumed his rubbing of the patient's back. He could not imagine how much longer the boy could go on breathing with such effort.

Then Mark raised his head and said to the priest, "What's it like to die, Father?"

It was the most explicit question the chaplain had ever been asked by someone who was dying. It was also a question he had had on his mind. His own father was nearing death in a hospital across town.

Trying to guess what a fifteen-year-old would fear most about dying, Father Carroll decided that Mark would probably fear the aloneness of the experience, being cut off from other people and going solitary into the unknown.

The priest leaned close to the boy. "Mark, as far as I know, dying is only a moment. It passes very quickly. When it does, you will be with Jesus. There will be lots and lots of people who will welcome you and love you. One day you will see your mother and father there, and you'll all be back together."

After a few moments, Mark nodded his head and gasped, "Okay."

He said nothing further until the priest was preparing to leave.

In order to see people before they went to surgery, Father Carroll made rounds every morning beginning at 6:00. Ordinarily when he was up with patients at night, he left them by 6:00 to observe this aspect of his ministry. Mark's great need for a comforting presence had caused the priest to stay on with the boy. But at 7:15, when daylight had broken, Father Carroll felt he could delay his rounds no longer.

He explained this to Mark. He offered to say a prayer. The youngster nodded and folded his hands. The priest folded his.

"Dear Lord," he said, "our brother Mark is in great distress at this time. He believes in you, trusts you, loves you, and he asks you now for your special help. We ask you . . ."

The priest cleared his throat. "We ask you to relieve him of his suffering. We ask you to never abandon him but to bring him safely home. We ask you this, Lord, in the words of the One who taught us to pray, Our Father, Who art in heaven, hallowed be Thy name . . ."

The boy had joined with him, gasping at nearly every word.

"Thy kingdom come, Thy will be done, on earth as it is in heaven. Give us this day our daily bread, and forgive us our trespasses as we forgive those who trespass against us. And lead us not into temptation, but deliver us from evil. Amen."

The priest rose. For a long moment he stood looking down at the boy. *O Lamb of God, that takest away the sins of the world . . .*

Words failing, he bent and kissed the pale cheek.

He could not have done otherwise. The moment would stand as one of the most poignant in his chaplaincy.

"Thank you, Father."

An hour later, before going to work, Bob Price drove to the store and bought some sliced ham and fresh rye bread for sandwiches for Mark, who had been eating very little else.

Ellen prepared a sandwich, dressed, and at 9:30 called Mark to tell him she was on her way.

His voice on the phone was very weak.

"Honey, I'm sorry, did I wake you up?"

"Yeah."

"Well, go back to sleep. I'm just about to leave. Can I bring you anything?"

"No."

When she arrived he was awake and extremely anxious, lying upright on his side, very short of breath, very pale, obviously feverish, apparently exhausted. He could scarcely talk. Ellen had been thinking in terms of weeks or months. The moment she laid eyes on him she knew he would die in a matter of days.

She kissed him, took her coat off, kissed him again. She felt as if she were moving in a dream. "How are you feeling?"

"Mom, I'm doing everything the doctors ask me to do, and it doesn't help."

Numbly she straightened his bedding. "Just do the best you can, honey," she said. "That's all you can do. Do you need something, can I get you something?"

He shook his head. "I'll see if I can go back to sleep."

Ellen walked into the hall and saw Dr. Asher on the telephone at the nurses' station. As she approached, he nodded to her and held up a finger. He was a short man with dark brown hair and what Ellen had always thought of as spaniel eyes. A soft-spoken person, and very caring, she felt.

Replacing the receiver, he said to her quietly, "I've been waiting for you. I'm sorry to tell you this, but his blood gases are very bad."

"Meaning what?"

"Meaning that the only thing left to do for him is to put him on a respirator."

"No. I don't want him on a respirator." Thank God, Ellen thought, for the conversation she and Bob had had about respirators last month with Dr. Earnshaw. It would have been awful to have to make that decision on the spur of the moment.

"I understand," Asher said sympathetically. "But I want you to understand that if we don't do it, he can't go on a great deal longer."

She was firm. There wasn't a doubt in her mind. "No heroics."

She called her husband and was told by Bob's secretary that he was already on his way. She called her former husband, Mark's natural father, who said he would get to St. Michael's as soon as he could.

Then Ellen sat with her son while he slept and tried to get a grip on herself. She had been preparing for his death for fifteen years. At times she had prayed for it. Now that it was upon her, she felt rattled, frightened, angry, grief-stricken. She couldn't bear the thought of losing him, of letting him go. Her tears came freely.

Yet how could she wish for him to stay? He had no color left.

His body had wasted away to little more than a skeleton. He could hardly breathe. He was in acute distress. She realized as she sat with him that he wasn't coughing. He didn't even have the energy to cough.

He awoke a little before noon. Going to him, she offered him some soda from the can on his bed table. He was not strong enough to sit up without her help. After a few sips, he sank back against the pillows. His face was hot. Ellen stroked his blond hair back from his forehead. He was terribly agitated.

After a moment he said hoarsely, "I'm sorry, Mom. I can't fight it anymore. I want to die."

Her hand froze at his temple. Their eyes locked.

"I'm not afraid," he gasped. "I have faith in God, and I'm ready to go and be with God."

Dazed, Ellen bent and touched her lips to his face. "Honey, you don't have to apologize for anything. If anybody deserves a rest, you do."

"Will you please ask Dr. Asher to give me something to help me?"

"I will."

But Dr. Asher had gone off the floor. Ellen left word with one of the nurses that she wanted to see him as soon as possible.

When she got back to the room, Mark was asleep again. Bob arrived minutes later. Seeing him in the doorway, Ellen jumped up from her chair and led him into the hall. There, holding him, she said, very lovingly, "He's dying."

Confusion filled him, a tangle of relief and disbelief. My God, was it actually happening? Was it finally coming to an end? A week, then? A few days?

"He told me," Ellen said, "that he was ready to go. He made a beautiful confession of his faith." She repeated the conversation.

Bob was overjoyed. His prayer had been answered. "Strengthen his faith," he had asked, and the Lord had done so. What a lift. What a lift.

Dr. Asher found them in the solarium. Ellen told him what Mark had said and what he had requested.

The physician spoke carefully. "You realize, of course, that that would hasten things. There would be no going back from that step."

"We know."

Wishing to make certain that Mark's parents understood the medical situation as fully as possible, wishing to forestall regrets, Dr. Asher went over with the Prices the three options open to them. The respirator was one. He discussed the pros and cons. Bronchodilators were another—drugs that would open up Mark's bronchial passages, ease his breathing, and conceivably buy time. The third option was to do nothing, in which case, the doctors told the Prices, Mark would surely die.

Neither parent would reconsider the respirator. Both agonized over bronchodilators. At length, hands shaking, Ellen took from her purse a copy of the Conversation and handed it to Dr. Asher, saying, "Most of all I want to do what Mark would want, and I think he has already told us."

The doctor read the three pages with full attention. Returning the document to the boy's mother, he said with no discernible reluctance, "I see what you mean. I understand your position. Insofar as the medication goes, I will give him the maximum I can under the law."

"Thank you," Ellen said tearfully. "We want him to be comfortable. It's the only thing left we can do for him."

There was nothing simple about their request. The parents were talking in the realm of euthanasia. Giving Mark a narcotic to make him more comfortable would depress his respirations and might very well hasten his demise. The legality of taking such a step even when the patient was requesting it was highly questionable. Asher felt himself between a rock and a hard place. What could he give that would satisfy the boy's request and the parents' wishes as well as the demands of his own conscience and the law?

Ordinarily such dilemmas are resolved through painstaking deliberation. This case did not offer that luxury. There wasn't time.

At last Asher decided on an unsatisfactory compromise. He would give Mark two milligrams of Valium. Given the level of the patient's anxiety, the amount was too small to calm him very much. But it was also too small to depress the boy's respirations. Though Asher didn't feel comfortable giving it, he could square the decision with his ethics.

He entered Mark's room. The Prices were with the boy. The doctor stepped to the bedside.

"Mark, I have something here that should make you a little more comfortable. I'm going to squirt it into your IV line."

The patient opened his eyes. "What is it?"

"Valium."

"How much are you giving me?"

Under any other circumstances, Ellen would have had to smile. Even now he had to know every detail.

"Two milligrams."

The patient closed his eyes without comment. The doctor infused the drug. A short time later, Mark drifted back into a fitful sleep.

But he kept waking up.

"Mom?"

"Yes, honey. I'm right here, Mark."

"Mom, I love you very, very much."

"Oh, Mark, I love you so much. We all do."

"I think I'm going back to sleep now."

"Bob?" His eyes opened, searched.

"Yes, Mark." Bob leaned over him.

"I want you to know that I love you very much."

"Markie . . ."

"Mom?"

"I'm here, darling. What can I do for you?"

"Please tell Dad I love him very much."

In the course of an hour, he named his sister, his brother, his step-siblings, and several of his nurses at Children's Hospital, beginning with Kate.

At about 1:45 he came awake and told his parents that the end was near. He said he was in pain. He asked for morphine.

This time Dr. Asher called the respiratory specialist who had seen Mark Wednesday night. At first the specialist recommended against giving the patient anything, on the grounds that the issue was legally unclear. But Asher felt anguished. The boy was distraught. If morphine was too strong, wasn't there *something* they could do to help him?

The specialist reconsidered. At last the two physicians agreed on a small dose of Thorazine, a drug somewhat more potent than the chloral hydrate Mark had been accustomed to taking for sleep. Again with reservations, Dr. Asher injected the drug into the patient's IV line. Again Mark questioned him as to the identity of the medication and the amount being given. This time when he went back to sleep, he slept soundly.

Seeing that his death was inevitable, the nurses disturbed the family as little as possible, as the Prices seemed to want. Of course they let it be known that they were available. Yet the nurses could see that not much could be done for the boy beyond what his mother was already doing. She seemed to know his needs by looking at him. He seemed well prepared for dying. The nurses attributed his acceptance to his good relationship with his mother.

They stood by feeling utterly helpless. The nurse in charge finally went into the medications room and cried.

Father Carroll returned to Mark's room as often as he could. In a few hours, with their own pastor out of town, the Prices had come to think of the priest as their friend. When he was with them, they felt swathed in a balm of peace. They found him an exceptional man.

Bob had arranged for Denise and Randy to be brought to the hospital after school by family friends. At 3:30 Ellen began watching for the car in the drive below Mark's window. By this time the Prices had been joined in Mark's room by the children's natural father and his wife.

Ellen saw the car turn in at 3:35. The two fathers went to meet Denise and Randy at the elevator. Right after they had gone, Mark emerged from sleep and acknowledged his mother with his eyes. For several minutes he dozed, oxygen prongs in place. A nurse noted in the chart that his hands and feet were bluish, and Dr. Asher wrote below that entry that the patient's respiratory distress was severe.

Suddenly the boy sat bolt upright in bed and cried, "Help me! Help me!" His tone was not fearful. He was making a request. Ellen would not realize until some time later that he was not making it of her.

She flew up from her chair. Putting one arm around his shoulder, she grabbed his soda with her other hand, pure reflex, then set the soda down and pushed a pillow into his lap for support, but he fell forward against her, and as she stood holding him, and as the seconds passed, she became aware that his chest was still.

Ellen's eyes met the other woman's. "Please go and get the doctor," she whispered. "I think he's dead."

He was pronounced dead at 4:17 P.M.

Father Carroll came in and helped his mother lay him down and straighten his body.

He turned to the family. "I've known Mark a very short time," he said, "but he made such an impression on me."

It's an answer to prayer, Bob was thinking. The boy's faith was strengthened, and within four hours, God took him. You could say there was something beautiful in that.

At 7:30, back home, Bob called Adolescent and asked for Kate. Told that she was at home, he gave the news to the nurse who had answered the phone and asked her to please let Kate know.

Kate had only to hear her colleague's tone of voice.

She hung up and dialed the Prices' number. Bob answered. "We wanted you to hear it from us," he said. "You're part of the family."

"I'm so sorry," was all she could say.

"We all are, Kate," he said, "but his pain is over. In a way, we're celebrating. Just a minute, here's his mother."

Kate broke down. "Oh, Ellen . . ."

"I know, baby. I know."

They had called Daniel Earnshaw first. The phone rang while he and his wife were eating dinner. It was he who answered.

"Dr. Earnshaw, this is Ellen Price. I wanted you to know that Mark died this afternoon."

For an instant he thought he had not heard her correctly.

But then he knew he had.

But they had just lost Janet this week.

But he had been expecting that.

"He wants an autopsy," Ellen said.

Earnshaw thought suddenly of his father's funeral. As a boy, his father had loved fire engines. He had learned the number and location of every fire engine, battalion chief, lieutenant, and captain in the city, and he had known many of the firemen. Even as an adult, in practice as a doctor, when a fire engine would come down the street and Pop had no patients, he'd put on his coat and run after it.

Earnshaw had done no crying when his father died. Almost ninety years old, the man had been failing mentally and physically for several years. The failing had been more a grief to Earnshaw than the death. He had done no crying at his father's funeral.

But after the funeral, as the family came out of the church, as the pallbearers were loading the casket into the hearse, a fire engine had come roaring down the street, bells clanging, and Earnshaw's tears had flowed.

As they flowed now for Mark. In all his years of caring for children with cystic fibrosis, Daniel Earnshaw had never before had a patient request an autopsy.

Friday, January 25

The Adolescent nurses gathered for morning report were unusually quiet. Much of what little talking they did took the form of solicitous questions about how the others were doing. They were not doing particularly well. Mark's death on top of Janet's had hit hard.

It might have hit less hard had he died at Children's. But the thought of Mark nearing his end among people who scarcely knew him deeply hurt the Adolescent nurses and made one or two of them angry. The anger was directed primarily at Daniel Earnshaw. One nurse actually felt betrayed by the physician. She found it almost inconceivable that a doctor who had taken care of so many cystics over so many years would not have realized how near death Mark was, and she could not imagine why, if he realized it, he would have transferred the boy. Another nurse wondered about Mark's role in the transfer. Had he knowingly gone to St. Michael's to die? Had he arrived at a stage of acceptance while the nurses who loved him had remained in a stage of denial?

With all their hearts those nurses wished that they had been able to share with Mark and his family his final hours.

They faced an immediate problem posed by the two CF patients presently occupying the room opposite the nurses' station. One was a sixteen-year-old with relatively mild manifestations of the disease who was being discharged today after a routine admission. The other was Lisa Fletcher. Admitted last evening from the emergency room in acute respiratory distress and showing signs of the same grave heart complication for which Janet had been treated only days before her death, Lisa was already terribly upset. If the girls asked about Mark, what if anything should the nurses tell them?

Bruce Griffin was called to Adolescent to advise the staff. Griffin was not at all eager for Lisa to find out about Mark. "However," he said to the nurses, "my feeling about this is the same as Dr. Earnshaw's: you wait until you're asked, and then you always tell the truth."

Kate was asked within five minutes of walking into the room. Both girls burst into tears. Trying not to, Kate cried with them. Her attempts to emphasize the peacefulness of Mark's death and the fact that he had died with his family fell on deaf ears.

Lisa kept pointing out that she and Mark were both fifteen. She questioned Kate sharply on how exactly Mark and Janet had died. When Kate had to say that the doctors didn't know that yet, Lisa began to scream.

"Nobody knows how you die of this disease! You never know if the next thing you get is going to do it! You just die!"

"I know," Kate said miserably. "It must be very frightening for you." She felt as if a bomb had hit and she had dropped it.

Eventually she told them that Mark had asked for an autopsy. Lisa wanted to know why. Kate quoted Ellen, saying "He wanted the doctors to learn enough about cystic fibrosis to cure it or prevent it."

Lisa nodded. Her pale face was red from crying. Tears shone in her eyes. "I see." Her voice was trembling. "He did it for us, then."

Kate couldn't answer her.

"He was brave," said Lisa. "Mark was brave."

Ø

Toward the end of the morning, Freddy Eberly was transferred out of the Isolation Unit and back across the hall to Acute. Treatment and a change of environment had altered his bacterial picture so that he was no longer a threat to other patients. The doctors were hoping to discharge him upstairs to the Leverett House Annex for rehabilitation within a matter of days. The period of danger to his brain was just about over. The doctors were beginning to believe the patient needed hyperventilation somewhat less than he needed rehab. Colin Kendall now felt satisfied that Freddy Eberly had recovered his ventilatory ability and could perform the mechanical functions of breathing without difficulty.

The nurses in Isolation were sad to have Freddy leave their unit. They would all miss him. For most of January, Isolation had been unusually full of very ill children. In that environment, Freddy Eberly had been a bright spot. He'd never been the sickest patient in the unit, and he had improved greatly during his three weeks in Isolation, and he had become very responsive. Sick as he still was, the nurses could always get him to smile.

Ø

It was 3:30 before Sam Silver found a few free minutes to call the DeRose household with the results of the latest enzyme studies. They were good. Silver wanted to tell Marie DeRose she could keep Gina on the two Methotrexate tablets.

The patient answered. Her doctor gave her the news and then asked her how school was going.

"Fine! I got a hundred and a ninety-one!"

He couldn't resist. "How come ninety-one?"

She pretended for an instant to be insulted. "Ninety-one's okay! Hey, Sam, why do ducks and geese fly north in the springtime?"

"I'll bite. Why?"

"Because it's too far to walk!"

Sunday, January 27

In the morning, one month and one day after being struck down by a car and receiving severe multiple injuries that raised fundamental questions about the kind of future he could anticipate, Frederick Patterson Eberly, age nine, learned to suction his own mouth, helped Angie Bremness figure out that he had a charley horse by writing LEG on a pad of paper after letting her know he felt pain but then being unable to organize his thoughts enough to show her where, and ate one whole cherry popsicle which he fed to himself.

In the afternoon, as his mother was getting ready to leave for home, Freddy picked up the pad of paper and a blue crayon that lay beside him on the mattress and wrote for her, in ungainly letters that were nonetheless completely legible, HAVE A GOOD TIME.

In the evening he was taken off the respirator. He did just fine.

Monday, January 28

Colin Kendall and the two junior residents with whom he was making morning rounds stood at Freddy Eberly's bedside in Acute and listened to several nurses describe the patient's progress with enthusiasm. Freddy followed the conversation by shifting his gaze from speaker to speaker. Though his tongue still protruded, though saliva bubbles still collected around it, though he was still drooling, his eyes were bright and alert. He was getting oxygen mist from the mouth of a thick green plastic tube anchored in his tracheostomy. The mist rose in a column to the level of the child's nose, then dispersed and vanished.

"Freddy had a popsicle yesterday!" Angie Bremness boasted to the neurosurgeons. "He did great!"

"That's the sure sign of cure," Kendall teased. "Once they start taking popsicles, that's it!" He picked up from the mattress a short piece of leather strap fitted with several large sleigh bells. Jingling them, he addressed the patient. "What's this?"

A nurse replied. "Those came off a baby stroller! They're his pee-and-poop bells, right, Pro?"

The patient nodded.

The nurse prompted him. "That's your cue to laugh!"

He laughed. His shoulders shook. From the tracheostomy in his throat, free, now, of the ventilator hookup, came a soft gurgling sound.

"He's supposed to ring the bells to let us know when he has to go," Angie put in. "He doesn't always do it, but he's getting better, aren't you, Frederick!"

He laughed again.

Smiling, Kendall began a cursory examination. "Can you lift your left hand, Fred?"

The child stared at him.

After a moment, Kendall lifted the hand himself and let go of it. Freddy returned it slowly to the mattress.

"Swallow, Pro," the doctor ordered.

The child did.

"Listen, Fred," Kendall continued confidentially, "I've been hearing all kinds of rumors that you're scratching your ear with your left hand. Is that just a story, or can you really do it?"

The hand twitched. So hard did the child appear to be concentrating that those watching could feel his effort.

"I'll help you a little," Kendall said. He laid the hand on the patient's abdomen. "Okay, Freddy, try again."

The child applied ingenuity. He lifted his left hand with his right and held it forth. The small crowd watching broke up.

A nurse admonished him. "No cheating!"

The patient laughed.

"He can do it," Angie insisted, blotting Freddy's chin. "Yesterday he was moving it all over the place."

The neurosurgeons moved ten steps across the floor to check on a craniofacial patient. The nurses remained at Freddy's bedside, coaching and coaxing him. Exactly what they said to the child did not reach Kendall's ears. But just as he and the residents started out of the unit, the nurses called out, "Colin! Colin!" and the neurosurgeons turned to see Freddy Eberly lift his left arm clean off his mattress and into the air above his side rail. Unassisted.

The nurses' expressions were something to behold. It was to them as much as to the patient that Colin Kendall said, laughing, "Okay, Pro, I see you! I believe you!"

Ø

In his office two floors up, Daniel Earnshaw went through the mail on his desk and tried to pull himself together to start the week. Mondays were always tough for Earnshaw, and today was worse than most because the week had been so bad—a week in which Earnshaw had been reminded how glad he was to have a colleague, somebody he could talk to. He would never have wanted to treat children with cystic fibrosis in isolation.

On Saturday he had slept much later than usual and awakened tired, surprised by the hour. He hadn't realized how tired he was. In the afternoon he had stopped by to see his mother. After checking her blood pressure, Earnshaw had told her about Mark's death without the least bit of feeling that he needed to be careful. To his surprise, she had wept.

"What am I crying for?" his mother had said. "I never even saw the child."

Her son could not get the youngster out of his mind.

He was to be buried this afternoon. Earnshaw would not be present for the ceremony. Although he had made an exception of the burial service for Perry Smith, the doctor spared himself his patients' funerals.

He would have wanted to be present for Mark's dying, however. For Mark's sake. For the family's sake. For his own. Daniel Earnshaw had lost many patients in his long career in cystic fibrosis. All but four had died at Children's. If Earnshaw hadn't been present at the moment of their passing, he had come in directly thereafter and talked to the family on the scene. These conversations helped him to resolve his own feelings about the death.

So did seeing the patient. Always he took comfort in the serenity on the face of a child who had died of CF. In life those faces were tense from struggle. In death the muscles relaxed into a remarkable peacefulness. While there was typically a little discoloring around the lips, Earnshaw found this preferable to an undertaker's makeup, to the stuffing with which he knew undertakers packed the children's jaws to camouflage the gauntness.

But Janet had died at home. Mark had died at another hospital. About both youngsters Earnshaw felt an absence of resolution.

He was optimistic that resolution would occur when the parents returned for a visit. Usually parents didn't come back, in his experience, until they felt strong enough to tolerate the memories the place would inevitably trigger. It always did Earnshaw good to see families getting themselves together again.

Often parents come back to Children's to learn the results of an autopsy. Earnshaw expected these to be the circumstances under which he would next see Bob and Ellen Price. In one sense meetings of this nature were invariably difficult for Earnshaw. CF parents weren't interested in cause of death. They had lived with that knowledge for years. Parents wanted to feel that their child's life had not been fruitless. They wanted to know what information their child had left behind that would help other children.

In truth a single autopsy rarely yields much new information. Of course Earnshaw did not say this to parents. His best answer to their question was some version of "You never know." He could say in good conscience that the autopsies of a great many children who had died of cystic fibrosis over the years had contributed substantially to current knowledge about the disease. While none of these findings had yet resulted in a cure, Earnshaw could tell parents truthfully that they had shed light on the machinery.

Conceivably he would be able to tell the Prices a little more. Mark had had tetracycline poured into his chest. In that respect the boy differed from all other cystic children Earnshaw had ever taken care of. The drug had been introduced in the hope that it would produce enough scar tissue to hold the patient's lung up against his chest wall. That had been . . . how long before he died?

Earnshaw reached for his calendar. Bright sunlight coming in his window warmed his shoulders. He was aware of sharp winds tearing around outside. A beautiful winter day, among the bitterest Earnshaw could remember. He had walked from the train with gloved hands in his pockets and eyes watering.

He counted back fifty-one days. Mark's autopsy would give his doctors a chance to look at what the tetracycline had accomplished in that period. Ideally, good adhesions would have formed. But even if they had not, Neil Martinson could place the autopsy results against the results of his rabbit study and gain some insight into the validity of the animal experiments in humans.

Earnshaw imagined himself saying to Mark's parents, "Well, now we've got a better idea what the inside of a pleura looks like seven weeks after tetracycline." He wondered how such a statement could possibly satisfy them. It wouldn't satisfy him. He had been at this work a long time now, hoping for an answer for nearly a quarter of a century. He was as impatient as the parents were.

Yet Earnshaw had a feeling that a good tetracycline finding would satisfy Mark. Mark was a realist. He would be expecting no miracles. If he could not contribute to a cure for CF, he might just be satisfied to spare someone else a little of the pain and uncertainty that had so taxed his own spirits in his last weeks.

The boy had *asked* for an autopsy. Earnshaw couldn't get over that.

He wished he knew exactly why. Mark had *said* he hoped something could be learned from him that would help unravel the mystery of his disease, a perfectly reasonable and logical justification for his request.

But Earnshaw wondered whether there might not also have been emotional grounds for Mark's decision to offer his tissues for dissection. The boy was only fifteen. Maybe he had said to himself, "I've never really had an opportunity to make my presence felt in this world. Here's my chance to do something for somebody." A way of saying the same thing, perhaps. But Earnshaw felt that the one said a little bit more than the other.

He had loved Mark as he had loved few other patients.

Yet as he pulled from his desk drawer a sheet of his personal stationery, the doctor recognized within himself the beginnings of relief. Like all children who die of CF, Mark had clearly lived past the time when his life contained any joy. "Death is the old man's friend," a professor of Earnshaw's had been fond of saying. Years in the field of cystic fibrosis had taught Earnshaw that death is also the friend of the chronically ill child.

He wrote now his second letter of bereavement in a week:

Dear Mr. and Mrs. Price,

It is difficult to know what to say to you. You have lost a son.

I have lost a patient. The world has lost a fine young man. The loss saddens us all.

As I remember Mark, I like to recall the happy times, his bright eyes, his enthusiasm, his curiosity and his joy in learning. When Mark grew older we became more than doctor and patient; we became friends. I looked forward to seeing him as one anticipates meeting a friend.

His memory will be precious to me, as I know it is to you.

Sincerely,

Daniel B. Earnshaw

As the hour of his burial approached, Mark Price was on the minds of many people at Children's Hospital. Whatever their other reactions to the news of his death, almost all had felt surprise.

Anesthesiology resident Susan Carlson had been shocked and saddened. Surgeon Abe Weinberg had been moved to wonder whether the whole matter of surgery for Mark shouldn't have been discussed more thoroughly beforehand and to wish he had not put the boy through any discomfort whatever.

Alan Cavanaugh's first impulse had been to throw up his hands. Mark had survived the pneumothorax, survived the pain of the tetracycline and the discomfort of the chest tubes, survived surgery; they had gotten a hyperal line in him and gotten him up to where he could be close to his family; all that had happened, and the boy hadn't even lived a week. Cavanaugh found Mark's death ironic and a shame and very depressing.

Darryl Barth had reacted with gratitude and pain. In common with virtually everyone else at Children's who had known Mark well, the resident felt that over the past several months, the boy had lived through more than any one person should be asked to endure. Barth felt grateful that Mark had been delivered from this ordeal. He saw Mark's demise as perhaps the least traumatic of all the catastrophes to have befallen the boy. Barth wept less for Mark's death than for the life he had had to live, and for his youth, and for the limitations of a science which ultimately had failed him.

Social worker Dick Jacoby, too, felt relief and sadness. But thinking of Mark and of other kids like him who had died—nice kids, brave kids—Jacoby also felt frustrated and angry, knowing that what had happened to Mark was going to happen again and again.

He lay in an open coffin in a small room adjacent to the pale yellow sanctuary of the Lutheran church to whose congregation he had belonged. Around him, greeting people coming in to see him, were his mother, his two fathers, his natural father's wife, his brother and sister and step-siblings, his grandparents and step-grandparents, his friend Carl, and Carl's parents, Ellen's good friend Sandy and her husband. Though Ellen's eyes were moist, though Bob frequently blew his nose, both gave and accepted warm hugs and loving words with occasional smiles.

Mark wore a light blue blazer over dark blue trousers. He had his glasses on. Even under makeup his skin looked pallid. People who hadn't seen him recently could hardly believe how thin he was. But the peace on his face was unmistakable. The three nurses from Children's who had been able to switch their schedules—Kate, Julie, and Allyson—arrived just in time to see him before the casket was closed and rolled into the church to stand throughout the service at the head of the aisle.

The organist played a prelude. Sun came into the sanctuary through pastel windows of yellow, blue, and lavender. The oak pews were well filled. From the simple white altar Pastor Arthur Stroud read scriptural passages chosen by Ellen, including the Ninety-first Psalm, which she had read to Mark while the tetracycline smoldered in his chest. Ellen had also chosen the hymns. All were favorites of Mark's, especially the first. Most of the congregants sang it without needing to consult their programs:

> Have Thine own Way, Lord; Have Thine own way!
> Thou art the Potter; I am the clay.
> Mold me and make me after Thy will,
> While I am waiting, yielding and still.
>
> Have Thine own way, Lord . . .

At the back of the church, Clara Bowman entered the sanctuary and slipped into the last pew. Back in the city she had broken a heel off her boot. Two closed repair shops later, broken heel and all, she had hopped in her car and headed north at seventy miles per hour, nearly tearing up the highway. She had swerved once dangerously but had not slowed down.

"Lord, just keep the cops off me, but I got to get there," she had prayed.

The news had come to her Friday morning in report. Clara had been unable to move. All day she had been unable to go near his room. That night she had called his parents intending to comfort them and had cried on the phone.

> Have Thine own way, Lord; Have Thine own way!
> Wounded and weary, help me, I pray.
> Power all power surely is Thine
> Touch me and heal me, Savior divine!

From the church to the cemetery was a short walk across a dirt road and up a steep hill. A grave had been dug for Mark just over the summit. From the gravesite one could see for miles around. Bared winter trees had exposed factories and communities which in summer would almost disappear from view behind the variegated greens of lush foliage. The hill itself was grassy. It had begun to be used as a cemetery quite recently. Aside from a few other graves, it had been preserved in its natural state. Signs at the bottom forbade sledding, snowmobiling, minibiking, and hunting. But one could easily envision the hill as a place where children or adults could enjoy picnics and games of all kinds. It was not a somber place.

Near the top of this hill, in sun so bright that the mourners squinted and winds so bitterly cold that the mourners shivered and tightened their scarves around their necks, Mark David Price, age fifteen years seven months and five days, was laid to rest.

SPRING

Tuesday, January 29

At three minutes after ten on the morning after Mark's funeral, a certain dial was turned to zero on a certain ventilator in the Intermediate Unit at Children's Hospital, and Jody Robinson began breathing entirely on his own for the first time in his life.

The event occurred without fanfare. Most children who come off the respirator are given parties by their parents. Jody's family was not around to plan any festivities for him, and Marla Meyerle was afraid to put on a celebration that might prove to have been premature. Cautious as the doctors are in weaning, kids sometimes run into trouble and have to go back on the machine.

Besides, Jody was off only in the sense that the respirator was no longer taking breaths for him. He still required oxygen and positive pressure. He didn't have to get this support from the respirator itself; in fact, the machine would be moved out of Intermediate within a day or two, assuming all went well, and would be replaced by a smaller machine. However, the time to celebrate, in Marla's opinion, was when the child became free of respiratory support altogether, or even when he got through an illness without having to go back on the ventilator. Then Marla Meyerle would let herself get excited.

It turned out to be just as well that there was no party. Jody did not have a particularly good morning. He seemed to have developed a small cold. He turned blue after a sham feeding and again after a gagging incident. Indeed he was blue on and off for several hours. While his heart rate didn't change noticeably, his eyelids drooped, and he looked sickish.

Each time the cyanosis manifested, the young nurse taking care of Jody bagged him with extra bursts of oxygen. Each time he pinked right up. But the blueness recurred so frequently that finally one of the doctors increased the concentration of oxygen being delivered to Jody from thirty to forty percent.

This helped. It also distressed the child's caregivers. At one time

Jody had needed a concentration of only twenty-five percent. He'd been just four points short of being able to tolerate room air. The increase to forty was a real step backward.

Prompted by concern about these events and the child's general tendency to turn blue, Peter Crossin sat down shortly before noon and reviewed Jody's chart for the second time in a week. Last Tuesday the doctor had been assessing the patient's ability to get along with only one breath from the ventilator every two minutes. This time Crossin was specifically looking for evidence that the patient was or was not aspirating: that his lungs were or were not being chronically contaminated by bacteria from his mouth and saliva.

In the past few days Crossin had realized that this possibility had been nagging at him ever since he'd read the chart last Tuesday. The nurses' notes about Jody had contained a reference to cyanosis almost every day. Why? Jody turned blue when he gagged or was being suctioned, but he also turned blue when he wasn't gagging or being suctioned. Again, why? Crossin had never come up with a satisfactory answer to those questions. He'd been hoping the problem would diminish of its own accord as Jody grew and gained strength and control. Clearly that was not happening.

Until this past week Crossin had never seriously entertained aspiration as the explanation for Jody's cyanotic episodes. He'd been assured by ENT specialist Jim Palardy, who had done all the reconstructive surgery on the child's larynx, that those operations had left Jody with a sound upper airway. Last month's bronchoscopy had again left Crossin free to assume that aspiration was physically impossible for this patient: that everything entering Jody's throat came out his esophagostomy.

Now Crossin wondered whether he'd believed his colleague too readily. If the child was aspirating, there had to be leakage somewhere.

He reviewed the chart again with a sense of deepening dismay. By the end of an hour he had become absolutely convinced that Jody Robinson had been trying to tell the Intermediate staff something that the Intermediate staff had not wished to hear.

The child simply was not fitting into the pattern that would have been right for him at this point. He should have been improving faster than he was. By now his respiratory rates should have dropped into a safe range and stayed there. Instead Jody's were hovering in a gray area. His need for oxygen should have continued to decrease. Instead it was increasing. He was being weaned, but it had begun to seem that the cost of weaning him was the necessity to beef up his O_2.

He should not have been having cyanotic episodes now at all. In fact, according to the chart, those episodes had actually increased in number over the weekend. Furthermore, the cultures grown from his tracheal secretions read like a sewer. Most kids in Intermediate showed two or three organisms in their trach cultures. Jody was showing five to seven, and they were the kind of organisms one would expect to see not in the respiratory system but in the digestive tract. If the child were not aspirating salivary secretions into his lungs, what accounted for the presence of those bugs in his trach cultures?

Crossin suspected that the integrity of the esophagus had broken down and sprung a leak, or that despite or even because of all the laryngeal surgery Jody had had, he now had laryngeal incompetence somewhere as well.

It was so ironic, Crossin thought. Just as the child had achieved the milestone of taking all his breaths for himself, this brand-new problem had developed.

Yet in a way perhaps it was not so ironic. Conceivably Jody was aspirating now precisely because he was no longer being ventilated artificially. Crossin had never seen this theory discussed in anesthesiology literature, but he felt certain that the phenomenon had occurred in his unit. It stood to reason. When the machine forced air out of the lungs, it drove out secretions as well. Once the patient had been weaned down to a low level of support, the process could, at least in principle, reverse itself.

Peter Crossin closed Jody's chart and idly drummed with his fingers on the stiff cardboard cover. They'd all seen the signs. He had, the residents and fellows had, the nurses had. They'd seen the signs, but they hadn't added them up. Crossin thought that somewhere in his subconscious he had actually realized that the child was aspirating but had put off confronting that fact.

He did not need to ask himself why. He had only to think of a little blond boy named Chuckie. That child, too, had developed chronic aspiration in Intermediate. The disorder can actually liquefy cartilage. It typically produces a low-grade inflammation that predisposes a patient to such infections as bronchitis and pneumonia. Chuckie had gone through one infection after another. Finally he had become so run-down and sick as to be on the brink of death. It had been clear to all that the child could survive only if the aspiration were stopped.

With utmost reluctance Peter Crossin had sent Chuckie to the OR where the ENT specialist had closed off the route by which secretions found their way to the child's lungs. He had done this by tying a permanent suture around each vocal cord. At the age of four, Chuckie was home now and doing fine.

But he had no speech.

The thought of Chuckie going through life unable to talk was painful for everyone concerned at Children's. It was no easier to contemplate a similar fate for Jody Robinson, especially after all he'd been through already.

Crossin and the others had been pulling so hard for Jody that nobody had wanted to see any red flags. But they were moving the child forward under less than perfect conditions. It was urgent, now, to get to the bottom of his latest problem.

Right after lunch Peter Crossin discussed with several of the Intermediate nurses his belief that Jody was aspirating. Eager to find almost any other explanation for the child's problems, one of the nurses mentioned Marla Meyerle's theory that the secretions that collected around Jody's tracheostomy were somehow getting into his lungs around the trach tube.

"We can easily find out by giving him methylene blue," Crossin replied. "Let him drink it in some water. If you get any blue coming out through the trach, you can be reasonably sure that the secretions are going into the airway from the esophagus."

An hour later, after padding the child's neck very thickly and carefully with four-by-four gauze pads, the young nurse taking care of Jody handed her patient, in his favorite green cup, a mixture of methylene blue and sterile water. As he drank it down and it streamed out his esophagostomy, she blotted up the colored water with as many fresh towels as she could hold in her hands. She was as certain as it was possible to be that none of the blue fluid had trickled down Jody's neck and seeped into his trachea around the trach tube.

But when he'd stopped drinking, when she removed the trach dressings, she saw hints of blue on the white gauze. When she suctioned Jody's trachea, some of the droplets she pulled into the catheter were tinged with blue. A little while later she saw blue droplets in the tubing that still connected Jody to the ventilator.

The nurse gave the bad news to Jan Haver, who in turn reported it to Peter Crossin. His response was a remark she heard very rarely from the medical director of Intermediate. All he said was, "Son of a bitch."

A short time earlier, social worker Lynn Story had gotten word by telephone that Jody Robinson's mother was back in jail for violating probation.

Ø

Evening. Ignoring the other parents crowded up against her, Sharita Queen stood in the elevator laden with packages and feeling exhausted. She had worn herself out in the past hour trying to find a stuffed dog for Freddy. Though years had passed since she'd last bought a stuffed animal for him, it had occurred to her that in his present circumstances, a smiling dog might make him happy. But every dog she picked up had looked sad. So instead she had bought him a figure of Batman and a figure of Colonel Warrior from *Star Wars*.

She had something else for Freddy, something she was planning for him if he felt well enough.

At the fourth floor, Sharita Queen left the elevator and headed for Acute. She had not been pleased at first when they'd moved Freddy out of Isolation. He'd been used to his room there. He could have his pictures up around him and his times tables chart on the wall where he could see it. On Saturday his stuff had been in a box under his bed in Acute, and the nurses hadn't even known where his baseball cap was. He'd been quiet on Saturday.

But by Sunday somebody had found the cap and given him his baseball glove, and the nurses had hung up some of his cards at the foot of his bed on two long trach strings they'd tied to something on the ceiling. His mood had improved. He had even written his mother a note!

She entered the unit and walked to his bedside. A nurse was there whom Sharita Queen did not know. Freddy was sound asleep, the fingers of his right hand curled around his pee-and-poop bells. A gown covered him from neck to knees. He was also wearing his socks and sneakers.

The two women introduced themselves in low voices. "I was about to wake him up and give him a popsicle," the nurse told the patient's mother. "He's doing great!"

The visitor took a small plastic jar from her purse. Opening it, she began to rub pink cream very lightly into the diminishing pink scar above Freddy's left eye. "It's vitamin cream," she explained to the nurse. "I put it on to make his scars go away."

The nurse left to get the popsicle. Freddy stirred. His mother bent over him talking softly. "Your Mama is here, Freddy. She's a little late, but she was trying to find something for you that would make you happy."

He opened his eyes and looked at her. She thought his eyes seemed bright.

"Sometimes when Mama visits you, she runs out of words," Sharita Queen continued, rubbing cream now into the healing scrape marks on his knuckles. "When she runs out of words, we have to have something to make up for her not talking. So I've brought you a surprise, Freddy. The kids in the neighborhood came over last night and made up a beautiful tape for you. In a few minutes we're going to play it. Would you like that?"

He nodded. His eyes did not leave her face.

The nurse returned, tearing the paper off the treat she had brought him. "Hey, Pro, look! Cherry! Your favorite kind!" She handed it to him. "Show your mom how well you can eat a popsicle!"

He started off with apparent enjoyment. His lips turned red almost immediately, and red juice began to dribble down his chin to his neck. His mother and the nurse took turns wiping him up. After a few minutes, his energy seemed to flag. He let the popsicle droop in his hand.

His mother urged him on. "You have to eat your popsicle if you want to see the goodies that Mama has for you. Is it good?"

He nodded and took another bite.

Replacing the lid on her jar of vitamin cream, his mother told the nurse about the tape. She wondered if hearing the tape right now would distract Freddy's attention from his popsicle and cause him to gag. The nurse said she didn't know; she'd never taken care of Freddy before.

"Well," his mother said, "does he have to concentrate when he swallows?"

The nurse said he did. The two women agreed that it would be better to play the tape when Freddy had finished eating.

"Explain to me again about the green tube."

"It's oxygen mist," the nurse replied. "It just provides him with a little more than he'd get from room air. But he's breathing on his own."

Sharita Queen nodded. "He was on the breathing machine for one month and two days."

A few minutes later the nurse said she was going to read to another patient. She asked the visitor if she had any other questions. The answer was no. So many things were wrong with Freddy that his mother felt she would not be able to cope if she worried about all of them at one time. He was off the breathing machine. Next he would be off oxygen. She was satisfied with that. She was concerned about his left side but did not want to think about that now. If she started to worry about his arm and his leg and how his thinking was going to be, she'd be going around in circles. She was trying to be patient and to concentrate on one thing at a time.

She tucked some tissues under his chin. "Getting better, Freddy, eating that popsicle all by yourself?"

He nodded.

She pointed to the bed across from his. "See the baby? See that baby over there? If you're watching the baby, move your foot."

He responded with his right toe. He had stopped eating. His grip on the popsicle loosened.

"Are you through?"

When he didn't answer, she took the popsicle from him and threw it away. "Okay, Freddy, want to listen to the kids? They've got lots to tell you." She blotted his chin, disposed of the tissues, and cleaned his chin and neck with a paper towel she dampened at the sink. "Okay, now, do you want to hear the kids? If you do, move your foot."

He raised a finger.

"Close your mouth, Freddy."

He did.

She rested the tape recorder on the side rail and turned it on. For a moment there was no sound at all. Then came the tentative, self-conscious voices of children unaccustomed to talking for a microphone. "My name's Anita. Hi, Fred. I hope you get well. I live up the street from you on the block. My name is Kevin. How ya doin'? My name is George, and I live down the street." Polite prompting: "Ask him how he's doing." Obediently: "How you doin'?"

Then the children warmed up and pretended to choose up sides for a baseball game. "We want Freddy on our side! No, we want Freddy on *our* side! You're still on our team, Pro! Play ball, Pro!"

The patient appeared to listen attentively. At appropriate moments, his face broke into a smile. The tape continued through a whole mock inning and ended in hilarity. "You're out, Ricky! You're out! We finally got him out, Freddy! Yeah, Fred, we finally got him out! We got thirty-seven points, Fred, and they only got one!" The kids burst into laughter. The patient joined in.

"That's all, Freddy! See you, Fred! This is Kevin; don't forget me! This is Margaret; don't forget me! This is George; don't forget me! This is Anita; don't forget me. I loves you, Freddy, goodbye! Goodbye! Goodbye!"

Sharita Queen pressed the REWIND button. Her son watched her lay the tape recorder at the foot of his bed. Acute seemed suddenly quiet. Another parent smiled at Freddy's mother, but she didn't see him.

"Did you like that tape?"

He raised a finger. He gave her a smile.

"You ready for Mama to show you what I have for you? Move both your legs if you want Mama to show you."

He wiggled his sneakered feet.

"Good. Now move your arm. Good. Now straighten your fingers." He had become accustomed to lying with the fingers of his left hand curled into the palm. She worried that if they stayed balled up like that, they'd get stuck. "Does it hurt for you to lie with your fingers stretched out?"

He shook his head no.

She stood. From her shopping bag, she took a brightly painted

cardboard box bearing the legend WORLD'S GREATEST SUPER HE-
ROES—BATMAN. She removed from the box a blue plastic figure
about a foot high and held it up for Freddy to see. "If you like this,
move your whole body for Mama."

His body seemed to tense, but it did not move.

She placed the toy in the crook of his right arm. "Batman is to
keep you company," she explained. "Sometimes the nurses may
have to take him out, so don't get angry with them." She opened
another box and laid the second toy, Colonel Warrior, beside the
first. He smiled at her, but his thoughts seemed to be elsewhere.

She asked him for a favor. Could he hold Mama's hand with his
left hand?

The hand lay alongside him on the mattress. She extended her
own into the air just above it. He could see that the distance between hers and his was no more than a couple of inches. He tried
until his whole arm seemed to bristle. Sweat broke out on his face.

She helped him. She laid her hand on the mattress beside his,
touching his, and nudged with her fingertips. He rolled his hand
over just enough that she could begin to slide her fingers underneath it. She did not rush him. In soft, loving tones, she gave encouragement. She did not do all the work for him, nor did he do it
all for himself, but over the course of several seconds, like flowers
opening or closing before a slow-motion camera, the long, slim
hand of the mother and the shorter, stubbier hand of her only child
sought and finally found each other.

"Squeeze," she urged. Freddy gripped his mother's fingers and
held on tight.

Friday, February 1

A few steps behind her mother, Gina DeRose walked unsmiling into
the Oncology Clinic waiting room and responded without smiling to
the secretaries' greetings. Charmaine and Ellie noticed but had no
attention to spare at that moment. In the past half hour Clinic had
become a madhouse. The two women were so busy that their

phones were going unanswered until the fourth or fifth ring. As Gina took her coat off, Charmaine glimpsed a T-shirt proclaiming that EVERY GIRL LOOKS FORWARD TO HER FIRST KISS and did manage to inquire lightly, hand over the telephone mouthpiece, "Did you get your first kiss yet?" The corners of Gina's mouth went up slightly. She shook her head.

She was to have the needles in her back for the first time in three months. The spinal tap. The extraction of bone marrow.

On Tuesday morning she had come down for breakfast withdrawn and upset. "I don't want to go on Friday," she had announced at the table after five minutes of silence.

Marie DeRose had tried to defuse her daughter's fear. "Oh, Gina, you've had this so many times. You should be used to it by now. You know you don't feel anything once that push is over."

"Well, I can feel them pushing."

"I know. But why worry about it now? There's time enough to worry about it on Friday. Other people are worse off than you, Gina. Don't feel so sorry for yourself. You have to be tough in this world, or you'll crack up."

This morning Marie's stomach was in knots. She was feeling the child's fear and some of her own. On Monday Gina had been in to have blood drawn for studies of her liver enzymes. Yesterday Dr. Silver had called to say that the enzyme level had risen again. Even though she was now getting only two Methotrexate pills on Fridays instead of eight, her liver was still functioning abnormally. The doctor had told Marie to go ahead and give Gina the two pills this week. But he'd also said he might have to take the child off the MTX entirely and put her on a different anticancer drug.

Silver came into the waiting room and approached a mother standing not far from the DeRoses who was holding a little boy of perhaps three. Where his curls had once been were a few blond wisps. As soon as he saw the doctor, the boy began to fuss.

Silver laid a hand across the small shoulders. "No needles in your back today, Teddy," he said very gently.

The fussing broke into tearful pleading. "Not in my back!"

"Not in your back, I promise you."

Gina observed this exchange in silence.

He caught sight of the DeRoses a moment later and came over to them. "Hi. How are you doing?" His manner was as easy and pleasant as if he'd run into friends on the street.

Gina's "Fine" suggested anything but.

"What's the matter?"

She looked up at him dolefully.

Waiting for an explanation that never came, trying to divine what she clearly expected him to understand, he suddenly remembered Teddy. "Is that what's the matter?"

She nodded.

"We'll get it over in a hurry, okay?"

She lowered her gaze to a space behind him at the level of his waist.

"Angie's tied up right now, but why don't you go on back to Bonnie and get your finger stick, and I'll be with you in a few minutes."

She dawdled. When she got to the lab, Teddy was in there, and he was crying. As Bonnie rubbed alcohol on his finger, she and Teddy's mother tried to placate the child. Gina stood in the doorway watching. After a moment she became aware that another person had come up behind her.

She turned. The girl was a teenager, lean as a boy, with small breasts, a boyish haircut, boyish dress. In one arm she carried a pink plush elephant. She was looking into the lab over the head of the child in front of her.

Gina lifted her eyes to the older girl's face. She asked quietly, "What do you have?"

The question was half invitation, half appeal, and the answer was a rebuff on both counts. "Leukemia," the girl said with utter nonchalance.

Gina persisted. "So do I."

The girl looked away.

But Gina had never before met anyone who understood how it felt to have leukemia. "What are you going to get?"

With obvious reluctance, the girl named two medications.

Gina asked about the elephant.

At this the girl at last exhibited a little animation. She joked about how she took the elephant everywhere, even radiation, and then she even admitted that having the elephant along with her made her feel better.

No sooner had she said this than Gina was called into the lab for her finger stick. Months would pass before she saw the older girl again.

From the lab she went to Angie's office to get weighed. Angie sat at her desk wearing Gloria Vanderbilt jeans and a loose mauve shirt with big sleeves and greeted Gina by reading her T-shirt out loud. "'Every girl looks forward to her first kiss.' I'll drink to that—coffee, that is!" Angie cracked up. Gina giggled nervously. "Will you go back with me?"

"You bet I'll go back with you. I haven't missed a procedure of yours yet, have I?"

The patient sat down on the floor and took off her new beige jogging shoes. As Angie pushed the scale weights to zero, Gina stood, and when Angie said, "Okay, darlin', hit the scale," Gina stepped onto the platform bent like a boxer and faked an uppercut. "Hit the scale—get it?"

Both laughed.

Silver would do the spinal tap first. With Gina curled shrimplike to separate the bones of her spine, the doctor would insert a hollow needle into cartilage below the area of the spinal nerves and catch in a vial a single cc. of the clear cerebrospinal fluid that would drip from the external end of the needle like sap from a tree. The CSF would then be analyzed for evidence that cancer cells had or had not penetrated the central nervous system. Radiation has proved quite successful in preventing CNS relapse among children with leukemia, but it is hardly foolproof.

The second procedure would be done at exactly the same site. Its purpose was to scout Gina's bone marrow for evidence of either continued remission or the reappearance of malignant cells. Marrow is a concentrate of young blood cells found inside bone cavities. To extract what he needed, Silver would have to drive a rather large needle through Gina's bone tissue.

Her first bone marrow had been done in her hip. The substance can be extracted in larger quantities from that area than from the spine, and a relatively large amount is needed for diagnosis. Withdrawing from a big bone is also easier technically. In adult hospitals the hip is used routinely for bone marrow. Not at Children's. When protocols require a child to have a spinal tap and a bone marrow on the same day, they are virtually always approached through a single puncture at the base of the spine, thus sparing the patient a second jab of a needle.

Gina had been so frightened of that first bone marrow that sweat had broken out all over her body. When she'd had her first spinal tap in the hospital, she had screamed so hard and tensed her muscles so tightly that for two days afterward she had walked around like a little old lady.

Now when she got her needles in her back, she didn't scream so much, and her muscles didn't get so tense. The way Dr. Sam gave needles didn't hurt that less, but she felt safer with him, just like she felt safer with Angie and Cindy.

In the examining room Marie DeRose presented Gina's doctor with a package containing one of the rugs she had made, a brown horse's head on a white background. Gifts from parents always made Silver feel slightly embarrassed. Yet as tangible signs that what he did for patients was appreciated, they also made him feel good. The rug was one of the nicer presents he'd gotten from a family. He was distressed that Marie had given him something so nice on a day when he had to do something to Gina that would hurt her.

She sat before him on the examining table. He made an observation. "You seem a little happier now than you did earlier."

"You should have been at our house last night," Marie put in before the child could answer. "We heard her screaming on the second floor, so Tony goes running upstairs to find out what's wrong, and guess what she's doing? Singing in the bathtub! First time she's done that since she got sick! We said, 'If you keep this up, we're going to have to give you singing lessons!'"

Marie's efforts were rewarded by giggles from Gina, which in turn made Silver grin.

He proceeded with his usual examination. While checking her eyes he asked about her hair. She replied in good humor.

"Growing in! It's black at the roots. My whole head's black! My mom said in a few more months I'll have short hair."

"What about your wig? Are you wearing it all the time now?"

"Sometimes I take it off at home, but Sam, you know what? I hung upside down on the bars in gym with it on! I was afraid it would come off, but it didn't! The kids know I have a wig, but they don't believe me! I push it up and down, but they still don't believe me! I took it off with my girlfriend Michelle! I asked her to promise not to tell anyone that she saw me with it off, and she didn't!"

When he finished, Silver talked with his patient and her mother about the possibility of stopping the Methotrexate entirely for a few months and putting Gina on a different drug. *If* he did this—and he emphasized that it was not yet a definite plan—she might have to have shots in her leg. *If* they went ahead with this new medicine, Silver wondered, how would Gina feel about her mother giving her the shots at home?

Her response was a look of confusion. Realizing that she needed more information, he left the room and returned opening a small package from which he took a needle that was very slender and very light. He held it up.

"That's all?"

"That's the whole story." Touching a fingertip absentmindedly to the point, he told her again that they might not have to do it and that in any case she would not get the needle today. He was saying that she could go home and think about it when Gina interrupted him to say brightly, "Don't stick yourself!"

She postponed the inevitable as long as she could. First she asked Silver if he knew where he was going to do the bone marrow.

"Yeah," he replied, "on your back."

"Where on my back?"

"You know. The place where it doesn't hurt as much."

"Mom says it's only a pinch," Gina said by way of reminder to herself, and both she and her mother burst out laughing when the doctor replied dryly, "Your mom hasn't had it!"

Then when she was lying on the table with jeans unzipped and torso bared and Silver said he had to go find Angie, the patient announced that she had to tinkle. Pulling down her T-shirt, zipping her jeans, she jumped off the table and ran out in the direction of the bathroom. She returned a few minutes later to find no one waiting for her but her mother. Gina jumped back up on the table. Suddenly she dropped her face into her hands. When Marie went to the child and held her, struck by the tension in her daughter's body, Gina whimpered and half laughed against her mother's broad bosom.

A tray of wrapped instruments came through the door on a cart pushed by Angie. She was followed by Silver, head nurse Cindy Strickland, and a young woman who was introduced to the patient and her mother as a student nurse. Seeing this entourage, Gina attempted a moan. "Oh, no! Everybody's going to watch me!"

"Listen," Silver said, removing instruments from the blue-green cloths that covered them, "*I've* got the hard part. All you have to do is lie there!"

"No, *I've* got the hard part! I've got to feel it!" But without prompting she lay down on her left side facing the wall, back to the doctor, head cushioned on her left arm, and lowered her jeans to provide Silver with the appropriate patch of bare back.

"When I had my tonsils out, they put me to sleep," she said chattily to five people whose faces she could not see. "That's why I'd rather fall asleep when I get my needles in my back, but you won't even do it to me."

"That's because you're so good, and you don't move," Angie said. From the cart she picked up two plastic bottles and some gauze pads. "We only put kids to sleep if they fight us and we can't hold them down."

"Angie?" Her tone was anxious. "Are you going to be here?"

The aide pushed the examining table away from the wall and squeezed in behind it to stand directly in front of Gina. She rubbed the child's shoulder. "I'm here, sweetheart."

She bent over Gina and swabbed the child's back with Betadine, then told the patient that she was going to wipe off the Betadine with alcohol. Angie knew that Gina knew by now what to expect of these procedures. But Angie had also learned that sometimes a needle in the back is harder for a child when several months have intervened since the previous one.

She offered encouragement. "This is going to go so well, Gina, you know why? Because I feel really lucky today."

Silver donned rubber gloves. "Remember, Gina, you can scream all you want, but just don't move." This caution was more a matter of practicality than of safety. Clinic staff had heard any number of stories about uncles who became paralyzed from spinal taps, but Silver, amused that the stories always involved uncles, had never known it to happen. Anyone who knew how to do a tap knew how to do it safely, in his opinion. However, if a patient squirms at the wrong moment and the needle doesn't penetrate properly, it may have to be pushed through the child's flesh a second time.

Because these procedures are tangible, Silver had once enjoyed doing them. Now he preferred seeing children on days when he was not required to do something that caused them pain or anguish. The hardest part for the kids, he knew, was not being able to see. The doctor's satisfaction lay in winning the child's trust so a painful procedure was not also scary. Gina's insistence that her taps and marrows be done by him and only him told Silver that she trusted him, which made him feel good.

"Time to curl up, Gina," Angie said. She waited for the child to tuck herself into fetal position, then put a special hold on Gina's body intended to immobilize her and maintain the curve in her spine. Marie stood at the head of the table caressing her daughter's upper back. The mother's face was pale.

"Okay, Gina," the doctor said, "the first thing I'm going to do is put this thing on your back."

"What thing?"

"The paper sheet with a hole in it," Angie explained.

"Good tight ball," Silver urged. "This is just my fingers . . . Okay, honey, you're doing real well."

From a small bottle held by Cindy, the doctor drew a watery liquid into a syringe. The patient began to whimper. "Wait, I'm not ready for it yet. . . ."

"This is my finger," Silver said calmly, "and this is going to be the numbing medicine. Take a deep breath, okay?" As he inserted the needle, she screamed, and then her cry broke into a babble. "Mommymommymommymommymommymommymommy . . ."

"I'm here, Gina. I'm right here." Marie was blinking back tears.

But when Angie asked, "What do you feel?" the babbling ceased instantly, and Gina answered in a perfectly normal voice, "Nothing." Over the laughter around her she added, "My foot's asleep!"

Once the numbing medicine took effect, the patient would experience no further pain. Silver picked up the hollow tap needle. It was about three inches long, knobbed at one end. "Gina, can you bend your back a little more?"

"Sure. I can bend it any way you want."

"You're just going to feel some pushing. . ." He sank the needle deep into her flesh.

"Your hands are cold."

"Here come the drops." He held the vial under the hollow knob. Clear fluid formed slowly into bulges and fell one drop at a time. "Push down like you're going to have a bowel movement."

"Why?"

"Or cough," Angie suggested.

"I'd rather do that." She did. "Thank you! I had to cough anyway!"

"You're very good," Silver said. "Remember how you were at the beginning? You scared me more than I scared you!"

She remembered.

Removing the tap needle, Silver wiped a bit of blood from the wound in Gina's back.

"Okay, that's done, chickadee," said Cindy. "Just one more back there, and then you're finished."

Silver inserted the marrow needle into the existing puncture.

"Oooooooohhhhh. Mommy, are you still there?"

Angie laughed. "Are you jiving me, is she still there? Where do you think she'd be going?"

"Okay, Gina," Silver warned, "you're going to feel some pushing." He began to exert force, screwing the needle, pushing it, screwing, pushing until his forehead glistened. "Okay, we're in," he said finally.

"When you put it in," the patient told him, "I hear a sound like when you break a cracker."

As Silver connected a syringe, Cindy pounded on the wall as a signal to the lab. Marrow clots very quickly. It is important to begin analysis as soon as the substance has been drawn. Sure enough, within half a minute a technician walked into the examining room to receive the marrow in a plastic cup.

"Okay, all through," Silver told his patient as Angie released her.

She hoisted her jeans and turned carefully to lie on her back. "Already? I didn't even count to twenty-one yet." The lightness of her words was at odds with the tone of her voice.

"You okay?"

She lay as if drained. She still had to have blood drawn for the enzyme studies and a chemotherapy injection. "I'm sweating."

"You really worked hard," Angie said.

"I'm tired."

"I don't blame you," said Silver. "But just think. You won't have to do this again until May."

Gina regarded him. "Can I ask you a question? Why do you get so wet?"

He took a handkerchief from his pocket and wiped his brow. "I'm probably nervous. I've had these too—did I tell you? Somebody here needed some bone marrow once from healthy volunteers, so an English guy and I each gave each other two . . ."

The lab technician interrupted. "And Dr. Silver was crying the whole time!"

He looked hurt. "I was only crying a little!"

Gina laughed.

She was getting her vincristine in the treatment room when Sam Silver walked back to the lab for the results of the finger stick and learned that the child's white count was low.

Another forty minutes were to pass before he would learn the bone marrow results. Even so, Silver had worked in oncology long enough to know that relapse is not the likeliest explanation for a decrease in white cells. Gina was taking drugs that suppress cell production. As her body had already exhibited a somewhat idiosyncratic response to Methotrexate, conceivably the low count likewise reflected her own peculiar reaction to one or more of her medicines. Or there might be viral activity in her system. Counts occasionally drop during flu-like maladies which are sometimes silent. Gina could have a virus without necessarily manifesting symptoms.

But while the low white count did not alarm Silver in terms of her leukemia, it did constitute a potential danger to her health. White cells fight infection. Having too few of them could render Gina susceptible to a wide variety of illnesses and land her back in the hospital. The way to avoid such problems is to take the patient off all medications that affect blood count, giving the white cells a chance to flourish and multiply until they again reach desired levels. Such decisions are not uncommon in Clinic. At one time or another almost every child in treatment has meds stopped temporarily because of low counts or fevers.

However, Gina was already getting less than the optimal dose of Methotrexate. Stopping it and the 6MP altogether would mean one more delay in straightening out the meds situation and getting the child onto the Maintenance routine of Clinic visits only once a month. For these reasons Silver was more reluctant to hold her drugs than he would have been under different circumstances. But there was no choice. On the positive side, the doctor knew that so long as the problem wasn't relapse, the matter of Gina's white count would resolve itself in about a week.

Feeling dismayed but not alarmed, he stuck his head into the treatment room and delivered the news in a few casual sentences, asking Marie to make sure she didn't leave without talking to him again so he could answer any questions she might have and telling Gina he wanted her back in Clinic next week. He had to see another patient now, Silver said from the doorway. He'd just stopped by so he wouldn't forget to tell them about the low count.

If his words had not taken her by surprise, Marie would undoubtedly have realized that the doctor would not break truly bad news so offhandedly. As it was, she heard white count and thought relapse. From then on Sam Silver might as well have been speaking in tongues.

Gina bounced from the treatment room to the waiting room in apparent high spirits. Clinic was over. She would not need another needle in her back for three whole months. When Charmaine invited her to come behind the desks and try out a typewriter that wasn't in use, the child chattered away about their typewriter at home which *wasn't* electric and made you push down on the keys, which was hard on the pinkie.

Her mother, taking a seat by the window, waited for Dr. Silver unable to think straight and trying not to shed tears.

He walked through the waiting room, put a hand on her shoulder, and sat down beside her. "The bone marrow looks fine."

She nodded.

He faced her. "You're upset, aren't you."

She could not reply.

"Has she had a cold?"

"No." Marie dabbed at her eyes with a tissue.

"Well, sometimes kids have viruses that you don't see. That's what I think the problem is—that and the medicines. We'll get it taken care of. Try not to be too upset. Just hold the MTX and the

6MP and keep her away from crowds over the weekend. If she has any problems with fever, let me know. I'll be on call."

"Is it really low?"

"Pretty low. But it looks as if there are a lot of young cells coming up. This is not unusual. I'd be worried if the count stayed low a long time, but by next week it should be okay."

He emphasized the point. "It's not unusual. Just make an appointment for next Friday. I'd be much more concerned if her platelet count was low. The platelet count is fine."

Marie drove her daughter home thinking of words she herself had spoken during one of the parents' meetings at Children's. A father had expressed fears about the medicines his child was taking. How could anybody be sure that the medicines would work? How did the doctors know what the side effects would mean for his daughter when she got older? Knowing that her husband also worried about the medicines, however rarely he said so, Marie had sat watching Tony grow increasingly upset, and finally she had been unable to keep silent a moment longer.

"What can we do," she'd said to the other father, "except trust the doctors? Nothing in this world is guaranteed. We don't know if the medicines are going to work. We don't know what reactions the children will get from them. The doctors are telling us that these medicines have worked with other kids. We have to take their word for it. We don't know any different. I feel the doctors know more than I do, but even if they're wrong, how do you know they're wrong?"

By this time she had been talking to Tony. "We just have to believe them. If they told us to jump off the dam five times a day because it would help some, we'd do it, because we'd believe it. If you don't trust the doctors, who are you going to trust? I'd be in terrible shape if I didn't believe the things they tell me. I either have to believe them or go nuts."

The oncologists at Children's had gotten Gina into remission. But they hadn't stopped there. In a way they had adopted the child. They had made her comfortable, just as they had made her mother and father comfortable. When things went wrong, they felt as bad as the parents did. Certainly that was the impression they had given Marie. They had made her feel that Gina wasn't just her child and Tony's child; she was their child too.

Dr. Silver had told her that the low white count did not have him worried. Marie believed him. She trusted Silver. She trusted all the doctors she'd met at Children's.

And because she trusted them, she knew that the words out of their mouths could change the world for her.

Tuesday, February 5

Jody Robinson was wheeled into the Children's Hospital Operating Room at 8:00 A.M. As soon as the methylene blue test had established almost beyond doubt that Jody was leaking salivary secretions into his lungs, Peter Crossin had placed a call to ear-nose-and-throat surgeon Jim Palardy, and the two physicians had agreed to investigate the cause of the aspiration by scheduling Jody for another bronchoscopy. Permission had been granted over the phone by the child's mother, reached in jail by a Children's social worker. Wanting to look down the bronchoscope himself to see whatever Palardy saw, Peter Crossin had volunteered to assist.

Palardy approached the surgery wondering what he'd find this time that he hadn't found last time. He'd be looking specifically for signs that previous repairs had broken down or for a brand new opening between the trachea and the esophagus. Given what he'd seen through the scope in December, the surgeon honestly expected to find none of these problems. In December, however, he hadn't been looking at Jody's trachea with aspiration in mind. That examination had been more or less routine.

This bronchoscopy was over in less than fifteen minutes. At the end of it the surgeon also examined Jody's esophagus with a scope intended for that purpose. In neither duct did Palardy or Crossin see any evidence of tissue breakdowns or holes new or old.

What they did see in a larynx that was grossly abnormal in appearance was clear evidence of a condition known as tracheal malacia, or softening of the cartilaginous skeleton that keeps the passages of the airway open. The condition had not been evident in December. Its presence now was not particularly surprising in view of all the surgery Jody had had on his upper airway. Its cause, Palardy suggested, was chronic infection. Crossin proposed that the infection was due to chronic aspiration. He was distressed to see how far back the flaccidity appeared to extend.

The malacia represented a major new problem. Virtually everyone caring for Jody was working toward the day when the child could breathe without assistance from any machine and could have his trach tube removed and his tracheostomy closed. If the tissue of his bronchial walls softened so much that he couldn't keep his airway open, he would need more surgery at the very least. It was even possible that the airway would have to be kept open permanently with the trach tube and that Jody would have the tracheostomy for the rest of his life.

Something else disturbed Crossin as he peered through the bronchoscope. In normal anatomy the voice box closes off during swallowing. It was Crossin's impression that when Jody swallowed, his voice box never quite closed off completely, which would certainly explain the aspiration.

Peter Crossin returned Jody to Intermediate feeling greatly discouraged. He firmly believed now that while the child's larynx was anatomically sound and generally functional, while it might very well provide Jody with a voice at such time as his tracheostomy could be closed, it did not serve to protect him from aspiration.

While the patient was still on the operating table, the surgeon and the anesthesiologist had replaced the tube in his tracheostomy with one of larger size. Doubtful as he was that the aspiration resulted from secretions pooling around the tracheostomy, Crossin nevertheless hoped the bigger trach tube would diminish the problem somewhat. Back in the unit, he instructed the nurses to stop all sham feedings, even water. Jody would have to do without drinking from his beloved green cup.

Beyond these measures there was little the experts could do for Jody at this point. What they might do in the future would depend entirely on what course the patient took from here on out. He represented a dilemma not uncommon among the children of Intermediate. No one in the world knew what Jody's natural history either should or would be. Conceivably he could outgrow the aspiration and the malacia as well. But if he continued to aspirate, if he contracted a series of aspiration pneumonias, and became run-down, the doctors' next step would be to follow the path they had taken with Chuckie: to stop the flow of secretions to the lungs by sewing Jody's vocal cords shut.

Leaving Intermediate for his office, Crossin agonized. Would it be better to close the cords now, to pay the price and avoid the risk? The surgery would deprive the child of his ability to communicate orally. Loath to take that irretrievable step with Chuckie, the doctors had postponed and postponed it while the patient had become sicker and sicker, until it had become certain that if they didn't take it, the boy would die. So they had done the deed, and Chuckie had gotten better. Perhaps Jody, too, would profit from this approach.

But maybe he would get better without it.

All things considered, Crossin preferred to wait until the child declared himself one way or another. But waiting, too, had its price. It could take months. It could delay the colon surgery remaining to be done, which in turn would delay Jody's entry into a normal environment.

Fortunately or unfortunately, his family was not waiting for him anyway. The loss would all be his.

Other matters awaited Peter Crossin. He turned to them with a sigh. He supposed that he and the others would look at Jody and wring their hands over him until their course became perfectly obvious.

Thursday, February 7

After discovering that her white count was low, Sam Silver had told Gina that he wanted to see her back in Clinic in a week, meaning tomorrow. But on Friday Gina's class was going on a field trip to the science museum. Her mother had volunteered as a driver. So they'd scheduled the visit instead for today.

The week had not been without its problems. On the afternoon of her spinal tap and the extraction of her bone marrow, Gina had developed a headache, become very tired, and complained of soreness in her back. None of this had surprised her mother. Given

what the child had been through—not just the procedures themselves but all the tension leading up to them—Marie DeRose had
expected her daughter to feel somewhat punky afterward.

But on Saturday she'd felt no better. Ordinarily she was fine the
day after she got a needle in her back. Instead all she'd wanted to
do was to lie around on the couch or in bed. She'd eaten poorly.
Marie had tried not to get too concerned. But it had been hard for
her not to worry about the child's white count.

On Sunday Gina had run a fever of 101 degrees. Marie had
called Dr. Silver immediately. Saying it was probably a virus, he had
suggested Tylenol. By evening her temperature had returned to
normal.

On Monday she had insisted on going to school. At noon the
school had sent her home. She'd been tired, headachy, and a little
dizzy: "You know," she'd explained to her mother, "like when you
get tired and your head starts to turn?" Despite the tiredness, she'd
had trouble falling asleep. Marie had been thinking of calling Dr.
Silver again on Monday when, on Monday evening, he had called
them. Knowing that she and Tony were upset, he had just wanted
to know how they were, and how Gina was. He had also wanted to
make sure that Marie had remembered which medicines not to give
her and to say that he himself was a little concerned but not very
concerned.

Since then he had called every night this week, just to check in.
Marie had been extremely grateful to him.

She and Gina were sitting in his office now, and as Marie was
telling the doctor that Gina seemed fine again, one of the lab technicians walked in with a slip of paper showing the results of the finger
stick. The two DeRoses watched Sam Silver's face light up.

"Great! Oh, great! The white count's back to normal!"

He put Gina back on a limited dose of 6MP. Because the liver
enzymes were still high, he said he wanted to keep her off the Methotrexate and have blood drawn today and again next week.

But he was pleased. Very pleased.

When he'd gone in to examine her, she'd been absorbed in a
book. He'd asked what she was reading.

"Oh, this is for school. You get people to sign up, and every
book you read, they give you a dollar!"

"How many have you read?"

"I'm on my ninth!"

Impressed, he had let her see that he was. "What happens to the money?"

"We take it in, and the nuns give it to . . ." She had had trouble with the pronunciation.

He had had no trouble at all with the meaning. Two words. Multiple sclerosis.

Ø

Later in the afternoon, one day before his scheduled discharge to the Leverett House Annex, Freddy Eberly was transferred out of the Acute Unit on the fourth floor to a six-bed room on a sixth-floor surgical unit. He no longer required intensive care, and his bed was needed for another child.

Before he left, the Acute staff gave him a party. It featured one cherry popsicle and a special present. The child had a somewhat unpleasant odor about him from frequent sweats, a result primarily, the doctors thought, of his elevated carbon dioxide levels. Whenever the nurses teased him about smelling good, like a baby or a rose, he'd always laugh. So about noon, when they had him in a wheelchair ready to go, when everybody in Acute was standing around him saying goodbye, the nurses gave him a wrapped package containing a bottle of British Sterling aftershave.

"That's to charm your new nurses!" they told him as he opened it, "and so you can smell good whenever you want to!" When they wheeled him out of the unit, Freddy Eberly was smiling.

Monday, February 11

The Leverett House Annex on the fifth floor of Children's is small and self-contained. Located at the end of a short hall leading nowhere else, it is entered through double doors which are usually kept closed. In appearance the sixteen-bed facility is very little different from units within the hospital proper. A youngster coming in from Children's would recognize the layout, the furnishings, the views across the city, the overall tone. As in other patient units throughout the building, the walls, windows, and bulletin boards of the Annex are bright with color snapshots, printed posters, and artwork done by kids.

Freddy Eberly's transfer to the Annex had been delayed for a few days by an infection he developed around the pin sites in his right leg. After just one day on Six Surgical, he had had to return to Isolation on Friday. Over the weekend the infection had improved enough that Freddy was at long last scheduled for discharge from Children's this afternoon. Colin Kendall, finishing his morning in the Operating Room, visited him to make absolutely certain that the patient was ready to go.

The neurosurgeon was not very impressed with the amount of movement Freddy had on his left side at this stage. Kendall was pleased, however, by the increasing spontaneity of movement the boy had exhibited over the past few days, and he knew that the spontaneity was likely to increase dramatically once the patient was out of the ICU. Also on the positive side, the mysterious acid imbalance that had so puzzled the anesthesiologists in particular had finally resolved itself.

The child's long-term prognosis was still largely a matter of speculation. How the accident had affected Freddy's mental capabilities was impossible to assess with any precision. Kendall didn't know what his intellectual potential had been before the car hit him. The boy attended public school. His grades were mostly B's and C's, which in Kendall's observation was what everybody seemed to get in the city system. Freddy had probably never been formally evaluated. Given his improvement so far, however, the doctor's best guess was that the patient would eventually return to school having lost very little in the way of intellect—so little that in his environment the deficit might well go unnoticed.

His environment was a factor in his favor in this regard. Kendall had often observed that when a child from a middle- or upper-class family suffered a bad head injury, every little difference in intellect struck the parents or grandparents as a major disaster. Reintegrating those patients into normal life could be quite difficult. Someone was always looking over the child's shoulder and saying, "Before the accident you used to be able to write better. You knew more words. You used to do better in math."

In an environment such as Freddy's, where families were struggling for survival, not for slots at prep school and Harvard, people didn't care so desperately about school performance, in Kendall's experience, and a minimal loss of brain power was unlikely to seem disastrous. Freddy would undoubtedly have trouble getting back to normal when he finally returned home. Neuropsychological problems such as memory loss, learning disability, and emotional impairment are typical after brain trauma. But Kendall expected that he would be less handicapped psychosocially than a child surrounded by relatives who had time to spend the whole day worrying about him.

About the patient's physical prognosis the neurosurgeon felt less optimistic. He worried about Freddy's legs. Between a fractured femur on the right and poor recovery on the left, at least so far, the child was going to need a great deal of physiotherapy. Even so he might end up in a wheelchair. Whether and how well he would be able to speak were questions that would not be answered until the tracheostomy tube was out and the hole in Freddy's throat was closed. At the very least he would probably need speech therapy.

The best to be hoped for was that Freddy would recover well enough to walk and talk without too much difficulty. Most likely he would not regain full motor function. He would probably be left with a mild spastic weakness on his left side. Insofar as life's basic routines are concerned, such a handicap is rarely limiting in children physically. Dragging a leg does alter self-image and affect the attitudes of others, of course, thus adding to the psychosocial problems of recovery.

Freddy might need special classes for a time. The right help could be difficult to arrange, a problem arising with increasing frequency in part, in Kendall's view, because the social system had yet to catch up with medical advances. At least in this case there would undoubtedly be an insurance settlement to help Freddy get what he needed. But for the boy to recover as much as he was going to recover would require many months.

Colin Kendall had been taking care of Freddy Eberly for nearly seven weeks. In a sense his involvement with the child had just begun. So long as the patient remained upstairs, the neurosurgeon or the residents would continue to see him daily. At some point the boy would probably move from Leverett House Annex to the main facility in the country. There the neurosurgeons would visit him every few weeks.

Once Freddy had been discharged from the rehab center, Kendall would continue to follow him in the Head Trauma Clinic at Children's. He would almost certainly be involved with the patient's lawyer when suit was filed against the driver of the car. He would also be involved with the patient's mother as she went about re-establishing the boy in whatever school might prove most appropriate for him. He would continue to run tests on Freddy and to see him at regular intervals at least until the boy finished high school.

But the period of Colin Kendall's intense involvement with Freddy Eberly had come to an end. In other beds at Children's, fifteen or twenty much sicker patients awaited the neurosurgeon's close attention. In the past couple of weeks, this boy had needed that kind of attention less with every passing day. Kendall had reached a point in this case that he reached sooner or later in all cases: the moment of distilling the lessons learned. What would he say about this child in lectures? in teaching rounds?

Reviewing the facts in the case, the doctor realized that Freddy was a patient who could rather easily have dropped between the cracks—the sort of patient neurosurgeons needed to see again and again so they were not tempted to become too confident about their cleverness. The doctors at Children's felt they treated head injuries very well. They were marvelous at taking out blood clots, at controlling high intracranial pressure, at putting patients into barbiturate comas and waking them up again. Here was a child who hadn't needed any of those things.

Here was a boy who had arrived at Children's with a head injury from which it had seemed almost certain he would recover. His major belly surgery had been done. He'd had no dramatic surgical problem in his head. He had never had intracranial pressure problems or hydrocephalus.

Meanwhile a number of patients on the neurosurgical service had seemed far more ill than Freddy. Several had needed exceptionally close monitoring. Several had died. With those children to worry about, it had been easy enough for the neurosurgeons to think, *Well, Freddy doesn't need the surveillance these other kids do. This guy's okay.*

Yet in fact the boy had had a very bad head injury. He'd had a long course and a lot of troubles. He'd had respiratory difficulties that had never been explained. He'd had an acid imbalance that had never been explained. Twice the doctors had extubated him in preparation for taking him off the ventilator; both times he'd been unable to keep his own airway open. There'd been one weekend when his carbon dioxide levels had drifted upward unchecked because the neurosurgeons had been involved with two emergency patients. Had Kendall not caught that problem when he had, additional injury might have occurred to Freddy's brain. It was even conceivable that the child might have died, and without anything very dramatic ever having happened. All this in a youngster whose outlook from the beginning had seemed—and actually was, in view of how badly he'd been hurt—rather good.

The case of Frederick Eberly had provided Colin Kendall with an excellent and rather humbling example of how important it was to take nothing for granted. To remain continuously fastidious.

Ø

The child's medical expenses upon discharge that afternoon amounted to $52,400. Virtually the entire bill would be paid through commercial insurance policies held by Freddy's mother.

The paperwork would be done in the Children's business office on the ground floor and would be overseen by the business manager, who had been at Children's for ten years and who kept on his desk several color photos of his wife and two young daughters.

The business manager had gotten his first taste of hospital billing while employed in a collection agency. There he had learned that there are people in any business who for one reason or another don't pay their bills. However, hospitals differ from other enterprises in one respect, he had found: because injury is sudden and illness usually unexpected, services are often rendered before a financial agreement has been struck. Debts not contracted for can be difficult to collect.

Those responsible for billing in a hospital for children escape entirely the intricacies involved in Medicare reimbursements. Nonetheless, the task of exacting payment for the care of a sick child carries its own challenges. Unlike their counterparts in adult hospitals, the Children's business manager and his colleagues never deal with a patient directly. As the manager has put it, "You don't dun a child." All financial transactions are conducted with parents or guardians. Many parents are young and without substantial economic resources. Some have no medical insurance of any kind. In counseling his colleagues about talking to parents, the business manager cautions staff members to keep in mind that "We're not collecting a bank loan."

Most parents whose children are treated successfully are only too happy to pay for that treatment. "Thank God my child came here and everything went well," they'll say to the business manager. They feel they have gotten their money's worth.

When a child dies, however, the parents may not have that feeling. "It's been a tough experience," a father might say to someone in the business office, "and even though your bill is due, you're going to have to wait for it." In this situation the business manager tells the parent that he understands and would feel the same way himself. He then attempts to convey that the hospital did its best, that though unfortunately its best was not good enough, the effort was made, and now it must be paid for. The business manager will suggest to parents who are strapped financially that they pay the bill a little at a time. Most often an arrangement can be worked out that is agreeable to all parties. Some cases must eventually be turned over to a collection agency.

Perhaps the hardest part of the job of billing at a children's hospital is to exact payment when a child has died. But in other ways the job is easier now than it used to be. When he first came to Children's, the business manager had many encounters with parents who owed huge bills for the treatment of children with cystic fibrosis. Now state or organizational programs have lifted some of those financial burdens from parents' shoulders.

When he first came to Children's, the business manager met often with parents owing huge amounts of money for the treatment of children with hemophilia, because insurance policies did not cover the cost of the blood they so frequently needed. Now the blood is paid for through state programs. Furthermore, youngsters with hemophilia used to be in and out of the hospital all the time, and their parents were always in panic, not only about the child they were bringing in but about the children they'd had to leave suddenly in someone else's care. Nowadays the children administer a clotting factor to themselves at home and are rarely admitted to the hospital. When they do come in, their parents are much more relaxed.

In the business manager's early days at Children's, he would look at the family of a child diagnosed with acute lymphocytic leukemia and think, almost panic-stricken himself, "Well, that's a lost child. I have to collect the bill for a child who is not going to live." Today the business manager knows that most of those children will be cured.

Friday, February 15

"Boy, your knees are a mess!"

"I know! They're all bruised, because when the sun came out and it got warmer, I went out on the new roller skates I got for Christmas, and I fell down all over the place!"

The nurse took supplies from a cabinet. She was about to draw a little of Gina's blood for yet another enzyme study. Cindy was at home sick. This was another nurse Gina knew named Becky. She had long red hair that Gina loved to braid.

Becky tore open a new syringe. "What's happening in school?"

"We just found out today about the procession we're having in May to crown the Blessed Mother. You know what, our class doesn't even get to crown her! The eighth graders do! It's no fair!"

"What's no fair?" Sam Silver had appeared in the treatment room doorway. "It's no fair that I don't get to see you today, that's what, but I've got to be at a meeting three minutes ago, so I just wanted to say hi."

"Which hand today?" the nurse asked the patient.

She whipped them out of sight behind her back. "Neither one!"

"Oh-oh," Becky said. "You know, Dr. Silver said I had to get some blood out of you today or he'd get mad at me."

"He can! He can get mad, yell and scream, pull his pants down . . .!"

Becky burst out laughing. The doctor, pretending to be shocked, said he was just leaving anyway and he'd see Gina next week. The nurse and the child got down to business. Gina held the gauze on her arm while Becky tied a tourniquet above it. "You'll be seeing Dr. Lassiter after you see me. You've met him, haven't you?"

"Yeah, when I had to get my checkup one time, he felt for lumps, and I was ticklish under my neck, and he goes, 'Oh-oh, we have to do an operation.' I go, 'What, a lump?' He goes, 'No, we have to take the tickle out!'"

The nurse laughed. "You know," she said, rubbing the back of Gina's hand with alcohol, "I think the last time I saw you, you were talking about becoming a nun. Are you still planning to do that?"

"No, see, when my girlfriend Michelle and I grow up, we're not going to go in college first, okay? We're going to work in either an ice cream shop or a pizza place or a sandwich bar, like, in the eleventh grade, and we're going to stay there and raise money plus our allowance, and we're going to put it all together until we have . . . ow, ow, ow!" She watched the tip of the needle disappear into her skin. "Shall I take the tourniquet off now?"

"Thank you. I think . . . This looks like a good one."

"Yep, the blood's coming. So anyway we're going to put all our money together until we have enough for the two of us to go in college, and then we're going in college together, or we might work as a secretary or a hairdresser, and then we'll go out and be a nun or whatever we want to be by ourselves."

"Sounds like you have it all planned out." Becky pulled slowly back on the syringe.

"I really want to go to college."

"Do your mom and dad talk about your going?"

"They don't even know! This is our idea! Even when we had . . . See, we were going to make a little, what do you call it, a little clubhouse right next to her house, like on the side between the two. There's this big open space? We were going to pretend it was our own clubhouse. There were already two sides. All we did was we put some sticks and leaves around it, and we were going to put a board up on top so the rain didn't come in, and nobody even knows! Her mother doesn't even know! It's her property, and we didn't even tell her!"

The blood samples drawn from Gina for enzyme studies had to

be sent out to another lab for analysis. Ordinarily the results came back to Children's three or four weekdays later. Ordinarily Sam Silver made a point of looking up those results and of calling the family.

The most recent analysis had not arrived until this morning. Rushed as he'd been, Silver had not had a chance to look for the report before leaving Clinic for his meeting.

So it was Dr. Lassiter who told the patient and her mother that the enzymes were more nearly normal than they had been at any time since Gina's liver had begun to show signs of malfunction.

Furthermore, Dr. Lassiter told them, her white count was still normal.

Marie DeRose left the Oncology Clinic walking on air.

Later that afternoon Sam Silver called her and asked her to start Gina back on two Methotrexate tablets every week.

Wednesday, February 20

Toward the end of the morning, Jody Robinson's mother called the Intermediate Unit at Children's, asked to speak to Marla Meyerle, and, when the nurse came on the line, told Marla that she had turned over a new leaf.

She would be out of jail soon, Sabra said. The Welfare Department had decided to give her another chance. This time she would be getting her own place to live. Jody and his little sister could come and live with her. She would learn Jody's trach care. How was Jody? She couldn't wait to start taking care of him.

After lunch social worker Lynn Story called the Welfare Department. Neither she nor the Intermediate nurses could believe that the Department might actually be considering giving Sabra a second chance.

Indeed the Department was. If Sabra could demonstrate for an extended period of time that she could keep out of jail, stay off drugs, and settle down, Gladys Wexler said to Story, the woman could certainly have her children. They would certainly be better off with her than with strangers.

Story could scarcely believe her ears. The last time she had talked to the social worker from Welfare, Wexler had stated flatly that Sabra could in no way be deemed a fit guardian for her son. She had assured Story that the Department was at last filing for formal custody of Jody. Now she had done a complete about-face. She sounded so spacey to the worker from Children's that at one point Story actually interrupted the Welfare worker to ask her her name.

Had the stakes been low, Wexler's total change of heart would have seemed almost comical. But Jody was to all intents and purposes alone in the world. He almost never had outside visitors. Of the love and support that only a family could have given him he'd had virtually none. The nurses he'd known in Acute he'd left behind when he'd come over to Intermediate. His first primary nurse in Intermediate had ceased to serve that function for him when she'd become the unit head nurse.

Now the child was losing his second primary nurse. Marla had found a job in a hospital across the city. She would be leaving Children's within a few weeks. Sooner or later his friends moved on. Jody needed someone who would not move on.

The Welfare Department had the power to take responsibility for Jody and to find him a foster parent or parents who could begin to visit him right away, who could love him while he was still in the hospital. So long as the Department was willing to wait for his mother to prove herself, the child would be denied that opportunity to be cherished. So long as the Department put the mother's rights above the son's, Jody would continue to be alone.

Ø

Hours after the social workers' conversation and forty miles from Children's, Robin Gregory drove alone through the darkness on a quiet country road, taking a shortcut home, weeping.

She had been to a nearby town for her first Twins Club meeting. Halfway through it, one of the women had suggested that the Club contribute again this year to Children's Hospital. Robin had felt herself starting to fight back tears.

Then a woman she had once talked to about becoming a counselor for nursing mothers had come up to ask whether she'd ever signed up for the classes. Without thinking, Robin had replied, "No, because I was pregnant."

And the woman had said, "You're not pregnant now, are you?"

"No," Robin had had to say then, "I had the baby, but he died." She had been unable to stay for refreshments.

Five weeks had passed since Brandon's death. Some days Robin was okay. Some nights she'd cry herself to sleep.

The twins helped. They required a lot of their mother's time, and they had reached a stage now when taking care of them was fun. Robin appreciated them more now too. She'd look at them remembering all the trials and tribulations of those difficult months after their births and thank God for the boys and for their health.

In other respects the Gregorys' lives remained difficult. Tom and Robin were fighting frequently. Robin thought her husband was drinking too much. The money pressures had eased very little. Last week Tom had taken his shotgun off the wall and threatened to blow himself away. Robin had been mad enough to yell at him, "Go ahead, pull the trigger and leave me here with all these bills!"

Because Brandon had died and they no longer needed medical assistance, Tom had started looking for work at some of the factories in the area. He wasn't looking at construction because those jobs paid only five dollars an hour with no benefits and because Tom hated working outside in the cold. On the other hand, he hated working inside when the weather broke. Even if he got a factory job, he kept telling Robin, he'd probably wind up quitting or getting fired anyway when spring came.

"You can't build up benefits that way," she'd reply. Robin wanted her husband to look harder for a job. Tom kept telling her he had to be in the right frame of mind. Sometimes, he told her, he'd sit talking to somebody about a position thinking, *Wow. What am I doing here?*

What he really wanted to do, he said, was train to become a truckdriver. This was fine with Robin. Driving was steady work. It offered good pay and good benefits. But when she'd encourage Tom, he'd say the trouble with driving was that he'd be away a lot and would worry about her and the kids.

Routine had long since resumed in the Infant ICU, of course, but Brandon Gregory had left his mark on his caregivers at Children's.

His death had hit the ICU staff quite hard. It had also caused, temporarily, a certain amount of discord. Some nurses felt strongly that the baby would not have developed necrotizing enterocolitis if his feeds had not been pushed. A few people were bitter about the matter of pushing feeds. However, Lea Bowersox had noticed that the bitterest was someone who hadn't taken care of Brandon much. The nurse wondered if perhaps her colleague was a person who had to go through anger in order to accept death.

For Bowersox herself, Brandon Gregory's death had been very depressing. She was still depressed about Brandon. Though life went on the same as always, Lea Bowersox did not feel quite the same. Saddened about the baby, she was also disappointed in herself. She had vowed never to become so deeply involved with another patient that if the patient died, she'd grieve. She had broken that vow. She had let Brandon Gregory become special to her, and she had lost him. Bowersox realized that she was going to have to start teaching herself protection all over again.

Brandon's death had prompted Dory Hatfield to take inventory—to look at herself and what she was doing, to look hard at what counted and did not count. Brandon's death had readjusted her perspective. It had reminded her that she and her colleagues were only human beings, that while people in the Infant ICU believed they were doing wonderful things for babies, they were not in charge. Dory Hatfield was not a churchgoer. But she did read the Bible and acknowledge a higher power in the universe. Somebody was running the show, in Hatfield's view, and not for no purpose. The nurse did not imagine that little babies were put on earth to suffer for the professional growth of Dory Hatfield and Logan Sadler and the neonatology fellow.

Hatfield could never remember the names of patients she'd taken care of who'd done well and gone home. She never forgot the names of babies who died, nor did she ever forget what she'd learned from them. Every one of those babies stayed with her, as Brandon would stay with her. He had taught her to be a little more careful in how she personally pushed kids. He had reminded her how important it always was to step back, to take a second look, to make sure that her judgments were truly objective and her rationales truly valid. Brandon Gregory had also reminded Dory Hatfield how suddenly life could end, and how important every day really was.

The baby's death had taught Logan Sadler a harsh lesson in medical reality. It had taught her exactly how fast and devastating necrotizing enterocolitis can be.

But Brandon's fate had also had subtler effects on his resident. He had made her a little more negative than she had been about the merits of supporting tiny premies at all. Every time such a patient was admitted to the Infant ICU now, Sadler would remember Brandon Gregory and think, *Why?* This week she was treating a baby even smaller than Brandon had been. Every time she looked at that little girl, Sadler thought about how much the baby would have to go through before they could declare her safe. Should they be subjecting her to any of it?

Were they trying to keep alive babies who were just too small? Neonatologists all over the country kept pushing back the barriers and saving premature infants of lower and lower birth weights. Logan Sadler wondered now whether they might all not be pushing just a little too fast.

For Roger Forbes, Brandon's demise had renewed the doctor's respect for the fragility of tiny premies, especially for the fragility of their digestive function. The baby's death had also driven home to Forbes how much mystery remained in the field of neonatology. He and the others had advanced this patient on tube feedings exceedingly slowly. Just when the baby had gotten past the rough spots and was making good progress, he'd developed NEC. So slow pace was no guarantee of success. But what was? The patient's primary physician had no better an answer now than he'd had before the baby was admitted. Brandon Gregory had taught them all more about their ignorance.

Wednesday, February 27

Because Mark Price had died at St. Michael's Hospital, his autopsy had been done there by a St. Michael's pathologist whose report to Dr. Daniel Earnshaw, along with some of Mark's tissue fixed in formalin and embedded in paraffin, was mailed under a covering letter dated February 25 which included the following paragraph:

> In speaking to Mrs. Price, Mark's mother, it becomes apparent that this young man carries his bravery beyond his demise in having wished that a post-mortem examination be carried out following his demise and that his badly damaged tissue be used to its maximal extent for study, education, and research. We have completed our studies, and at the request of Mrs. Price, I forward to you this material which I am sure you can process in your histopathology department and use for study and teaching.

The pathologist had done a number of autopsies on children with fibrocystic disease. He thought all those youngsters brave. Waking up every morning to the knowledge that they were unlikely to survive to adulthood built very courageous constitutions, in the doctor's opinion.

Yet he also believed that no one could fully realize while they lived how genuinely sick these kids really were. Only after their deaths did the extent of their bravery become apparent, and then only when a pathologist reported on the physical devastation wrought by years of progressive disease. Only then could one appreciate how terrible the child must actually have felt most of the time.

The St. Michael's pathologist had found the condition of Mark's body to be fairly typical of children with his illness. Certain parts of his system had been totally destroyed, most notably his lungs and his pancreas.

In mid-February, the pathologist had received a call from the boy's mother. Mrs. Price had wanted to know why her son had died when he did. She had expressed some anguish over decisions she had made on his last day of life.

The pathologist had assured her that her decisions had served Mark well.

Sitting against the radiator under the window sill in his office, Daniel Earnshaw read the pathologist's report with the amazement he always felt on these occasions, particularly when perusing the observations made about the patient's lungs. Alive, a person maintains his or her lungs somewhat inflated. In death, the lungs deflate and compress and, in a cystic child, squeeze mucus into the air passages. Mark's air passages on autopsy had been completely filled with mucus—a column of mucus reaching right up into the larynx. Earnshaw was always impressed by how much of that stuff there really was. He knew the child had been breathing right up until the moment of his death. How could that have been possible? How could this boy have lasted so long?

Regarding Mark's cystic fibrosis, the autopsy report was unexceptional. It was the tetracycline finding that interested Earnshaw most, and that news was good. Between Mark's lung and his chest wall on the left side, firm, well-established adhesions bound the two surfaces together so closely that another lung collapse had the patient lived would have been extremely unlikely if not impossible. Had Mark's doctors felt confident that good scarring took place so quickly, they would have been less hesitant to remove the chest tubes, and the boy would have been spared some of the pain and suffering the tubes had caused him. The autopsy confirmed the effectiveness of the tetracycline treatment in one human being. It left open the question of whether the adhesions were worth the pain. Of course, as Earnshaw would point out to Mark's parents, that question could not be answered by an autopsy.

He had not talked to Ellen Price since the night Mark died. Listening to her then, he had felt optimistic about her ability to recover. She had seemed to be spelling out to herself that evening that while Mark's life had been short, it had been a balanced life, good in many ways, which had come to a well-rounded conclusion. Some days later she had sent Earnshaw a copy of "A Conversation with Mark" with a letter saying that while she found it difficult to write, she was feeling better. Her letter had fortified his optimism.

He himself was not in especially good spirits. For most of the month just past, in fact, Earnshaw had been in depression. Only in the last few days had he finally understood that the cause of his depression was the deaths of Mark and Janet.

Furthermore, he faced in July the end of his career at Children's Hospital. A new chief of medicine had decided to abolish Earnshaw's Division of Respiratory Disease and bring its function under a larger division with a director already in place. This posed no professional crisis for Earnshaw. From an excellent hospital across town he would direct full-time the state-run health maintenance program for children and youth that he already directed half-time. He believed in the effort and looked forward to the challenge. Still, he could not feel happy about having his job abolished. Moving would be a hassle. He had been at Children's a long time.

The biggest change to result from the move was that he would no longer take care of children with cystic fibrosis. About this he had truly mixed reactions. He would miss his patients and miss also the kind of responsibility he had had for patients who were on their way to dying.

But he could also foresee that it would be a great relief to be spared the agony of losing all those youngsters.

Friday, March 14

Tammy Torrence gave Candy Rudolph a bear hug and lifted her onto the counter of the Six Surgical nurses' station. Other nurses gathered around. The child was dressed in pink tights, a pink skirt, a white jersey printed with pink hearts, her patent sandals. Her wig was loose on her head, though not so loose that it would fall off when her father held her upside down by her ankles.

"Tell Tammy what the boys did with your wig," the child's mother prompted. They had come in from Long Island for a checkup with Dr. Lorimer.

"They took it off!" She fingered the new engagement ring safety-pinned to the pocket of Tammy's blouse. Yvonne had been thrilled by the news.

"How did you feel about that?" Tammy asked.

"I was mad." A little shyly. Nearly three months had passed since Candy's discharge. At home she had stopped talking about the nurses until reminded by her mother that she'd be seeing Tammy again soon, which had made Candy very excited.

"I don't blame you."

Silence.

"She couldn't wait to come up here," Yvonne said, laughing, "and now she won't say anything! Tell the nurses what you said to the boys when they took your wig off."

"'Put it back on!'"

Tammy: "Did they?"

"No!"

"What did the teacher say?"

"The boys had to stand in the corner!"

She had returned to kindergarten in late February. Notwithstanding her mother's desire to protect her from ridicule by the other children, Candy had grown so bored at home that she had begged to go back to school. When the other kids had asked her where she'd been, she had told them that she'd had an operation. Taking her wig off, she'd shown them where the doctor had cut. There had been teasing. Candy had reported on it and had apparently taken it in stride.

Her teacher had remarked that the child was not as bubbly as she had been, causing the mother, by no means for the first time, a bout with guilt. Had the surgery ruined the child's personality?

Yet Yvonne could see that Candy still wasn't herself physically either. Nearly four months after surgery, her scalp was still tender. At the very top it still had a tiny crust. Candy tolerated shampoos but wouldn't let her mother touch the spot. Often after very busy play, she complained that her head or her chest hurt.

Asked at these times what she'd been doing, Candy would reply that she'd been playing on the swings. Yvonne had been puzzled about how mere swinging could cause discomfort at the rib graft site until she'd happened to glance out the window one day in time to see Candy going monkey-like across the bar from which the swings were suspended.

Nonetheless, the child was not to be her old self until late spring.

Wednesday, March 19

Toward the end of his thirty-ninth day as a patient in the Leverett House Annex, Freddy Eberly spoke the first comprehensible sentence he had been able to get out since stepping off a bus on the twenty-seventh of December. The nurses were ecstatic.

Those assigned to care for Freddy the first day or two he spent in the Annex had seen a child in such bad shape that at least one nurse had thought he stood no chance of ever leading a normal life.

He drooled constantly. His jaw hung open. His tongue protruded. Along with a tracheostomy, he had tremendously heavy secretions which he handled poorly. He was still on oxygen. The pin sites in his leg were infected. He appeared only slightly aware of what was happening around him. He seemed unable to look anyone in the face. His balance was so poor that he couldn't even sit up in bed, let alone stand.

He exhibited little spontaneous movement. He wasn't communicating well. He had trouble eating. At first the nurses thought this was because he had trouble swallowing. However, the speech therapist who began working with Freddy almost immediately had attributed the problem not to his swallowing mechanism per se but to nerve damage which prevented him from being able to move his tongue out of the way to let food pass.

By Freddy's fourth day in the Annex the staff had begun feeling much more optimistic about him. Though knowing Freddy would never go home the child he had been before the accident, the nurses had nevertheless begun to appreciate that certain aspects of what they had construed as the child's condition were actually accounted for by his mood. Given a couple of days of adjustment, Freddy's whole demeanor had changed.

He had begun communicating. The nurses had given him bells to ring when he needed to go to the bathroom or wanted to go to the playroom, and while he tended to forget to ask for a urinal or a bedpan, he had gotten very good very fast at letting people know he was ready for play. He'd responded to questions or jokes in a way that made the nurses realize he could understand everything they said to him. He had begun to point to things he wanted and to want more things. He had let it be known that his favorite food was chocolate pudding.

He had become more active. He had drawn on a pad with crayons. He had shown off his knowledge of multiplication tables. He had made a model racing car by gluing the parts together. With the play therapist fingering the chords, he had strummed the strings of a guitar. He had learned to play a card game called Crazy Eights. Though he had never been too interested in books, he had begun to read the Hardy Boys. He had smiled at people who passed his room. He had exhibited playfulness, pretending to give his nurse a needle and laughing when she pretended it hurt.

He had even become somewhat better physically after his first few days in the Annex. He had drooled less. He had begun tolerating short periods off oxygen. In fact, once the newness of the place had worn off a little for him, Freddy had made so much progress that the head nurse had begun talking about him as "one of our best."

By the ninth day he had been improving so rapidly that each time he'd added an accomplishment to his repertoire, one of the nurses would run out to the nurses' station saying, "Come look at what Freddy can do now!"

His progress had by no means been miraculous. Now, in mid-March, the boy continued to have trouble eating. Though he could hold clay, he lacked the strength to work it. Though he had learned a few signs from the speech therapist, signing required two hands, and Freddy could really move only his right hand well enough to do it. He had little or no feeling on his left side. In some ways he reminded the nurses of a stroke patient. Almost everything he did he did slowly and often with great difficulty.

In the past few weeks, however, he had learned to sip through a straw on either side of his mouth. He had gotten so he could lift his left arm slowly and bring it down again. His left fingers had begun to move more freely. His drooling had continued to decrease. More and more, he kept his tongue in. Though he would have to go back on again once or twice before finally coming off for good, Freddy was now able to get along without oxygen support for the first time since being injured.

Furthermore, with every passing day he was becoming more alert and more eager to enter into the life around him. Some Annex patients like to stay in their beds and watch TV. Freddy would watch TV if nobody was with him, but he was much more interested in people. He was constantly pointing toward the playroom. At first his interaction with the other kids had been somewhat difficult. Perhaps because he'd still had his tracheostomy and could not talk, the others apparently had had the impression that he was not of normal intelligence. But whenever a child or a parent would say hi to him, he would respond with a big smile. In time he had become so interested in playroom activities that now he always wanted to at least observe what the other patients were doing even if he couldn't participate. Gradually the kids had gotten the idea that Freddy was one of them.

With the staff his interaction was good. He played a running game of War with one nurse and had a running joke going with another who kept saying she was going to have her dog sic him if he didn't hurry up and do this or that. Sometimes he'd cock a finger at her as if to say, "Oh, no!" Or he'd show her a fist. But either way, he'd have a smile on his face. Sometimes if a nurse suggested he do something he didn't want to do, he'd tease her by giving her a dirty look, but he'd always try anyway. Gradually he had learned to communicate his thoughts by pointing to words on a language board.

At the end of the first week in March, Freddy had been sent to the Operating Room to have his tracheostomy closed. Afterward he had spent a day or two on a surgical floor. As this had been his first time away from the Annex in the four weeks he had been a patient there, the nurses had worried in advance that the separation would upset him. He had not been at all upset. His whole approach had been "Just give me my toothbrush, and I'll be back" in a few days! The staff had taken this as a sign of the child's growing independence.

Last week he had "gone back" to school. Elsewhere on the fifth floor of Children's is a classroom presided over by a teacher paid by the city school system. The teacher holds classes in that room for patients well enough to get there. If patients are well enough to study but cannot leave their rooms or their units, the teacher goes to them. For now the teacher was coming to Freddy. Eventually he would go down the hall to her classroom.

His progress was a daily adventure for the Annex staff. With some kids needing rehab, the nurses wait three months to see any evidence of improvement. With Freddy they were seeing something new every day. They had come to think of him as "hardheaded." Some children with similar problems remain in a state of what the staff calls "do for me." Freddy didn't want people doing for him. He wanted to learn how to do for himself. His hardheadedness pushed him further than he might have gotten otherwise and made him fun to take care of.

On top of that his spirits were good. He was a happy kid who had maintained his sense of humor during the long weeks of hard work. He could turn a dressing or diaper change into a funny experience. He had acquired a lot of crazy facial expressions that made the nurses laugh. Just as had been true in Isolation and Acute, the Leverett House nurses kept saying to Freddy, "You're a riot!" Long after the child had left the Annex, the staff there would remember his humor.

Yet there were times when they also felt deeply affected by the boy's constant struggle to do all the things he wanted to do. This was especially true for one nurse who had a child Freddy's age. Some days after working eight hours to help her patient learn all over again the things he had mastered as a baby or preschooler—to sit up, to feed, bathe, and dress himself—this nurse would go home and collapse, too exhausted to even speak except to make a special point of saying to her children, if they happened to be going outside, *"Watch before crossing the street."*

If Freddy had changed a lot during his early weeks in rehab, his mother had also changed noticeably during that period, in the nurses' view. At first it had seemed to the Annex staff that Sharita Queen only wanted to play tapes for Freddy when she came in, or to play short games with him. She hadn't appeared to express a lot of affection for the boy. She hadn't asked to learn any of his care or sought other ways of interacting with him. While this had distressed the nurses, they hadn't wanted to push Mrs. Queen. After all, she worked a forty-hour week. It wasn't as if she spent whole days at the hospital with time on her hands.

Soon, however, Freddy's mother had begun encouraging the boy to do certain exercises the staff had taught him. When the nurses taught her new ones, she had worked with him on those. She had become extremely good about bringing in pictures of friends and neighbors and talking about them with Freddy. She'd help him work on his memory by showing him a photograph of someone he knew and asking him to write down the first initial of the person's last name. She'd take him to the playroom window in a wheelchair and explain things that were going on outside. If a bus went by, she'd relate it to the accident. In these and other ways Sharita Queen was working to help her son regain his grasp of reality. Freddy liked praise and liked being able to please. His mother had gotten very good at making him do things in exchange for warm words from her.

Within the past week, now that his tracheostomy was closed, Freddy had begun to make sounds and to form words. His mother was not present to hear the first understandable thing he said on the afternoon of March 19, because she was at work. Instead he said it to a nurse: "I want my mommy." When Mrs. Queen arrived a few hours later, the nurse tried to make him say it again. All he could get out was "Mommy." That the word was misshapen because of nerve damage in one vocal cord, that the child's voice was deep and croaky and wheezy could not have mattered less to his mother at that moment. Her son was talking. She had expected him to die.

She felt terribly proud of him. For the boy to be recovering the way he was from the kind of accident he had had told Sharita Queen that Freddy Eberly was an outstanding child.

Friday, March 21

Jody Robinson's primary nurse left Children's Hospital for good at the end of the day shift. Marla Meyerle had worked in Intermediate for two years and two months. After a week off, she was to begin a new job at a large hospital in the heart of the city. She would have a two-part assignment. Though assigned full-time to a small pediatric intensive care unit much like Acute, she would also "float" to either a general pediatrics or an adolescent floor when either of those units was short-staffed. This arrangement would permit Marla to broaden her experience in several directions and would strengthen her application, ultimately, for a master's program in nursing instruction. She was delighted for the opportunity.

She said goodbye to Jody with very mixed feelings. Marla had been quite upset about the softening of tracheal tissue turned up by the February bronchoscopy. Deep down she thought it likely that the child would never be able to have his tracheostomy closed. Though convinced that Jody needed the larger trach tube that had been inserted in February, the nurse devoutly wished that he had not needed it, because if the trach ever were to be closed, the bigger tube would leave him with a bigger scar.

She'd been distressed about the ban on sham feedings. That, too, she knew, was absolutely necessary. But it deprived the child of oral stimulation. Marla wondered when and if Jody would ever learn to eat. She hated it that he couldn't even drink water, that he had to be refused something that any normal child could have for the asking.

On the positive side, he had been breathing on his own for nearly eight weeks. Not only had he not needed to go back on the ventilator, but his need for oxygen was again diminishing. His episodes of cyanosis had not increased. He was continuing to gain weight. Developmentally he was a joy.

Marla left Jody feeling good about the roles he and she had played in each other's lives. He had taught her a great deal about respiratory and gastrointestinal problems. She had also reaped the slow but steady rewards of his growth and development. Because he was not free to explore the world outside the unit, Marla and others had brought as much as they could of that world to his bedside, exposing Jody to sensations and experiences he would not have gotten had they not been so diligent. In that sense Marla had reaped the rewards of her own contributions.

She left him in the care of a nurse she respected. She left him knowing that she would come back to visit him from time to time and that wherever she went, Jody Robinson would in some way stay with her.

Insofar as the child's own future was concerned, Marla had always felt that it was out of her hands.

Monday, April 7

Putting her nose out the front door to sniff the first nice day of spring on Long Island, Yvonne Rudolph found in the mailbox a long envelope for which she had been waiting with some apprehension. In the closing days of winter, Candy had taken a battery of aptitude tests given to all new students at the school she had attended since her father's transfer to Long Island in the fall. Fortifying herself with a fresh cup of coffee, Yvonne read the results at the kitchen table.

The fortification proved unnecessary. The tests had shown Candy to be a few months behind her age group in arithmetic but right where she should be in spelling and half a year ahead of herself in reading.

In the afternoon, instead of meeting the school bus by car, as they usually did, Yvonne and her younger daughter, Amy, went on foot down the long, unpaved road from their subdivision to the highway. Walking back slowly, the girls scampering ahead of her, the earth warming, the days getting longer, and Candy looking better with every week that passed, Yvonne knew as she had not known until that moment that the surgery had been worth all the anxiety and pain and suffering and frustration her family had gone through, that the Rudolphs had been truly lucky, and that God was good.

She would be struck again by these thoughts the first week in June when, bubbliness returned, Candy would perform perfectly her role in the kindergarten production of the "Operetta from the Three Bears."

Then in mid-June, when Candy's hair had grown long enough, Yvonne would take the child to a beauty shop for a professional pixie cut and would hear the hairdresser say pleasantly, nodding at the child, "Okay, I understand. Is it Down's syndrome?"

Reporting this conversation to Rolfe Lorimer a week later during Candy's scheduled checkup, Yvonne would still feel sick. Three months thereafter, when the Rudolphs returned to Children's for a routine visit to Craniofacial Clinic, the comment would still be smoldering in the mother's heart.

This would be obvious to the plastic surgeon. It would also be obvious to Rolfe Lorimer that with her face only partly fixed, Candy still looked abnormal enough to not escape the teasing and the psychological fallout that her surgery had been meant to forestall. Lorimer was well aware of parental sensitivity to the concept of having a Down's child. He also considered the psychological fallout of teasing to be a very important matter. The whole purpose of reconstructing a face, after all, was to foster a healthy psyche. Only incidentally did the surgery correct any function.

It was time, Lorimer would tell the Rudolphs in clinic, for them all to revise their thinking about the second operation.

That operation would be performed the following June. Candy Rudolph would by then be eight years old. The field of craniofacial reconstructive surgery would be older too, and Rolfe Lorimer would operate on Candy's midface expecting that the changes he made then would not have to be remade several years later.

This time, working through the patient's mouth, the surgeon would advance her nose and upper jaw, build up her cheekbones and the sides of her face, and soften the upward tilt of the right eye. This time there would be no complications. Candy would be discharged from the hospital after one week. Her jaw would remain wired for an additional nine weeks. For most of that time she would be physically comfortable and very bored.

The operation on her midface would improve Candy's speech somewhat. It would do nothing to improve either her eyesight or the ease with which she pronounced words. No surgery could alter the fact that Candy Rudolph had been born with Crouzon's syndrome. She would very likely be saddled with poor vision and imperfect speech throughout her life. Certainly in principle these problems would be manageable with corrective lenses and, if Candy chose to have it, with speech therapy.

But if surgery could not spare this little girl all the troubles ordained for her by her genes, it would spare her the worst of them. It would spare her the brutality of rejection at first glance.

For the second reconstructive procedure Rolfe Lorimer would perform on Candy Rudolph would come off better than the surgeon had dared hope. While the first operation had obliterated the dominant defect, it had also accentuated the remaining abnormality. The second operation would bring harmony and coherence to the patient's face. The second operation would put an end to questions from strangers about Down's syndrome and all but put an end to the stares.

Lorimer would still see details he wanted to fiddle with at some later date. But when the child walked into his office for her first checkup after that second operation, the surgeon would realize he had accomplished something he could not have sworn would occur in this case. Candy Rudolph's face would look normal.

Would the child herself perceive a change? Nothing she said to her family after either operation would suggest that she thought of herself as any different.

Frequently and for some time after her first operation, Candy would instigate doctor play with her little sister. Shots would be given and references made to needles hurting. Whenever Yvonne or Bill would look at their eldest and tell her how much prettier she was now, Candy would invariably agree.

This would be all. Admitted to Children's for the initial procedure as a six-year-old, immature for her age to begin with, the child was perhaps just too young to understand or to care what her hospitalization was all about.

Or so her parents would be left to surmise. If Candy did understand and did care, she chose to bear that burden alone.

Saturday, May 3

After a stay of eleven weeks and five days, Freddy Eberly was discharged from the Leverett House Annex and taken into the country to Leverett House proper. The ambulance traveled at normal speeds and without sirens.

The discharge summary that accompanied the patient from the Annex described a child with significant motor deficits. In some form those deficits will plague Freddy as long as he lives. In this respect the summary stands as a tragic document. Because a car hit him as he was heading off to spend a vacation day with Grandma Baker, Frederick Patterson Eberly will never again be whole and sound.

On the other hand, he left the Annex able to walk a few steps with assistance. He could get himself unassisted from his bed to his wheelchair. To a very limited degree he was able to express himself in words to someone who made a real effort to understand him. To a degree limited by the fact that he'd never been a super speller, he could express himself on paper to someone willing to make guesses about what he was trying to get at. He could converse a little in sign language.

He was continent when he left the Annex. He had good control over his secretions. He was able to feed himself and had improved his eating skills enough that he was no longer in danger of aspirating when he swallowed. He could bathe himself using a long-handled brush on his back. He could put on clothes that did not snap, button, or zip. He had become a very demonstrative child—a great kisser and hugger who was very friendly toward the other children and openly emotional with his mother and the staff. Having arrived in a funk, he left the Annex a child whose sense of humor could make a nurse's day.

Freddy was to continue his rehabilitation at Leverett House in the country for fifteen and a half weeks. Six weeks after his arrival, he would make his first visit home. He would go home for good, finally, on the seventeenth of August, almost a full eight months from the day of his accident. Months of rehab would still lie ahead of him.

In the company of his mother, who took time off her job at the Springfield Hospital laundry for the purpose, he would begin to visit Children's Hospital two days a week. There he would see speech, physical, and occupational therapists. The speech therapist would work with him on ways of using his breath, his tongue, and certain throat muscles to produce the best possible voice and on speaking slowly and carefully so people could understand him. She would also work with him on keeping his tongue in and his mouth closed when he wasn't speaking.

The physical therapist would work with Freddy primarily on using his back muscles to stand up straight, on developing more mobility in his trunk, on walking more steadily, and on his endurance. At first he would get short of breath doing exercises for the therapist, a consequence, she thought, of the fact that he'd had a tracheostomy. Though his endurance would improve gradually, a year after the accident he would still be puffing and wheezing during physical therapy.

The occupational therapist would be especially interested in helping Freddy increase the function in his left arm and shoulder, make the left hand a better assist to the right, improve the overall stability and balance of his trunk, and further develop the skills he needed for daily living, such as buttoning buttons and tying shoes. Finding the child reticent with strangers, hesitant to talk in part because it was sometimes hard for people to understand him and in part just out of shyness, this therapist would also work with Freddy on socialization.

Several months after moving back home, Freddy was to enroll in a public school for children with orthopedic handicaps. He could have returned to his old school if he'd wanted to. However, he would not have been able to get from a regular school the support offered by the special school, specifically occupational and physical therapy. It would be the opinion of people at Children's and of Sharita Queen that the boy would be better off in an environment focused on addressing precisely such problems as he had.

Because Freddy could walk and do many things for himself, school district administrators would be a little reluctant at first to assign him to the special school. Mrs. Queen would have to plead her case. She would do so in the company of a Children's Hospital social worker, who would go along as child advocate. The social worker would find Sharita Queen to be a remarkable person. Though clearly overwhelmed by all that had happened to her son, though possessed of few supports either psychological or financial, she was very committed and incredibly strong. Going up against the school system was terribly difficult for her to do. It made her feel very small. But she did it beautifully, and the administrators said yes.

Since he had missed so much of it while recuperating, her son would repeat the fourth grade.

A special bus would pick Freddy up at home each morning and drop him off at home each afternoon. At school he would function intellectually below normal, according to his teacher. This would not worry the teacher very seriously because she would have learned that he had performed similarly at his old school before the accident. Though a whiz at his times tables, though sometimes on a spelling test now he would spell every word perfectly, schoolwork would not emerge as his greatest strength.

His greatest strengths would lie in the direction of cooperation and effort. When his teacher asked who wanted the job of watering plants, Freddy would raise his hand high. Instead of playing out in the schoolyard, he'd come into the classroom early every morning to discharge his responsibility. Whenever there were chairs to be straightened up, Freddy would be right there. His teacher would find him a willing, reliable, emotionally stable child whose dress and grooming showed a family that was concerned about him and took care of him. At the end of the year Frederick Patterson Eberly would receive a Certificate of Achievement, signed by the principal, commending him for making an outstanding adjustment in a new school.

The therapy available to him there would take the place of the hours he had been spending with the physical and occupational therapists at Children's. This meant he would return to the hospital only to see the speech therapist and Colin Kendall. Approximately a year from the date of the accident, the doctor would conclude on the basis of testing that Freddy was functioning intellectually about two years below age level—not two years below normal, but two years below average—and in that respect had recovered from his accident rather well.

Kendall would also see a child who remained quite compromised physically. Freddy would still have a lot of coordination problems. His gait would be disjointed. Because of interference between his brain and his muscles, he would have trouble getting words out. Knowing that his speech, walk, and posture would improve with work, Kendall would also judge—wrongly, it would turn out—that Freddy would never run again, and that he would never regain full use of his left hand. What kind of job he could cope with would have to be determined in vocational counseling. He would not be able to earn a living from manual labor, nor would he ever be the sportsman he had once dreamed of becoming.

However, the neurosurgeon would be able to assure the child's mother one year post-injury that Freddy would finish school and would certainly be able to marry, to support himself, and to lead an independent life.

Such issues would remain far back in Sharita Queen's mind. She would be mainly concerned with the here and now. She would look at Freddy and see that everything about him was getting better Though he still had a limp, he walked better with each month that passed. He was more active: he'd go outside and play ball. His speech was improving: she could hear him better and understand him better. If she asked a question and didn't understand the answer, he'd say, "Never mind," or he'd write it down on paper for her.

His handwriting was better than before the accident. Though he used his left hand less than before, knowing he could do what he needed to with his right, his left could nevertheless pick things up again. He had no trouble eating. He was pretty well up to date with his memory, from what his mother could see. Like most people, he remembered some things and not others. He got along well with his friends—just as he had before, Sharita Queen would tell her friends.

He liked his new school better than the old school. Freddy liked to help people, and at the new school he got lots of chances. One boy did not know how to take six from five, so Freddy showed him how to borrow. The teacher asked Freddy to help a little girl who was having trouble with her spelling, so he spelled some words for her. He was enjoying reading for the first time in his life.

He never complained. The only time he got depressed was if he wanted to go someplace. His mother did not allow him to go anywhere by bus by himself or walk places by himself, because he didn't look when he walked. Otherwise he was happy. Sometimes it would seem to Sharita Queen as if nothing had ever happened to him.

She would feel so proud of him. Almost a year to the day of his accident, he would be an usher at church. At breakfast she would remind him to stand straight and tall. He would stand up at the back of the church for one whole hour! Every time she'd look back at him, he'd be standing straight and tall as could be.

Whenever he'd go back to see them, Freddy's old friends at Children's would share his mother's pleasure in his progress. "Every time you come up here you look better!" one of the nurses in the Annex would tell him. He'd be so improved physically, so much more confident about being able to talk to people, that to the occupational therapist the improvements would seem "drastic." He'd have gone from being a nonambulatory person with no speech, severe balance problems, and a useless left arm to a child who could walk, talk, be independent in all the activities of daily living, and was well on his way to being a functioning member of society.

"Well, he still has his great sense of humor!" the nurses would say to each other after Freddy and his mother had left. They might also comment on the changes in Sharita Queen, who when they'd first met her had seemed so quiet and now just loved to talk about how her son was doing.

Freddy would always get very excited about his trips back to the hospital. He'd talk for days about going to see his "girlfriends"—all his favorite nurses in Acute and Isolation and the Annex. In fact, he'd refuse to go to Children's unless his mother would promise him he could see them. One day he'd even want to wear a suit for the occasion. "Not now," his mother would reply. "But when you finally get released from there, definitely."

Nonetheless, he would always dress very carefully for his visits back to Children's. Every time he went, until the bottle was finally empty, Freddy would stand in front of his mirror and splash himself lightly with the British Sterling cologne given to him as a farewell present and a token of their affection and esteem by the nurses in Acute.

Tuesday, May 6

Barefooted, dressed in shorts and a halter, Robin Gregory sat on the trailer steps enjoying the sun and watching the twins. They were playing in a sandbox with the little boy next door. The boy's mother had recently gone back to work. Seeing a chance to pick up some cash to help out with bills, Robin had offered to take care of the child. This was the first week she had tried it and also, she had decided, the last.

The child was not fully potty-trained. He was rough with Tommy and Keith. All three needed a lot of attention individually. Together they were a real handful. More money might have made the job seem worth doing to Robin, but she was only getting twenty-five dollars a week and feeding the child lunch and dinner every day.

So when the twins got potty-trained and could stand to be away from her, Robin would start looking for a job. After divorcing her first husband, she had gotten a two-year degree in social work and had loved working with foster children. If she couldn't find anything in that field, she'd go to a big corporation nearby that trained people for all kinds of jobs, gave full fringe benefits, and let employees work their way up. Robin wanted a job in which she could prepare for the future.

Tom had signed himself up for sixteen Saturdays of training to become a truckdriver. Having this work would mean he'd be traveling a lot, but Robin thought it would be good for them both to have some time apart.

Life was settling down a little for the Gregorys. What made Robin feel bad was realizing that Brandon had had to die in order for things to get back to normal.

She went through her days in sadness and with little inner peace. For one thing, she felt guilty—guilty about having gotten up too soon after she had hemorrhaged and the doctor had told her to rest, guilty about what had happened the night before her water had broken. If she and Tom hadn't had sex that night, would Brandon still be alive?

Robin also had many unanswered questions about her baby's treatment at Children's Hospital. Why had the male nurse insisted on her holding Brandon that one time, when the mother's common sense would have told her that someone that small should not be held? They had moved him from one room to another shortly before his death. Had he caught the virus that killed him from another baby? How could he have gotten so sick so fast? What had the autopsy shown? Robin had expected someone from Children's to call her about the autopsy. Since no one had, she'd concluded that they'd probably learned nothing from it. She herself still had questions about the findings.

She had questions about the doctors who'd treated her before her delivery. Brandon had been a normal baby. That's what Robin couldn't get over. Everything that had gone wrong with him had gone wrong after his birth. If her placenta had been in the normal position, she'd now be raising three sons. Did medical science, advanced as it was, have no way to fix placentas such as hers so that the mothers could carry the babies to term? Robin found it almost impossible to believe that a perfectly normal baby had had to suffer and die because of a mistake in nature that had had nothing at all to do with him.

If she had called Children's and expressed these concerns, staff members there would almost certainly have responded with compassion to the mother's guilt and would almost certainly have been able to ease her mind to the extent that her questions had answers.

Unfortunately, the Gregorys had never come to appreciate the staff as a resource for themselves. In this sense Robin and her husband had slipped through the cracks at Children's. Short on money, they could visit Brandon only infrequently. When they did go in they were passive souls in an aggressive environment that can intimidate the most sophisticated parents. Because the Gregorys communicated with some difficulty, staff found it difficult to communicate with them. Because the staff was undeniably busy with other patients and other parents, they did not spend the time it would have required to draw the Gregorys out. Trust had never developed on either side. Nor had understanding. The nurses had always been puzzled as to why Robin Gregory had consistently refused to hold her baby. Robin had always been puzzled as to why the nurses would suggest that she hold him.

Therefore, though her heart continued to be troubled, Robin never even thought of calling Children's Hospital. While she remembered Dr. Sadler telling her on the day of Brandon's death to call at any time, Robin Gregory did not think her questions could be answered by anybody at Children's, or by anybody at all.

Thus she did not ask them. Thus was Brandon Gregory's mother left with her questions and her guilt.

Tuesday, May 13

In a cluttered laboratory which smelled of chemicals, Dr. Neil Martinson and a research associate took positions on either side of a narrow stainless-steel table and proceeded to open and examine the chests of four of the last half-dozen New Zealand white rabbits to be sacrificed for Martinson's tetracycline study.

These four rabbits corrected a control group imbalance in the research but yielded no news about the value of the drug as a sclerosing agent in patients with pneumothorax. That point had already been well established by all the rabbits sacrificed previously. In fact, Martinson and his associate had already drafted the article they would eventually publish on the study. The key sentences in the draft read as follows:

> There was a spectrum of results with the [various] sclerosing agents, but with concentrated tetracycline solution (Group E), there was uniform pleurodesis [scarring] and thickening of the pleura by histologic [tissue] evaluation. . . . We conclude that tetracycline is an effective agent in causing pleurodesis and can be used during an active pulmonary-to-pleural air leak without untoward effect. Tetracycline pleurodesis should be attempted as the method of choice in patients who are poor risks for thoracotomy [surgery]. We also feel that tetracycline pleurodesis may be offered as an alternative to patients who are candidates for operative treatment because of recurrent spontaneous pneumothorax.

Along with reporting on their laboratory findings, the authors included in their article a case study of a "severely cachetic 15-year-old white male with cystic fibrosis." (Cachexia is a term used to describe the general ill health and emaciation of persons with chronic illnesses.) But when the article was submitted to the prestigious professional journal *Chest,* editors there felt that a single case study did not belong in the article, and the discussion of Mark Price was dropped.

However, in the months to come, Neil Martinson would stand

before audiences at several major cardiothoracic conferences and describe to colleagues from all over the country his experience with tetracycline as a sclerosing agent in thirty-two New Zealand white rabbits and one fifteen-year-old white male with cystic fibrosis. Mark's autopsy had extended the validity of the research findings one critical step from animals to humans. For that reason, Martinson had begun to use tetracycline routinely for spontaneous pneumothorax in his own practice and from the podium urged his colleagues to do the same.

Thus did the lesson of Mark Price's lungs, a lesson purchased by his severe pain and by the daily agony of wondering whether today would be the day his lung collapsed again, begin to be spread to members of the healing profession whose patients were likeliest to profit from it.

Furthermore, alerted by Mark's experience, Neil Martinson and his associates had begun to search for ways to spare other pneumothorax patients getting tetracycline the pain Mark had endured. Eventually the surgeons would find their solution in a drug called ketamine. Though a general anesthetic, ketamine does not depress respirations, and its effects last three or four hours. In CF patients, Martinson would discover, it would work like a charm. The kids would get ketamine before getting tetracycline, and they would wake up with no memory of pain.

These, then, are Mark Price's legacies to medicine and to the human race—small contributions, perhaps, but hardly insignificant ones.

Friday, May 16

Sitting quietly in his crib, a syringe wrapper clutched in his fist, Jody Robinson watched a familiar figure come through the doors of the Intermediate Unit at Children's: a slight man with a short beard wearing the white uniform of Central Supply.

Vanderbilt stopped his metal cart beside the nurses' desk. The shelves of the cart were full of small packages, all different sizes, all wrapped in sky-blue paper. After leaving some of his packages on the desk, he picked up the charge slips that verified new orders and made straight for Jody's crib.

"Hey, baby." Vanderbilt reached a hand over the side rails and knuckled the nappy head. "Hey, Jody! How ya doing?"

Pleased, Jody looked up into Vanderbilt's face.

The man presented his open palm through the side rails. "Hey, Jody, gimme five!"

Dropping the syringe wrapper, Jody slapped his hand down hard against Vanderbilt's, his body bouncing slightly on the mattress. He laughed.

"Hey, great! Do it again!"

This time Vanderbilt caught Jody's hand and held it. He began stroking it with his thumb. Bending, he spoke softly through the side rails.

For a moment, Jody listened carefully, seriously, watching Vanderbilt's lips and eyes. But he had noticed the pens in the man's pocket. With Vanderbilt stooping as he was, they were well within the child's reach.

Jody withdrew his hand. Reaching through the rails, he closed his fingers around one of the pens and began to draw it slowly out of the pocket. He stopped, searching the face in front of him.

"Now, you know you're not supposed to play with that stuff." The man's voice was tender.

Jody slowly replaced the pen. He looked back at Vanderbilt's face. Receiving no negative signals, he grasped another pen. Watching Vanderbilt's face, proceeding slowly, he drew the pen out of the pocket and brought it back between the side rails. Hugging it to himself, he smiled triumphantly at Vanderbilt, who beamed concession.

"You be careful with that!"

The child's future was no more apparent now than had been true in December. His doctors weren't even speculating on a likely date of discharge. Jody was still biding his time at Children's Hospital. He was waiting for a decision to be made about his colon surgery, waiting for the doctors to learn what if anything they would need to do about his chronic aspiration, waiting for a decision to be made about custody, waiting to grow enough that his body could tolerate what remained to be done to it, waiting, ultimately, for a

home to be found. So far as the staff at Children's knew, Welfare
Department social worker Gladys Wexler was still hoping that Jody's
mother would eventually agree to provide for him. What staff did
not know was that in August Gladys Wexler would be reassigned
within the Department. Children's social worker Lynn Story would
have to begin all over again with Wexler's replacement.

"Okay, Jody," Vanderbilt said finally. "I gotta go. Put the pen
back, okay? Right here."

He leaned over and positioned his pocket.

Jody listened, but his face was preoccupied.

Vanderbilt leaned closer. "Right here, baby," he said. He tapped
his pocket.

Jody replaced the pen, point down.

"Hey! You did it!"

Gleefully Jody clapped his hands together and pressed them
over his eyes.

Vanderbilt laughed. "Listen, you, I gotta go," he repeated.
"Okay? I'll come back tomorrow or the next day. Promise. Okay?
Right now I really gotta get out of here. Okay?"

He stooped. "Jody. Gimme some sugar." Between two side rails,
the man offered his pursed lips, eyes closed. When nothing happened, he opened his eyes again.

"Come on, Jody. Gimme some sugar." Vanderbilt made kissing
sounds.

Jody watched the man's lips, concentrating. When they stopped
moving, he looked up. Again Vanderbilt's eyes opened.

"Like this." He demonstrated again.

Sitting where he was, Jody tried to imitate what Vanderbilt was
doing. He couldn't make his lips purse like Vanderbilt's, but he discovered that if he smacked his lips, he could make a similar sound.

For a few seconds he practiced his sound. Then, as soon as he
was sure of it, he leaned forward, still smacking, until his lips
touched Vanderbilt's and smacked against them.

Vanderbilt kissed. A strand of saliva stretched fine between them
and broke, and then Jody's visitor was gone.

Ø

Early evening. A mild, fair evening, bringing into the Children's

Hospital Emergency Room more cases than appear when rain is falling, among them the cases typical of spring: the asthmatics, the youngsters who have been bumped or cut or fractured during exuberant play outdoors.

Most were brought in by parents or other kin. New arrivals were directed immediately to a triage booth where a nurse checked them over quickly. Those needing attention right away were sent into one of three big rooms designated for acute patients just beyond the triage booth. The others either were led across a hall to one of seven single examining rooms or were asked to have a seat in the waiting room. Also sitting in the waiting room were a handful of parents or grandparents distracting or ignoring or reprimanding bored youngsters whose siblings were being treated somewhere inside.

At 7:15 a woman and a small boy walked together through the ambulance entrance of Children's and reported to the triage booth without being instructed to do so. The boy wore sneakers, jeans, a brown sweater with a picture of a train captioned CHOO-CHOO on it, and, around his forehead, a yellow headband. He told the triage nurse he was five years old. He said a door had fallen on his left arm, and he couldn't move it. He was alert and chatty and did not seem to be in pain. But a traumatized arm is an acute problem, and the nurse asked the mother to take her son into the first room on the left. There, inviting the child to sit on a chair, another nurse began a more thorough examination.

The boy's interest was almost instantly engaged by the other people in the room. On a litter a few feet from him lay an older boy who had hit his head earlier today but was telling a resident that he couldn't remember how. The youngster's grandmother was telling the resident that Marshall had vomited four times and gotten very weak. On a chair nearby sat a teenaged girl who had stepped on a broken bottle. Her foot was wrapped in bloody gauze. Her mother had just arrived. Instead of offering consolation, the woman was complaining loudly about the ride down on the bus and scolding the girl for getting hurt. On another litter a younger girl sat taking oxygen for asthma, heaving for breath as her mother dabbed tears from the child's face.

The nurse asked the five-year-old about his headband. He was so busy watching the others that his mother had to answer for him. "He wants to be an Indian," she explained.

At this the boy looked at the nurse as if to confirm his mother's story. Removing a denim blood pressure cuff from his arm, the nurse said to him with just a hint of teasing, "I think you're healthy enough to be a chief."

The thought pleased him. He looked up at his mother to see if she, too, was pleased. She responded with a look that wavered somewhere between skepticism and concern. The nurse said a doctor would be right with them.

On an average day some two hundred youngsters visit the Children's Hospital Emergency Room. Nearly a quarter of these visits are of an acute nature: asthma; seizures; lacerations; ingestions; foreign objects such as keys, crayons, erasers, spitballs, or roaches in noses or ears; respiratory arrest, including perhaps twenty cases a year of sudden infant death syndrome; rape in children under twelve (by contract with the city, older victims are taken to rape crisis centers); and major trauma, including breaks, bumps, bites, multiple injury, and injuries resulting from child abuse. Half of all these youngsters are sick enough to be admitted to the hospital at least overnight.

The great majority of patients seen in the Children's ER, however, present problems of a nonacute nature: rashes, minor dehydration, old cuts and bruises, low-grade fevers, earaches, sore throats. As in adult hospital emergency rooms, there are occasional "turkeys," as they are sometimes called by staff members—patients who don't need to be there but must be checked out anyway, just to make sure. Cancer and brain tumors are among the diagnoses that have been made at Children's on youngsters showing up in the ER with seemingly minor complaints.

Several residents now entered the big room and consulted with their colleague who was attempting to ascertain whether Marshall had amnesia. One of the newcomers was Darryl Barth, finishing his first-year residency and no longer thinking of quitting medicine. For some minutes he and the others conversed intently in low voices about how they were going to proceed with Marshall. When they had made their decisions, Barth detached himself from the group and stooped beside the Indian.

He began very gently to manipulate the boy's left arm. The boy watched. As Barth worked, he questioned the patient. "Was it a big door or a small door that fell on you?"

The boy nodded.

"Did somebody pull your arm?"

Again the youngster nodded.

"Did somebody punch you in the nose?"

Another nod. The boy's mother smiled ruefully, and Barth caught her eye. To her son he said, "Do you want to be an actor when you grow up?"

The boy nodded once more, very solemnly.

"This is my third time in here with this arm this year," his mother told the resident apologetically. "Sometimes I think he just likes to come here and see what's going on."

"How did it happen?"

"Playing with the dog. That's what his grandmother said."

Barth assured her that she was right to bring the boy in if she was worried about him. He said he'd like one or two of the other doctors to look at the child, but they couldn't do it right away because they were busy with other patients.

The Indian and his mother were in the ER for nearly three hours. During that time Marshall had x-rays and became less groggy and remembered that he had fallen from a railing. The girl who had stepped on glass had the glass removed and the foot stitched. She was sent home on crutches. The asthmatic became more comfortable and stopped taking oxygen but stayed on the litter while the doctors decided whether to admit her.

The staff remained very busy with dozens of other patients, among them a seven-year-old with a broken femur, a toddler who had swallowed a mothball, another who had put pieces of a Pamper up her nose, a teenager who had had an odd episode at school which the doctors thought might have been hysteria, a four-year-old with ringworm, a six-year-old with a fever and seizures, and a twelve-year-old whose mother said he just didn't have the energy a boy his age should have.

In the midst of it all Lisa Fletcher came in, carried by her father who had driven her from home because she was very short of breath. Lisa arrived looking terribly frail, and she was crying, begging the staff to tell her what they would do if she stopped breathing altogether. Someone called Daniel Earnshaw at home. At his recommendation, Lisa was given a dose of chloral hydrate, the drug Mark had used for sleep. Eventually she calmed down enough to go home.

Meanwhile the Indian was examined by three more residents. The first, like Barth and the nurses before him, found nothing wrong with the child's arm. But the Indian still insisted he could not move it, and no one had seen him move it since he'd arrived.

The second resident came in with a finger puppet from *Sesame Street*. "How do you feel?" he made the puppet ask the Indian.

The child beamed at the puppet. "Great!"

"Get Ernie," the resident urged. He aimed the puppet at the patient's left arm and began to zero in. The boy grabbed Ernie with his right hand.

Between the second resident and the third, an hour passed. The third noticed the Indian's interest in all the activity around him and began to tell him about those other patients. The boy listened as if to a wondrous bedtime tale he was hearing for the first time. Suddenly the resident held out his palm to the patient's left and said to the Indian, "Gimme five!"

The boy slapped the palm.

"Oho, you're strong! Can you do it harder?"

He could. He did. He did not notice the sheepish smile on his mother's face.

"Harder!"

This time the Indian raised his left arm as high as he could and smacked the resident's palm with all his might.

The resident laughed. The Indian laughed. His mother laughed in spite of herself.

The resident told the patient's mother that she could take her Indian home and put him to bed.

Bright lights would burn all night in the ER complex. They would burn all night in all the nurses' stations at Children's, in one or two operating rooms, in certain hallways, in the vending machines in the cafeteria and the lobby, and over certain patient beds in units throughout the hospital. Bright lights would burn past midnight in a laboratory or two and an office or two and would burn at McDonald's until 11:00 P.M.

Night was well established at Children's by the time the Indian and his mother left by the ambulance door. The sky above the stepped glass roof was black. In the big lobby, though individual trees were lit softly by spotlights, and though soft light came up through the clear fountain floor, casting in dark relief the countless pennies tossed in for luck, a restful dimness prevailed—dimness and the music of water splashing into water.

A few people stood in line at the one cash register open at McDonald's. Except for a resident studying, the seating area was vacant. Here and there in the molded chairs around the lobby, perhaps ten adults sat alone or in pairs, a few dozing, a few staring into space or smoking, one or two attempting to quiet young children who sat with them. A uniformed security guard walked through the lobby with a radio on her hip. Two more guards bantered at a desk near the elevators. Soon the elevators would fill with nurses about to report for night-shift duty.

Up on the fourth floor in the semidarkness of Intermediate, Jody Robinson slept on his back in a diaper. His chest rose and fell according to the dictates of some inner impulse, every breath his own doing. One hand curled loosely around the fuzzy arm of his wind-up monkey. Next door in Acute, which had received Candy Rudolph after her surgery and Freddy Eberly after a car had hit him, cardiothoracic surgeon Neil Martinson, dressed in a suit, checked on a patient he had operated on at 7:00 A.M. The attention of the staff was focused on a three-year-old who had fallen out a second-story window this morning. Most of the other patients were asleep. Across the hall in Isolation, where Freddy had gradually emerged from his coma, all the patients were asleep.

The hallways between these intensive care units and the Infant ICU were still lit but were even more silent than they are in daylight. Overhead lights blazed in the ICU nurses' station and in one of the five glassed-in patient rooms, and a small light burned over the baby in the warmer bed once occupied by Brandon Gregory. A resident in a scrub suit stood at the foot of that bed. Elbows on the edge of it, chin propped in hands, she gazed down at the baby as if caught in time, as one gazes at the sea.

One floor up in the Oncology Clinic, a cleaner in a blue uniform dusted the tops of cabinets in preparation for running the orange vacuum cleaner she had brought in with her. Though most lights were off in the Clinic waiting room, the caged birds chattered quietly. The illuminated fish tanks are never turned off. Their inhabitants surfaced and dropped, foraged and huddled on schedules of their own. Most of the toys that clutter the room in daylight had disappeared into toy boxes. On one chair, however, left, perhaps, by a latecomer to Clinic, lay a doll in a strawberry dress.

Upstairs on Six Surgical, the room in which Candy Rudolph had spent two weeks battling a complication of her surgery was dark, and the door was closed. The room in which Freddy Eberly had spent his last night at Children's before being discharged to the Leverett House Annex for rehabilitation was likewise dark. Two nurses sat at the nurses' station talking about their weekend plans and working on charts.

Several nurses at the Adolescent nurses' station on the other side of the sixth floor were engaged in similar activities. Yards away, in the unlit head nurse's office, two residents discussed a patient. Mark's room lay some yards in the other direction. The door was closed and the shades drawn, but the lights were on, and so was the television set. Out in the darkened hallway, the parents of a patient in Adolescent sat holding each other's hands. The mother wore a hospital blanket around her shoulders. She had obviously been crying.

At the center of each main hallway at Children's, the space widens to form a small balcony which, like some of the playrooms, juts out into the atrium. From this vantage point now, one could look down into the lobby and watch a woman pace slowly around the fountain, or look into a third-floor lounge and see a parent reading, or look into the fifth-floor Stepdown Unit and see nurses tending an infant, or look across the atrium into the lights of a city otherwise invisible in the darkness.

Ellen Price had stood in this spot many times during Mark's last admission to Children's. Marie DeRose had escaped often to this spot the week Gina was a patient on the Oncology Unit right after her diagnosis. Yvonne Rudolph had composed herself here during the hard days on Six Surgical when Candy had seemed to be getting no better. Generations of parents had preceded these mothers in this small niche. Generations will follow them.

Downstairs in the chapel off the lobby, a young father prayed alone. The chapel is a modern oval room of blue and gold and wood with seats for twelve. In a stained-glass ribbon that circles the room just below the ceiling is inscribed a passage from Genesis on the Creation. The altar is a table covered with a white cloth. Its only appointments are a Bible and a bouquet of dried flowers in a brass bowl. Christians sometimes notice and object to the absence of a cross or a figure. The chaplain has wondered if these parents' objections originate in fear that God has abandoned them.

After a time the young man rose and approached the chapel lectern. On it is kept an open spiral notebook and a ballpoint pen. Picking up the pen, the father glanced briefly at the most recent entries, then bent and added his own thoughts to those written in times of trial or thanksgiving by other parents of patients at Children's Hospital and by the professionals who have chosen to take care of those patients:

> Father, these days are long and hard on my heart. My sweet wife cries for our son who is suddenly in unexpected danger, and I've become fine-tuned to parents with similar sorrow. I pray for hope. I'm sensitive with new eyes. Please let the music grow, for joy of good news, in the future of these parents and afflicted children. Keep me wise and strong enough to protect my family; out of this challenge may my son through your blessing return home healthy, where I sing praises to the Lord, where I'll sing songs of hope for children. Amen.

Friday, May 23

The DeRoses were leaving town for the Memorial Day weekend. Tony arrived home from his construction job about 5:30, and the family immediately sat down to supper. As soon as the meal was over, they packed the car and got on the road, heading straight into the setting sun for the campsite Marie had thought they could not possibly rent this year because of Gina's leukemia. Forecasters had promised three beautiful days.

Gina sat in the back seat pretending that they were almost there. They didn't go in at the first sign but first passed a store and a house and a playground. Their campsite was Number 33. It was a lot of space with woods all around it. All you did was walk down the road, and there was a whole bunch of woods. The DeRoses had one tent. When they got there, Gina would help her mother unload the car while her dad put the tent up. There was a water hose at the campsite. There was also electric, but her family didn't use it. Tonight they would just probably get the tent up and go to sleep.

Tomorrow they would get to go swimming, fishing, get to play, get to eat, go to the candy store, all good kind of stuff! They swam down at this lake where there were little baby sharks and snapper turtles and bullfrogs and minnows and other fish. A lot of people swam there. When they were fishing, she and Little Tony would use their new poles with their names carved on them. Her dad always put the worms on. He was afraid that she and her brother would get hurt on the hook. Her chores were to set the picnic table, dry the dishes, and help with Little Tony. Probably after supper they would roast marshmallows over the fireplace.

Gina could not wait to get there! She was so excited! But it was always an hour and twenty minutes, no matter how you felt!

The children didn't fall asleep until after 10:00. By then most of the other campers had also settled down for the night. Except for a few lights burning here and there which occasionally moved or were crossed by shadows, the entire campground had become almost invisible in the darkness. The surrounding trees had blackened into shapes resembling clouds. Stars glittered all over the sky.

Marie and Tony looked up at the stars from a blanket on the grass not far from their tent. They lay side by side holding hands. Marie began telling Tony about a phone conversation she'd had this morning with one of the mothers from the parents' group at Children's. The mother had been describing how her relationship with her husband had been different since their son was diagnosed with cancer.

Tony turned his head to look at her. "I don't see any great difference in the way you and I behave toward each other because of what's happened to Gina," he said with surprise in his voice. "I haven't noticed any change."

"Really?"

"Why? Was there?"

"I don't know." She fell silent. A breeze passed through the trees, reshaping them, then letting them go. She said finally, "I feel like *I* changed."

"Do you?"

"Yes, I'm more mouthier to you than I was. Don't I tell you more now where to get off than I ever did before?"

He chuckled. "Yeah, now that you mention it! But I don't pay any attention!"

"I'm expressing myself, like it or not," she continued. "I'll say, 'Why did you do this or that? Why don't you take out the garbage? Why don't you hang up your clothes?' Or I'll say, 'From now on you're not going to get your clothes washed if they're not in the hamper! I'm tired of picking them up!' I'll holler at you. Before, I would never do that. Before, I would mother you and then curse you all day long. Now I come right out and say to you, 'Why the hell did you do this?'"

"How come?"

"I don't know what it is." After a moment she grinned at him. "Maybe I just flipped!"

But Marie had some theories. Though she had never been a picky person, Gina's illness brought her anger out. She was more short-tempered. Because she had big worries on her mind constantly, little things annoyed her more. She was impatient with other people's small complaints. She did not want to be bothered with such small inconveniences as a full garbage can or clothes thrown over a chair.

And maybe she was getting liberated as she was getting older, Marie told her husband as they lay talking under the stars. She had been brought up to believe that the man in the house was always the boss. For years she had never dared to speak out to Tony about certain things. Yet a change had been building up in her. Until Gina had gotten sick, it had built slowly. But having a child with cancer had given Marie a new understanding of what was important in this world. Much as she loved Tony, much as she respected him, she had learned that treating the man in her house as the boss was not as important as she had once believed. She simply felt more comfortable now saying to him what was on her mind.

She did not know whether she liked herself that way or not. She said so to Tony, adding, "I know *you* like me meek and quiet!"

He acknowledged this in a tone meant to tease. "I'd rather have you meek and quiet!"

But Marie knew that she would never be meek and quiet in the same way again.

She knew that Gina's illness had changed Tony too. The man who for years had been unable or unwilling to discuss the death of their first child could now say her name. He could talk about things he remembered from the five months she had lived. He could talk about Gina's illness. He didn't do it gladly, and in a way he had no choice, because Gina was taking medicines every day and going to Clinic once a month, and there was no way to forget what she had. But he talked. This time Marie was not going through an unbearable situation without him. This time they were together.

Saturday, May 24

The DeRoses had an early breakfast and went fishing.

The lake sparkled in front of them. Poles held out in four directions, they sat on rocks or on the grass in a place some distance from the beach where the water got deep very suddenly. Tony had offered four quarters to the person who caught a fish first. Within five minutes little Tony had landed a baby bass too small to keep. His father had given him the four quarters anyhow.

Marie sat enjoying the sun on her back and feeling more relaxed than she had since Gina's diagnosis. The child was feeling good, she looked very good, her hair had grown in, they were away from all the places they associated with her being sick, and they were back in woods. Here the kids could run and yell and pick wildflowers, and their parents were not constantly having to holler at them for being too noisy or for getting into things. The weather was perfect. Nine months had passed since they had begun to notice that something was wrong with Gina. Today Marie could almost forget that her daughter had cancer.

Would their lives ever be completely normal again? Marie thought not, unless the doctors came right out and said that Gina was cured. Even then she and Tony probably wouldn't believe it. Her disease was a fact that they could not escape. It took them to Children's once every month for Clinic, which she and Gina were both getting tired of; it made them uncertain about the future. But

Marie believed now that they could learn to live with what had happened so long as the child stayed the way she was.

She glanced over at her daughter. Gina was sitting on a rock in her bathing suit watching her bobber, completely absorbed. In three weeks she would be nine years old. As yet her body showed no signs of womanly development. But within the past few days she had let her mother know that a boy at school liked her—a boy she couldn't stand, of course—and had gotten silly at the supper table about a subject she had never before mentioned: making out.

She had seen something about it on *Happy Days*. Actually, she'd told her parents, she already knew all about it. Wanting her to feel comfortable confiding in them about such matters, Marie and Tony had played along. "Oh, really, Gina? What's making out? This must be something the younger generation has that we don't know anything about. Teach us. We want to learn from you in our old age."

Making out, she had informed them, meant that you kissed somebody on the neck and ear in the dark between nine and nine-thirty at night.

She was growing up. Nine months ago they had expected her to die before Christmas.

Sitting on the bank between his daughter and his son, eyes on their bobbers as well as his own, Tony DeRose was also thinking of the difference between the past and the present. Specifically he was remembering what had happened at the end of last week when Gina had come home from school after finding out who her fourth-grade teacher would be in the fall. They'd been talking about this at the supper table. All at once the child had disappeared into the living room.

Tony and Marie had rushed in to find her crying in an armchair. Questioning her, it had dawned on them that Gina had first started to feel sick at the beginning of the school year, and that she must have known how sick she was.

"That was last year, Gina," her father had kept saying to her until finally her tears had stopped, "and this is this year."

He had spoken with utter conviction. Tony DeRose had begun again to measure time in terms of weeks and months, not days.

He had no special powers. He could not possibly know that Gina would still be in remission and doing beautifully a year from now, or that two years from now his family would be back at this same campsite still intact, still whole. All Tony knew was that his daughter had gone through a nightmare and survived it. They all had. He had every expectation that Gina was going to be fine.

Ø

Two hundred miles to the northeast, driving in sunglasses with his elbow out the car window, Bob Price felt the skin on that arm begin to redden. He and Ellen had been on the road about an hour, heading north on a four-lane highway toward a small resort in a low range of wooded mountains along the uppermost border of the state. They'd be there four days: their first time away together in more than a year.

Beside him, curled sideways against the seat, Ellen dozed. Having agreed to an early start, she had stayed up reading till almost two. A sign, Bob thought, that she was still exploring her freedom, still feeling her way toward a new schedule. A new role, actually. For most of her adult life, an increasing portion of Ellen's time and energy had gone into caring for Mark. During his last hospitalization her life had been completely dictated by his illness. Suddenly those demands, that routine, had all ended, leaving huge holes to be assimilated.

Furthermore, in part because they had had to spend so much time without her over the past year, Ellen's other two children had grown increasingly less dependent on her. Randy had just graduated from high school. He would be going away to college in the fall. Denise was twelve, on her own more and more. Ellen had some big adjustments ahead. They both did: Bob's life, too, had revolved around Mark's illness that last intense year.

They had been able to bear up under his death better than Bob had ever thought they would. Ellen had borne up a thousand percent better than her husband would have expected her to. Much of the credit, he believed, belonged to Mark. Mark had prepared them for his death. That had made it so much easier. They didn't even feel any particular bitterness about what had happened. Though Bob sometimes looked back thinking what a shame it was that Mark had been so ripped off by life, he could not but remember that the boy himself had always made the best of things. Odd as it seemed, he had been happy. Except for the past year, he had been as happy a youngster as Bob had ever known.

For a while after Mark's death, Bob had felt guilty that they had let the boy transfer to St. Michael's Hospital. If Mark had stayed at Children's, where the doctors really had a bead on cystic fibrosis, maybe he wouldn't have died when he did. Maybe they could have gotten him home again. Not wanting to upset his wife, Bob had kept these thoughts to himself.

But then Ellen had talked to the St. Michael's pathologist, who had told her Mark's lungs were so terrible it was a miracle he hadn't died sooner. This had made Bob feel better. He'd been able, then, to mention his guilt feelings to Ellen, who it turned out had shared them.

A carload of kids passed them, with radio blaring. His wife stirred, blinked, looked at him, shook the sleepiness, stretched, smiled. "Hi."

"Hi."

"Where are we?"

"I'd say the hinterlands, based on the number of places I've seen in the last twenty minutes where a person could get a cup of coffee!"

Ellen surveyed the fields and woodlands which comprised the landscape. "I should have thought to bring a thermos. How long did I sleep?"

"Oh, half an hour." He rumpled her hair. "You were really zonked!"

She kissed his hand and took it into her lap.

"Hey. You trying to take my mind off my driving?"

"Now you know I'd never want to do that!"

They were going away in part to rejuvenate their intimacy. The whole time Mark had had chest tubes in his body, Ellen had found lovemaking unthinkable. Bob had been completely understanding. In recent months grief had inhibited them both. But Ellen felt sure that time alone in a relaxed setting would help their relationship get back to normal in this respect as well as others.

Four months had passed since Mark's death. Never once had she wished him back, not the way he'd been at the end. She could accept his death because he had accepted it.

His words that last morning went through her head a hundred times a day: "I'm not afraid, Mom. I'm going to see God." In his readiness to die, he had given her the greatest gift she could imagine receiving. Ellen felt she was going to be fine. As long as she could keep Mark's words in front of her, she expected to be okay.

Of course the hard memories would not disappear overnight, nor could Ellen stop thinking of Lisa's hell now that Mark and Janet were gone. She had also grown increasingly upset over certain things that had happened or not happened while Mark was at St. Michael's. His having to wait for percussion when he was sick enough to be dying. His having spent his last night in the company of strangers. If the nurses had thought Mark to be so badly off that he needed to be seen by a priest, why hadn't they called the family?

And why hadn't Mark called her himself?

These questions were to trouble Ellen for some time. Ultimately they would be resolved through a letter to the hospital administrator and a meeting between Ellen and Bob and the director of nursing. Both officials would take the Prices' complaints very seriously. Following the meeting, the director of nursing would write to the Prices detailing the steps being taken to assure that in future the hospital staff would be fully responsive to the "humanistic needs of patients and families." She would express deep regret that her professionals had erred in their responsibilities. Her letter would assure the Prices that their concerns had made an impact at St. Michael's and had renewed the staff's resolve to make sure that patients and families were treated with the greatest possible sensitivity. It would help Ellen to learn from the nurses that Mark had not wanted her called because he had not wanted to distress her. At least that would explain why *he* had not placed the call.

Ellen was also bothered from time to time by the fact that since Mark's funeral, she and Bob had had no contact with anybody from Children's Hospital. In February she had written to Kate and the other nurses who had been at the service sending each a snapshot of Mark taken before his last admission. The photo showed him sitting at the kitchen table holding Taffy on his lap. Wearing a light nylon baseball jacket so his skinny arms wouldn't show in the picture, he was smiling directly into the camera, and he looked good. None of the nurses had responded.

Dr. Earnshaw had written them a beautiful letter, which Ellen had deeply appreciated, but since then they hadn't heard from him, either. In a way Ellen could understand this better than she could understand not hearing from the nurses. While she had felt close to

Daniel Earnshaw for many years, it wasn't the kind of closeness that had developed with the nurses during Mark's last admission. By the same token, since she had known the man so long, Ellen just assumed that at one point or another she'd talk to him again. She was interested to find out what he had thought of the autopsy findings.

She had not called him. Nor had she called the nurses. She felt awkward about calling, thinking she might somehow put them on the spot. Bob thought the nurses hadn't called because *they* felt awkward, or would if he or Ellen broke down on the phone. Bob was not distressed by the lack of contact with Children's. He felt that everybody needed time to heal. Ellen certainly saw the wisdom in that.

She looked over at him. "Do you want a cookie, honey?"

He nodded. "I want a cookie in three minutes when I'm sitting down with my coffee!"

She laughed, gratified to see him so lighthearted again. Positive as he was, he had gotten very depressed before Mark died. That last night after Bob had spent the evening alone with Mark at St. Michael's, Ellen had been lying awake, heart aching, and realizing that Bob, too, was still awake, had said something to him. He had stunned her by replying, "I wish I were dead." She had never heard him so down.

Releasing his hand, she lit a cigarette for herself and said, teasing, "You really believe there's coffee up ahead, don't you."

He looked at her with a grin on his face. "Sure. Don't you?"

Her eyes held his. She grinned back. "Sure!"

Inhaling, Ellen let her head drop back against the seat. She exhaled very slowly. Hot sun blessed her skin. The breezes that whipped at her hair were cool and fresh. Bob was on the seat next to her. They were on vacation. The mountains were in view now— an uneven greenish band across the horizon. The kids were safe and healthy. They were spending the weekend with friends. Mark had been delivered from his misery. As the miles passed, Ellen became aware of feeling within herself a peace unlike any she had ever before experienced.

When they had stopped for coffee and were on the road again, she withdrew from her purse a letter she had kept there since receiving it in early February. The letter had come from the guidance counselor at Mark's and Randy's old school. Though they had received many wonderful letters after Mark had died, this one in particular had been a source of comfort to Ellen. She had taken to reading it to console herself in times of deepest grief. The counselor's message was happy. Ellen had often thought that the day she could read that letter feeling the same spirit, the same optimism the counselor had obviously felt in writing it, she would know that she had once again touched solid ground.

The letter had been handwritten on yellow stationery. In one corner was a printed drawing of a little girl sitting in a chair with a doll at her side, a book in her lap, and a bouquet of flowers in her hand. Ellen read, for the umpteenth time:

Dear Mr. and Mrs. Price,

Rather than send you a sympathy card with my condolences, I'd like to take this bright paper and tell you of the many ways in which I remember Mark.

When I first knew him, he was just Randy's little brother. And then I found he was little brother to the whole school, and he was teased and protected (fiercely) by all his classmates and friends.

Mark never took advantage of those friendships. He never tried to hide behind his illness. Those who didn't know him probably thought of him as a slight kid who must be terribly smart to get into high school at such a young age.

I often identify kids with "syndromes": the "George syndrome" who is always innocent while all around him are getting caught; the "Ralph syndrome" that everyone's out to get him; the "Tommy syndrome" that I'll get the world; the "Randy syndrome" that I'll run my heart out. (Could you get out and just run and run the day Mark died, Randy?)

Mark is so clear in my mind as "joyful courage syndrome." I have seen him so often in my mind's eye, standing with a group of boys just outside the Guidance door, his hair tossed, his face alight as he shared fully in their talk and plans. There stood a boy tuned into life, enjoying it perhaps more than we realized, putting away from him the pains and fears of his hospital stay just ended and facing the future unafraid.

I knew when I picked up the phone that Friday what the message would be. And I wept for one of my own who had so much to look forward to. And I wept for each of you in your loss and frustration. Why, oh God, why?

Then, as I was driving home, I saw Mark running and jumping—shouting to the breeze—no pain, no gasps, no hesitation—he's running at last like his brother. And so my tears are not for Mark. God bless you and comfort you.

Ellen read the last paragraph in a blaze of tears. Folding the letter, she turned her face toward the wind streaming in through her window. The wind drove the tears out of her eyes and dried them on her cheeks. In the near distance, in a huge field overgrown with flowering weeds, Ellen saw her son as the counselor imagined him, but in slow motion, running free, soaring like a deer over boulders and brush, his blond hair shining, lifting and falling in the sun.

Dry-eyed, glad at heart, Ellen turned to her husband and smiled.

Bibliography

Sources for Material on Pediatric Hospitals

Abt, Isaac A., M.D., ed., *Abt-Garrison History of Pediatrics,* W. B. Saunders, Philadelphia and London, 1965.

Ackerknecht, Erwin H., M.D., *A Short History of Medicine,* Ronald Press, New York, 1968.

Cone, Thomas E., Jr., *History of American Pediatrics,* Little, Brown, Boston, 1979.

Drake, Donald C., medical writer, *Philadelphia Inquirer,* interviews 6/28/79; 10/26/83; 10/27/83.

Garrison, Fielding H., *History of Medicine,* W. B. Saunders, Philadelphia and London, 1929.

Hardgrove, Carol B., and Rosemary B. Dawson, *Parents and Children in the Hospital,* Little, Brown, Boston, 1972.

Lindheim, Roslyn, Helen H. Glaser, and Christie Coffin, *Changing Hospital Environments for Children,* Harvard University Press, Cambridge, 1974.

Poynter, F. N. L., ed., *The Evolution of Hospitals in Britain,* Pitman Publishing, London, 1964.

Radbill, Samuel X., M.D., Philadelphia, interview 10/12/83.

Robertson, James, *Young Children in Hospitals,* Basic Books, New York, 1958.

Study to Quantify the Uniqueness of Children's Hospitals, conducted for National Association of Children's Hospitals and Related Institutions, 1978.

Sweeney, Robert, president, National Association of Children's Hospitals and Related Institutions, interview 10/12/83.

Sources for Material on Pediatric Illnesses

Abt, Isaac A., M.D., op. cit.

Amidei, Nancy, Washington, D.C., free-lance writer on poverty and hunger formerly of Food Research Action Committee, interview 9/21/84.

Anderson, B. J., associate general counsel, American Medical Association, Chicago, interview 9/28/84.

Arras, John, philosopher in residence, Montefiore Medical Center, New York, interview 11/15/84.

Baker, Susan, M.P.H., professor, Department of Health Policy and Management, The Johns Hopkins University School of Hygiene and Public Health, Baltimore, interview August 1984.

Behrman, Richard E., M.D., Victor C. Vaughan III, M.D., and Waldo E. Nelson, M.D., eds., *Nelson Textbook of Pediatrics,* 12th ed., W. B. Saunders, Philadelphia, 1983.

"Better Health for Our Children: A National Strategy," The Report of the Select Panel for the Promotion of Child Health, U.S. Department of Health and Human Services, 1981.

Birth Defects: Tragedy and Hope, National Foundation/March of Dimes, 1977.

Birth Defects: Tragedy and Hope, March of Dimes Birth Defects Foundation, 1983.

Cone, Thomas E., Jr., M.D., op. cit.

Cooper, Charles, assistant attorney general, U.S. Department of Justice, Civil Rights Division, interview 9/21/84.

"Court Backs Parents on No Surgery for Infant," *Philadelphia Inquirer,* 10/23/83.

"Cutting the Risk of Childbirth After 35," *Consumer Reports,* May 1979.

Facts/1983, March of Dimes Birth Defects Foundation, 1983.

Gill, Frances, M.D., hematologist, Children's Hospital of Philadelphia, interviews 10/18/79, 11/21/83, 12/1/83, 11/16/84.

Golbus, Mitchell S., "The Current Scope of Antenatal Diagnosis," *Hospital Practice,* Vol. 4, April 1982.

Goodman, Ellen, "Baby Jane Doe's Unfeeling Uncle," *Philadelphia Inquirer,* 11/12/83.

Gratz, Rene Resnick, "Accidental Injury in Childhood: A Literature Review on Pediatric Trauma," *Journal of Trauma,* Vol. 19, No. 1, Williams & Wilkins, Baltimore, 1979.

Haddon, William, Jr., M.D., M.P.H., "Advances in the Epidemiology of Injuries as a Basis for Public Policy," *Public Health Reports,* Vol. 95, No. 5, September–October 1980; interview 12/9/83.

Haggerty, Robert, M.D., president-elect, American Academy of Pediatrics, interview 11/9/83.

Healthy People, The Surgeon General's Report on Health Promotion and Disease Prevention, U.S. Department of Health, Education and Welfare, Public Health Service, 1979.

Healthy People, The Surgeon General's Report on Health Promotion and Disease Prevention, Background Papers, U.S. Department of Health, Education and Welfare, Public Health Service, 1979.

Historical Statistics of the United States, Colonial Times to 1957, U.S. Department of Commerce, Bureau of the Census, 1960.

Hughes, James G., *Synopsis of Pediatrics,* C. V. Mosby, St. Louis, 1975.

"'Infant Doe' Dies, Ending Legal Battle," *Philadelphia Inquirer,* 4/82.

Kantrowitz, Barbara, "U.S. Is Denied a Handicapped Baby's Records," *Philadelphia Inquirer,* 11/18/83.

Koop, C. Everett, M.D., surgeon in chief, Children's Hospital of Philadelphia, interview 8/18/80.

Krugman, Saul, M.D., Robert Ward, M.D., and Samuel L. Katz, M.D., eds., *Infectious Diseases of Children,* 6th ed., C. V. Mosby, St. Louis, 1977.

Lazaraus, Bill, "Judge Orders Medical Care for Deformed Baby," *Philadelphia Inquirer,* 6/24/81.

Leavitt, Richard, science information editor, National March of Dimes Birth Defects Foundation, interview 11/15/83.

Levine, Carol, ed., *The Hastings Center Report,* interview 11/21/83.

Mackey, Trish, executive assistant to the director, Office of Civil Rights, U.S. Department of Health and Human Services, interviews 1/5/84, 7/2/84, 9/18/84.

McKinley, Pat, Development Staff, Children's Memorial Hospital, Chicago, interview 12/6/83.

Monthly Vital Statistics Report, Vol. 33, No. 3, U.S. Department of Health and Human Services, National Center for Health Statistics, June 22, 1984.

Morgan, Lael, "On the Rise: Teenage Suicides," *Philadelphia Inquirer,* 1979.

Moriarty, Helene, R.N., counseling coordinator, Pennsylvania SIDS Center, Philadelphia, interview 11/9/83.

"Policy Options for Reducing the Motor Vehicle Crash Injury Cost Burden," Insurance Institute for Highway Safety, Washington, D.C., 1981.

Preblud, Stephen, M.D., Office of Immunization, Centers for Disease Control, Atlanta, interview 11/1/83.

Rashkind, William, M.D., cardiologist, Children's Hospital of Philadelphia, interview 8/16/79.

Rivara, Frederick P., M.D., M.P.H., "Epidemiology of Childhood Injuries, I. Review of Current Research and Presentation of Conceptual Framework," *American Journal of the Diseases of Childhood,* Vol. 136, May 1982; interview 11/10/83.

Robertson, John A., "Dilemma in Danville," *The Hastings Center Report,* October 1981.

Robertson, Leon S., *Injuries,* Lexington Books, D. C. Heath, Lexington, Mass., and Toronto, 1983.

Rudolph, Abraham M., M.D., and Julien I. E. Hoffman, M.D., eds., *Pediatrics,* 17th ed., Appleton-Century-Crofts, Norwalk, Conn., 1982.

Sasso, Joyce, information referral specialist, Spina Bifida Association, Chicago, interview 11/18/83.

Schraeder, Barbara, R.N., Ph.D., associate professor of nursing, Thomas Jefferson University, Philadelphia, interview 12/6/83.

Sewell, Edward M., M.D., chairman, Philadelphia Pediatric Pulmonary Center, interview 12/1/83.

Smith, David W., M.D., ed., *Introduction to Clinical Pediatrics,* 22nd ed., W. B. Saunders, Philadelphia, 1977.

"Spina Bifida: A New Disease," *Pediatrics,* Vol. 68, No. 1, July 1981.

Still, George Frederic, *The History of Paediatrics,* Oxford University Press, London, 1931.

Sweeney, Robert, president, National Association of Children's Hospitals and Related Institutions, Alexandria, Va., interview 9/26/84.

"Violence Is Leading Death Cause for First Half of Human Life Span," *Philadelphia Inquirer,* 9/5/80.

Winkle, Daniel, "Teenagers Who See Suicide as a Way Out," *Philadelphia Inquirer,* 5/2/82.

Zackai, Elaine, M.D., geneticist, Children's Hospital of Philadelphia, interview 11/22/83.

Miscellaneous Sources

D'Angio, Giulio J., "Pediatric Cancer in Perspective: Cure Is Not Enough," *Cancer,* Vol. 35, No. 3, March 1975.

———, "Perspectives of Pediatric Oncology Battlegrounds, Old and New," paper prepared for National Conference on the Care of the Child with Cancer, American Cancer Society, 1979.

Drake, Donald C., "Baby's Breath: Life on the Machine," three-part series for *Philadelphia Inquirer,* 9/24/78–9/26/78.

———, "To Put a Price on Life: A Medical Dilemma," *Philadeliphia Inquirer,* 10/5/80.

Evans, Audrey E., Patricia Borns, Milton H. Donaldson, C. Everett Koop, "Cure of the Child with Cancer," *Pennsylvania Medicine,* September 1973.

Henig, Robin Marantz, "The Child Savers," *New York Times Magazine,* 7/27/81.

Ledger, Marshall, "A Sense of Beauty," *Pennsylvania Gazette,* April 1980.

McBroom, Patricia, "New Faces, New Lives," *Philadelphia Inquirer,* 4/1/73.